DRUGS
FROM DISCOVERY TO APPROVAL

DRUGS
FROM DISCOVERY TO APPROVAL

Rick Ng, Ph.D.

Biopharmaceutical Manufacturing Technology Centre
Singapore

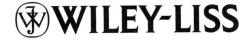

A JOHN WILEY & SONS, INC., PUBLICATION

For general information on our other products and services please contact our Customer Care Department within the U.S. at 877-762-2974, outside the U.S. at 317-572-3993 or fax 317-572-4002.

Wiley also publishes its books in a variety of electronic formats. Some content that appears in print, however, may not be available in electronic format.

Library of Congress Cataloging-in-Publication Data:

Ng, Rick.
    Drugs—from discovery to approval / Rick Ng.
        p. ; cm
Includes bibliographical references and index.
    ISBN 0-471-60150-0 (alk. paper : cloth)
    1. Drug development.
    [DNLM: 1. Technology, Pharmaceutical.   2. Chemistry, Pharmaceutical.
3. Clinical Trials—methods.   4. Drug Approval—legislation &
jurisprudence.   5. Drug Approval—methods.   6. Drug Design.   7. Drug
Industry—methods.   QV 778 N576d 2004]   I. Title.
RM301.25 .N5 2004
615'.19—dc22

                                    2003020804

Printed in the United States of America.

10 9 8 7 6 5 4 3 2 1

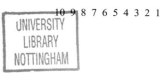

To

Cherry, Shaun and Ashleigh

CONTENTS

PREFACE

This book is written as a basic framework to introduce the concepts and processes from drug discovery to marketing approval by regulatory authorities. It is particularly suitable for undergraduates pursuing courses in medicine, pharmacy, science and life sciences. Professionals in the pharmaceutical industry will find this book useful as a quick reference guide.

There are eleven chapters:

- Chapter 1 provides a snapshot about the drug discovery and development processes, as well as the current status in the pharmaceutical industry.
- Chapter 2 describes the all-important steps in identifying disease targets and receptors for drug interaction and intervention.
- Chapter 3 explains the current technologies and methodologies for discovering new small molecule drugs.
- Chapter 4 introduces the various large molecule drugs and the methods for discovering and developing them.
- Chapter 5 summarizes the steps for drug development and preclinical tests.
- Chapter 6 details the processes and conduct of clinical trials with due respect for safety, risks and benefits.
- Chapter 7 describes the major drug regulatory authorities in selected countries such as the United States, European Union, Japan, China and some international organizations.
- Chapter 8 shows the basic procedures for applications to regulatory authorities for clinical trials and drug marketing approvals.
- Chapter 9 discusses the regulatory requirements for drug manufacture, with selected examples.
- Chapter 10 demonstrates the controls required to manufacture drugs that meet the regulatory requirements.
- Chapter 11 gives perspectives about the future events for drug discovery and development.

Some background concepts are introduced in four appendices together with acronyms and glossary.

In writing this book, I am indebted to many friends and colleagues. I am grateful to Dr. Choon Onn Wong, Dr. Dinesh Khokal, Dr. Wang Sijing and Dr. Paul Baker who painstakingly read the entire draft and provided insightful and invaluable suggestions. For the artwork, I thank Mr Jadish Kuchibhatla and my brother-in-law Mr Yong Kit Song. My thanks to Mr Tim Badgery-Parker who worked on the copyediting and Ms Jessica Teo and Ms Stephanie Chiang who helped with proofreading the drafts. I sincerely thank Ms Luna Han of John Wiley & Sons for seeing potential in this book and agreed to publish it.

I thank my family for the encouragement and support that they have provided me.

Rick Ng

CHAPTER 1

INTRODUCTION

1.1   AIM OF THIS BOOK

The process from discovering a new drug to registering it for marketing and commercialization is very complex and lengthy. The intention of this book is to provide an overview about how a drug is discovered, the amount and types of laboratory tests that are performed, and the conduct of clinical trials before a drug is ready to be registered for human use. The role of regulatory authorities in these processes and their control over safety evaluation, clinical trials, manufacturing and marketing approval of a drug are also explained. This book aims to integrate, in a simplified manner, the interrelationships between all these complex processes and procedures.

To establish a frame of reference, it is appropriate to commence with a definition for the term 'drug'. Generally, a drug can be defined as a substance that induces a response within the human body, whether the response is beneficial or harmful. In this context, toxins and poisons can be classified as drugs. However, the term 'drug' used in this book is strictly reserved for a medicinal substance, which provides favorable therapeutic or prophylactic pharmaceutical benefits to the human body. Readers are referred to Exhibit 1.1 for a definition of drug according to the Food and Drug Administration (FDA) of the United States.

It should be noted that the descriptions in this book on discovery and regulatory processes are mainly for ethical drugs, as opposed to over-the-counter (OTC) drugs. Ethical drugs are prescription drugs that require prescriptions by physicians, whereas OTC drugs can be purchased from

Treatment TB   ex: moxifloxacin was first new treatment for more than 40 years

---

Exhibit 1.1   FDA Definition of a Drug

'An active ingredient that is intended to furnish pharmacological activity or other direct effect in the diagnosis, cure, mitigation, treatment, or prevention of a disease, or to affect the structure of any function of the human body, but does not include intermediates used in the synthesis of such ingredient'.

---

pharmacies without prescription. The OTC drugs are mainly established drugs that are deemed safe enough to be taken without supervision by a physician.

There is a further differentiation of ethical drugs into new drugs (those covered by patents) and generics (copies of drugs that have expired patents). Most of the descriptions in this book apply to new drugs.

1.2   AN OVERVIEW OF THE DRUG DISCOVERY AND DEVELOPMENT PROCESS

Although human civilization has been experimenting and consuming drugs for many centuries, it is only in the past 100 years that the foundation was laid for the systematic research and development of drugs. Readers are referred to Appendix 1 for a brief description of the history of drug development since the ancient times.

Teams of scientists, clinicians, and statisticians, as well as regulatory, marketing, medical practitioners, and even economists and legal attorneys, are involved in the process of drug discovery and development. Previously, the main scientific personnel in the discovery process have been the synthetic chemists. Now molecular biologists, biochemists, microbiologists and even computer scientists play equally important roles in the drug discovery and development processes. The reason for this is that drug discovery and development has made a quantum leap forward in the past decade with progress in genomics and biotechnology. In addition, advances in laboratory equipment automation and high-speed computing have assisted in analyzing and processing of large data sets. Personnel with different disciplines and expertise are needed to contribute to discover and develop drugs targeting diseases at the cellular and molecular levels.

It is estimated that, on average, a drug takes 10–12 years from initial research to reach the commercialization stage. The cost of this process is estimated to be more than US$500 million. From discovery to marketing approval of a drug, the following stages are involved (Figure 1.1):

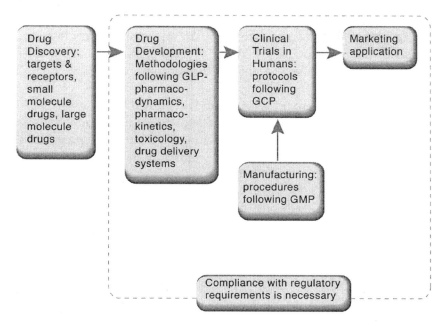

Figure 1.1 The stages from drug discovery to marketing approval

Drug Discovery: The process involves finding out the target that causes the disease. Next, chemical or biological compounds are screened and tested against these targets or assays, which are representative of these targets, to find leading drug candidates for further development. Many new scientific approaches are now used to determine targets (most targets are receptors or enzymes) and obtain the lead compounds; including the use of genomic technology, synthetic chemistry, recombinant DNA (rDNA) technology, laboratory automation and bioinformatics.

Drug Development: Tests are performed on the lead compounds in test tubes (laboratory, *in vitro*) and on animals (*in vivo*) to check how they affect the biological systems. The tests, often called preclinical research activities, include toxicology, pharmacodynamics and pharmacokinetics, as well as optimization of drug delivery systems. Many iterations are carried out, and the leading compounds are modified and synthesized to improve their interactions with the targets, or to reduce the toxicity or improve pharmacokinetics performance. At the end of this process, an optimized compound is found and this becomes a potential drug ready for clinical trial

Prozac: Controversial cure

0787151927 0

in humans. The development work has to follow Good Laboratory Practice (GLP) to ensure that proper quality system and ethical considerations are established. Only compounds that satisfy certain performance and safety criteria will proceed to the next stage of clinical trial.

Clinical Trials: These are trials conducted on human subjects. The pertinent parameters for clinical trials are protocols (methods about how trials are to be conducted), safety and respect for human subjects, responsibilities of investigator, institutional review board, informed consent, trial monitoring and adverse event reporting. Clinical trials have to follow regulations and guidelines from the FDA, the European Agency for the Evaluation of Medicinal Products (EMEA) of the European Union (EU) or European Member States, Japan's Ministry of Health, Labor and Welfare (MHLW), or regulatory authorities in other prospective countries where the drug is intended to be registered and commercialized. Clinical trials are conducted in accordance with Good Clinical Practice (GCP).

Manufacturing: The drug designated for clinical trials and large-scale production has to be manufactured in compliance with current Good Manufacturing Practice (cGMP; the word 'current' denotes that regulations do change from time to time and the current regulations have to be applied) following US FDA requirements, EU Directives or International Conference on Harmonization (ICH) guidelines. Regulatory authorities have the rights to conduct inspections on pharmaceutical manufacturing plants to ensure they follow cGMP guidelines so that the drug manufactured is safe and effective. A quality system has to be set up such that the drug is manufactured in accordance with approved procedures. There must also be traceability of materials as well as appropriate tests being conducted on the raw materials, intermediates and finished products. The emphasis is that drugs should be safe, pure, effective, and of consistent quality to ensure that they are fit to be used for their intended functions.

Marketing Application: A drug is not permitted for sale until the marketing application for the new drug has been reviewed and approved by regulatory authorities such as the US FDA, the EU EMEA or Japan's MHLW. Extensive dossiers are provided to the authorities to demonstrate the safety, potency, efficacy and purity of the drug. These are provided in the form of laboratory, clinical and manufacturing data, which comply with GLP, GCP and cGMP requirements. After the drug has been approved and marketed, there is continuous monitoring of the safety and performance of the drug to ensure that it is prescribed correctly and adverse events (side effects) are investigated. The advertising of drugs is also scrutinized by regulatory authorities to ensure that there are no false representations or claims for the drugs.

The subsequent chapters will elaborate on each of these processes. An example of the complexity, time and cost of developing a new drug is shown in Exhibit 1.2.

Exhibit 1.2 Did You Know?

Total drug development time grew from an average of 8.1 years in the 1960s to 11.6 years in the 1970s, to 14.2 in the 1980s, to 15.3 years for drugs approved from 1990 through 1995. Pharmaceutical companies and regulatory authorities are working together to reduce this time span.

The cost of developing a new drug is more than three times the price of a Boeing 747-400 airplane.

Typically, tens of thousands of compounds are screened and tested, and only a handful make it into the market as drug products. The statistics are such that, of 5000 compounds that show initial promise, five will go into human clinical trials, and only one will become an approved drug.

SOURCE PhRMA (Pharmaceutical Research and Manufacturers of America), http://www.phrma.org/ [accessed Mar 28, 2002].

A recent report puts the cost for developing a drug at US$802 million, although this figure has been challenged by various groups.

SOURCE Ezzel, C., The price of pills, *Scientific American*, July, p. 25 (2003).

1.3 THE PHARMACEUTICAL INDUSTRY

The pharmaceutical industry as we know it today started in the late 1800s. It started with the synthetic versions of natural compounds in Europe (refer to Appendix 1).

Drug discovery and development are mainly carried out by pharmaceutical companies, universities and government research agencies, although there are increasing activities in the start-up and smaller companies that specialize in particular fields of research. A substantial number of the research findings and potential drugs from the start-ups, smaller companies, universities and research organizations are, however, licensed to the multinational pharmaceutical companies for manufacturing, marketing and distribution. Alternatively, alliances are formed with the multinational pharmaceutical companies to develop or market the drugs, because of the huge cost involved for drug development and commercialization.

In 2002, the combined worldwide pharmaceutical market was around US$400 billion. The distribution of the market (in US$ billion) is shown in Table 1.1. From these data, it is evident that the US, Europe and Japan account for more than 85% of the worldwide pharmaceutical market. The regulatory authorities in these countries are hence very important to the pharmaceutical companies to ensure their products are approved for commercialization.

Table 1.2 shows the top 10 drugs in 2002, according to IMS *World Review 2003*. Exhibit 1.3 provides an explanation of cholesterol and the mechanism of action for Lipitor and Zocor. Exhibit 1.4 gives more information about Prilosec.

Table 1.1 Global pharmaceutical sales by region, 2002

World	2002 sales (US$bn)	% Global sales	% Growth market
North America	203.6	51	+12
European Union	90.6	22	+8
Rest of Europe	11.3	3	+9
Japan	46.9	12	+1
Asia, Africa and Australia	31.6	8	+11
Latin America	16.5	4	−10
Total	**400.5**	**100**	**+8**

SOURCE IMS *World Review 2003* and IMS Consulting, http://www.ims-global.com/insight/ news _story/0302/news_story_030228.htm [accessed Mar 25, 2003].

Table 1.2 The top 10 best-selling products, 2002

Product	Therapy	Company	US$ (bn) (% growth from 2001)
Lipitor (atorvastatin)	Cholesterol reducer	Pfizer	8.6 (20%)
Zocor (simvastatin)	Cholesterol reducer	Merck	6.2 (13%)
Prilosec (omeprazole)	Antiulcerant	AstraZeneca	5.2 (−19%)

Table 1.2 *Continued*

Product	Therapy	Company	US$ (bn) (% growth from 2001)
Zyprexa (olanzapine)	Antipsychotic	Eli Lilly	4.0 (21%)
Norvasc (amlopdipine)	Antihypertensive	Pfizer	4.0 (6%)
Erypo (erythropoietin)	Anemia	Johnson & Johnson	3.8 (18%)
Prevacid (lansoprazole)	Acid reflux disease treatment	TAP	3.6 (3%)
Seroxat/Paxil (paroxetine HCI)	Antidepressant	GlaxoSmithKline	3.3 (13%)
Celebrex (celecoxib)	COX-2 inhibitor and anti-inflammatory	Pharmacia	3.1 (−1%)
Zoloft (sertraline)	Antidepressant	Pfizer	2.9 (12%)

SOURCE   IMS *World Review 2003*, http://www.ims-lobal.com/insight/news_story/0302/news_story_030228.htm [accessed Mar 25, 2003].

Exhibit 1.3 Cholesterol and Cholesterol-lowering Drugs

Cholesterol is a fatlike substance (a sterol) that is present in our blood and all the cells. It is synthesized within the body or derived from our diet. Cholesterol is an important constituent of the cell membrane and hormones.

Cholesterol is carried in the bloodstream by lipoproteins such as low density lipoprotein (LDL, or 'bad cholesterol') and high density lipoprotein (HDL, 'good cholesterol'). LDL carries cholesterol from the liver to other parts of the body. LDL attaches to receptors (see Chapter 2) on the cell surface and is taken into the cell interior. It is then degraded and the cholesterol is used as a component for cell membrane. When there is excessive cholesterol inside the cell, it leads to a reduction in the synthesis of LDL receptors.

The number of active LDL receptors is also affected by a condition called familial hypercholesterolemia, in which there is a defective gene coding for the receptor. In either case, the reduction of active receptors means that the LDL carrying cholesterol is unable to enter the cell interior, instead it is deposited in the arteries leading to the heart or brain. These deposits build up over time, and may block blood supply to the heart muscle or brain, resulting in a heart attack or stroke. In contrast, HDL transports cholesterol from other parts of the body to the liver, where it is degraded to bile acids.

An enzyme (see Section 2.6) called HMG-CoA reductase is involved in the biosynthesis of cholesterol. Drugs such as atorvastatin (Lipitor) and simvastatin (Zocor) are competitive inhibitors of HMG-CoA reductase. They inhibit cholesterol synthesis by increasing the number of LDL receptors to take up the LDL.

Exhibit 1.4 Prilosec

Omeprazole (Prilosec, AstraZeneca) is a drug termed as proton pump inhibitor. It turns off the secretions of acid into the stomach. When less acid is produced, there is a reduced amount of acid that can flow back up from the stomach into the esophagus to cause reflux symptoms.

It should be noted that there are normally three names associated with a drug: the trade or proprietary name (for example, Prilosec), generic or non-proprietary name (omeprazole) and a specific chemical name for the active ingredient. In the case of omeprazole, the active ingredient is a benzimidazole: 5-methoxy-2-[[(4-methoxy-3,5-dimethyl-2-pyridinyl) methyl] sulfinyl]-1H-benzimidazole. It has an empirical formula of $C_{17}H_{19}N_3O_3S$.

SOURCE AstraZeneca, http://www.priloseconline.com/ [accessed Apr 15, 2002].

The top 10 pharmaceutical companies in 2002 are shown in Table 1.3. These 10 companies account for almost half of the global sales of drugs. In the same period, they spent in excess of US$20 billion in research and development, which is around 10% of their sales revenue.

Table 1.4 shows the R&D investments into drug research by research-based US pharmaceutical companies and the National Institutes of Health (NIH) for the period from 1991 to 2000. The enormous spending on R&D has escalated in recent years. According to a report, PhRMA Annual Report 2000–2001, US pharmaceutical companies have almost double their R&D spending every five years since 1980. Out of every $5 in sales, $1 is put back into R&D.

Pharmaceutical firms have to ensure that there is a pipeline of new and better drugs to return the substantial investments made. It is estimated that large pharmaceutical firms need 4–5 new drugs approved every year to maintain their premium positions. However, most firms are far short of this target, with only about 1–2 new drugs approved per year.

According to the May 2003 report by IMS Health, the sales of pharmaceuticals through retail pharmacies in 13 major world markets for the 12 months to March 2003 grew at 6% to US$284.4 billion. Biopharmaceutical products make up to about 7% of the total pharmaceutical markets of US$400 billion. However, the growth rate for biopharmaceuticals is high, and it is expected that half the total pharmaceutical market will be biopharmaceuticals within the next 10–20 years.

The top five biopharmaceutical companies are listed in Table 1.5.

Table 1.3 The top 10 pharmaceutical companies, 12 months to September 2002

Company	Rank	Market share
Pfizer	1	7.3%
GlaxoSmithKline	2	7.1%
Merck	3	5.1%
Johnson & Johnson	4	4.6%
AstraZeneca	5	4.6%
Novartis	6	4.0%
Bristol-Myers Squibb	7	3.7%
Aventis	8	3.6%
Roche	9	3.1%
Pharmacia	10	3.0%

SOURCE   IMS *World Review 2003*, http://www.ims-global.com/insight/ news_story/0302/news _story_030227htm [accessed Mar 25, 2003].

Table 1.4 R&D investments by research-based US pharmaceutical companies and the National Institutes of Health (NIH)

Year	Companies (US$ billion)	NIH (US$ billion)
1991	10.0	8.9
1992	11.5	9.6
1993	12.4	10.8
1994	13.2	11.3
1995	15.2	11.8
1996	17.0	12.4
1997	19.0	13.5
1998	21.0	14.3
1999	24.0	16.0
2000	26.4	17.8

SOURCE   Zoon, K.C., FDA CBER: Update — 100 years of biologics regulation, *FDA Consumer Magazine* (2002).

Table 1.5 The top five biopharmaceutical companies, 2002

Companies	Sales (US$ billion)
Amgen	4.0
Genentech	2.2
Serono International	1.4
Biogen	1.1
Immunex	1.0

SOURCE Contract Pharma, http://www.contractpharma.com/JulyAug 022.htm [accessed Sep 18, 2002].

1.4   ECONOMICS OF DRUG DISCOVERY AND DEVELOPMENT

The pharmaceutical market is very competitive. It is imperative that pharmaceutical companies (including biotechnology companies), large or small, discover and develop drugs efficiently and within the shortest time span to remain competitive.

Figure 1.2 shows the expenses versus revenues to a company's investment in developing a new drug. Up until the clinical stage, the investment is substantial in the discovery and development processes. The largest cash demand is in the clinical trial stages, where hundreds and thousands of human subjects have to be recruited to test the drug.

A positive return of revenue only occurs after the drug has been approved by regulatory authorities for marketing. The overall profitability of a drug is the difference between the positive returns and the negative expenses within the patent period of 20 years. After that period, if the patent is not extended, there is no further protection on the intellectual rights for the drug.

After patent expiry, generic drugs from other companies are unencumbered by patent rights infringement and can encroach into the profitability of the company that developed the original drug. It is thus crucial that drugs are marketed as quickly as possible to ensure there is maximum patent coverage period and to be 'first to market', to establish a premium position. When cimetidine (Zantac, GlaxoSmithKline) came off patent in the US, it lost almost 90% of sales within four years (from $2085 million in 1995, to $277 million in 1999).

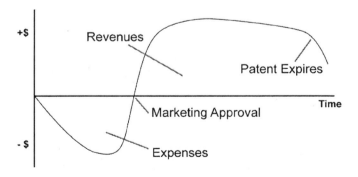

Figure 1.2 Expenses and revenues curve for a new drug

Exhibit 1.5 provides a brief explanation of patents. Patents are the pillars that support the drug industry. In contrast, traditional medicines, which are mainly derived from natural products of plant or animal origins, are not patentable. This is because traditional medicines consist of a multitude of compounds and it is difficult to establish patent claims based on varying quantities of materials.

Exhibit 1.5 Patents

A patent is a right granted by a government for any device, substance, method or process that is new, inventive and useful. The patent discloses the know-how for the invention. In return for this disclosure, the owner of a patent is given a 20-year period of monopoly rights to commercial returns from exploiting the invention.

There are two ways to register patents: either through applying in individual countries, which means multiple applications for different countries, or through designating the desired countries in a single application using the Patent Cooperation Treaty (PCT) mechanism. There are more than 90 member countries belonging to the PCT, including major developed countries.

PCT does not grant patents. Application with PCT goes through two phases: an international phase and a national phase. The international phase is where the application is searched, published and subjected to preliminary examination. Then the application enters into the national phase in each country. The application is subjected to examination and granting procedures in each country.

Another important item for a patent is the priority date. The priority date is established when a patent application is filed for the first time. If the invention is known before this date, then the patent is not granted. Most countries are first-to-file countries, which means that the patent is awarded to the person with the earliest filing date. In the US, patents are awarded to the first person to invent. The inventor can attempt to show the invention was made before another person's filing date to claim priority.

SOURCE The Patent Cooperation Treaty, http://www.wipo.org/ pct/en/index.html [accessed Oct 8, 2002].

1.5 TRENDS IN DRUG DISCOVERY AND DEVELOPMENT

The approach to drug discovery and development can generally be classified into the following areas:
- Irrational Approach
- Rational Approach

- Antisense Drugs
- Biologics
- Gene Therapy
- Stem Cell Therapy– both somatic cell and germ cell.

Irrational Approach: This approach is the historical method of discovering and developing drugs. It involves empirical observations of the pharmacological effects from screening of many chemical compounds, mainly those from natural products. The active component that gives rise to the observed effects is isolated. The chemical formula is determined, and modifications are made to improve its properties. This approach has yielded most drugs available today.

Rational Approach: This approach requires three-dimensional knowledge of the target structure involved in the disease. Drugs are designed to interact with this target structure to create a beneficial response. This is an emerging field in drug discovery.

Antisense Therapy: This is a relatively new approach and it requires the modifications to oligonucleotides that can bind to RNA and DNA (refer to Appendix 2 for a description of cell structure, genes, DNA, RNA and proteins). The antisense drugs are used to stop transcriptional (from DNA) or translational (from RNA) pathways from proceeding, and so interfere with the process of disease.

Biologics: These are mainly protein-based drugs in the form of antibodies, vaccines and cytokines. Their discoveries generally start from an understanding of the biological mechanistic pathways that cause specific diseases. Manufacturing of these drugs is based on recombinant DNA technologies using living organisms such as bacteria, yeast and mammalian and insect cells.

Gene Therapy: The basis of this therapy is to remedy a diseased gene or insert a missing gene. This is a hot new topic that raises many ethical considerations to resolve. The diseased gene is taken out from a patient, fixed outside the body (*ex vivo*) and then reinserted back into the body. In the case of missing gene, a copy of the new gene is inserted into the patient. The aim is for the inserted gene to influence the disease pathway or to initiate manufacture of the missing proteins or enzymes.

Stem Cell Therapy: With stem cell therapy, the aim is to grow body parts to replace defective human organs and nerves. The stem cells are harvested from very early embryos or umbilical cord blood. Because of the very young age of these cells, they can be directed to grow into organ tissue to replace diseased tissue. The stem cell technology can provide an alternative to organ transplants with perhaps less rejection problems than the current practice of obtaining parts from another donor person. Stem cell therapy using germ cells involves cloning, and there are strict regulatory guidelines on how research is to be conducted.

Human genomic research has discovered many novel disease targets, which can be utilized to develop better and more effective drugs. Regardless of the approach used for discovering new drugs, pharmaceutical and biotechnology companies are now using a full suite of technologies to discover new drugs. These enabling technologies include:

- Microarray for Disease Target Identification
- High Throughput Screening
- Combinatorial Chemistry
- Structure–Activity Relationships: X-ray Crystallography, Nuclear Magnetic Resonance, Computational Chemistry
- Bioinformatics: Data Mining
- Recombinant DNA Technologies.

Detailed discussions of these technologies are presented in Chapters 2–4.

1.6 FURTHER READING

Center for Drug Evaluation and Research, *Drug Information: Electronic Orange Book,* FDA, Rockville, MD, http://www.fda.gov/cder/ob/default.htm [Jul 21, 2002].

Center for Drug Evaluation and Research, *New Drug Development and Review Process,* FDA, Rockville, MD, http://www.fda.gov/cder/handbook/index.htm [Jul 21, 2002].

Food and Drug Administration, *From Test Tube to Patient: New Drug Development in the US,* 2nd edn., FDA, Rockville, MD, 1995.

Food and Drug Administration, *The Drug Development Process: How the Agency Ensures that Drugs are Safe and Effective,* FDA, Rockville, MD, http://www.fda.gov/opacom/factsheets/justthefacts/17drgdev.pdf [accessed Jul 10, 2002].

Harvey, A.L. (ed.), *Advances in Drug Discovery Techniques,* John Wiley & Sons, New York, 1998.

Jurgen, D., *In Quest of Tomorrow's Medicine*, Springer-Verlag, New York, 1999.

Pharmaceutical Research and Manufacturers of America, *Why Do Prescription Drug Cost So Much?*, PhRMA, Washington, DC, 2000.

The Pharmaceutical Century: Ten Decades of Drug Discovery, November 17, 2000, http://pubs.acs.org/journals/pharmcent/ [accessed Jun 8, 2002].

Wermuth, C.G., Koga N., Koning H., Metcalf B.M. (eds.), *Medicinal Chemistry for the 21st Century*, Blackwell Scientific Publications, Oxford, 1992.

CHAPTER 2

DRUG DISCOVERY:
TARGETS AND RECEPTORS

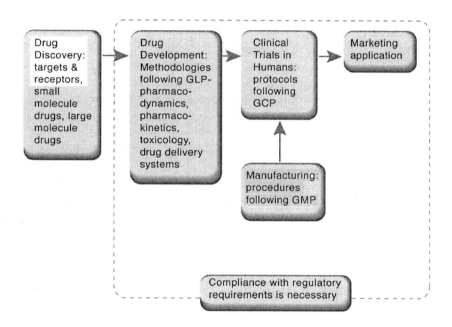

2.1 DRUG DISCOVERY PROCESSES

For a drug to work, it has to interact with a disease target in our body and intervene its wayward functions. An analogy is the lock and key comparison, with the lock being the disease target and the key representing the drug. The correct key has to be found to turn the lock and open the door to treat the disease.

The conventional method for drug discovery under the irrational approach is to scan thousands of potential compounds from natural sources for a hit against specific assays that represent the target (more about this in Chapter 3). This procedure has been compared to finding a needle in a haystack. In our analogy, it is like trying out many keys to find a fit to a lock. As we can imagine such a process is somewhat random and cumbersome. The chances for failure are high, although it should be borne in mind that most drugs on the market today were discovered in this manner.

Further advances in drug discovery led to the rational approach. This approach starts with finding out about the structure of the target and then designing a drug to fit the target and modify its functions. A comparison to the lock and key concept is to determine the construction of pin tumblers in the lock first and then design the key with the appropriate slots and grooves to pick it and open the door. The latest progress in drug discovery is contribution from genomics and proteomics research. Here the emphasis is to identify and validate targets *a priori* to drug discovery. This approach is to find out the target that causes the disease as the first step in drug discovery. After that, the rational approach would proceed. The analogy is to find out the exact diseased lock and then discover a drug to unlock the correct door.

With the foregoing in mind, the typical current drug discovery processes would proceed according to the flow chart in Figure 2.1. This chapter focuses on the medical needs, identification and validation of disease targets; followed by discussions on receptors, signal transduction and assay development. Chapters 3 and 4 focus on lead compound generation and optimization, for small, synthetic drug molecules and large, protein-based macromolecules, respectively. In Chapter 5, we cover drug development and preclinical studies.

2.2 MEDICAL NEEDS

A pharmaceutical organization has to determine which medical area has an unmet clinical need for an effective prophylactic or therapeutic intervention.

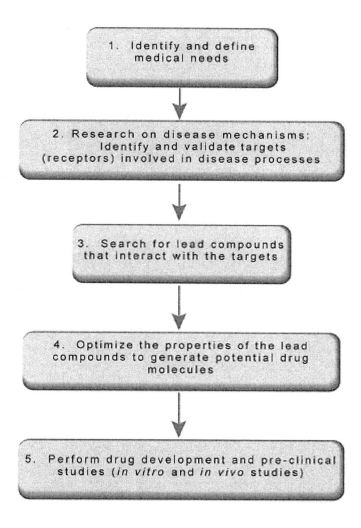

Figure 2.1 Flow chart of drug discovery processes

Next the organization has to evaluate its core competency, technological advantages, competitive barriers and financial resources before committing to develop a drug to fulfill the unmet need. As discussed in Chapter 1, for a monetary outlay that averages US$500 million for each drug development, the organization has to weigh its options carefully. The important factors to consider are:

- Market potential
- Patent, intellectual property portfolio
- Competitive forces and regulatory status
- Core competencies.

Overall, the organization needs to project the expected returns from such an investment and assess the competitive factors and barriers, including government regulations, before deciding which drug to develop.

Table 2.1 shows the therapy classes in terms of global sales in 2001. The top three therapy classes are antiulcerants, cholesterol and triglyceride reducers, and antidepressants. They account for 49% of sales in these top 10 therapy classes. There are significant changes to the growth of some therapy classes within a single year. This is especially true when new and more effective drugs are introduced; their sales can increase dramatically within a short time span and surpass the sales of more 'established' drugs.

Pharmaceutical companies have to be continuously vigilant and forecast the future directions of drug developments and regulatory requirements. They have to use their core competencies to deliver a pipeline of products to remain competitive and profitable in the long term.

2.3   TARGET IDENTIFICATION

2.3.1   Genes

Most diseases, except in the case of trauma and infectious diseases, have a genetic connection. Genetic makeup and variations (see single nucleotide

Table 2.1 Leading therapy classes, 2001

Therapy class	2001 sales (US$ billion)	Global sales	Growth
Antiulcerants	19.5	6%	+14%
Cholesterol and triglyceride reducers	18.9	5%	+22%
Antidepressants	15.9	5%	+20%
Antirheumatics (non-steroidal)	10.9	3%	+16%
Calcium antagonists (plain)	9.9	3%	+4%
Antipsychotics	7.7	2%	+30%
Oral antidiabetics	7.6	2%	+30%
Angiotensin-converting enzyme (ACE) Inhibitors (plain)	7.5	2%	+5%
Cephalosporins and combinations	6.7	2%	0%
Antihistimines (systemic)	6.7	2%	+22%

SOURCE   IMS *World Review 2002*, http://www.ims-global.com/insight/news_story/0204/news_story_020430.htm [accessed Jun 8, 2002].

polymorphism in Section 11.5) determine a person's individuality and susceptibility to diseases, pathogens and drug responses.

The current method of drug discovery commences with the study of how the body functions, in both normal and abnormal cases afflicted with diseases. The aim is to break down the disease process into the cellular and molecular levels. An understanding of the status of genes and their associated proteins would help to pinpoint the cause of the disease. Drugs can be tailor-made to attack the epicenter of the diseases. In this way, more specific (fewer side effects) and effective (high therapeutic index, see Section 5.2) drugs can be discovered and manufactured to intervene or restore the cellular or molecular dysfunction.

From the Human Genome Project, we know that there are approximately three billion base pairs that make up the DNA molecule (refer to Appendix 2). Only certain segments of the enormous DNA molecule encode for proteins. These segments are called genes. The estimate is that there are about 30 000–40 000 genes that encode proteins. Exhibit 2.1 provides some information about the number of genes and the complexity of life forms.

From these 30 000 to 40 000 genes, many thousands of proteins are produced. Drug targets are normally protein or glycoprotein molecules

---

Exhibit 2.1 Genes and Molecular Complexity

The number of protein-coding genes in an organism provides a useful indication of its molecular complexity, although there is as yet no firm correlation between the number of genes and biological complexity.

Single-celled organisms typically have a few thousand genes. For example, *Escherichia coli* (a bacteria commonly found in the intestines of animals and humans) has 4300 genes, and *Saccharomyces cerevisiae* (a fungus commonly known as baker's or brewer's yeast) has 6000 genes. *Caenorhabditis elegan* (a small soil nematode about 1 mm long) has 19 000 genes. *Drosophila melanogaster* (a 3 mm fruit fly) has 13 600 genes. For human beings, the number of genes is estimated at around 35 000.

It was initially thought that the number of human genes was of the order of 100 000. The smaller number of 35 000 was surprising considering the complexity of human beings compared with smaller organisms. The latest view is that, although the number of genes indicates complexity, there is more involved in determining complexity. Each gene may code for more than one protein, to account for human complexity.

SOURCE   Ewing, B. and Green, P., Analysis of expressed sequence tags indicates 35,000 human genes, *Nature Genetics*, 25, pp. 232–234 (2000).

because proteins are the ingredients for enzymes and receptors, with which drugs interact. To date, only about 500 proteins have been targeted by the multitudes of drugs in the market. The opportunities that are opened up by the genomics and proteomics research have paved the way for many more targets and new drugs to be discovered.

Exhibits 2.2, 2.3 and 2.4 provide examples of genetic causes of diseases, for example cancer, sickle cell anemia and cystic fibrosis.

Exhibit 2.2 The p53 Protein in Cancer

The p53 gene is a tumor suppressor gene, which means that its activity stops the formation of tumors via the production of p53 protein. As shown in the picture below, the p53 protein has four identical chains, which are joined together by a central tetramerization domain. The p53 protein molecule wraps around and binds DNA. This wrapping action then turns on another gene, which codes for a 21-kDa protein that regulates DNA synthesis.

Normally a cell grows by cell division and then dies through a process called apoptosis—programmed cell death. The p53 protein triggers apoptosis, which is a 'stop signal' for cell division, to arrest cancer growth.

In the case of cancer growth, the gene that codes for p53 is mutated. The mechanism for programmed cell death becomes inactivated and no longer functions. Cancer cells then just keep on growing and dividing at the expense of surrounding cells, thus leading to tumor formation.

SOURCE   Campbell, M.K., *Biochemistry*, 3rd edn., Harcourt Brace College Publishers, Orlando, FL, 1999.

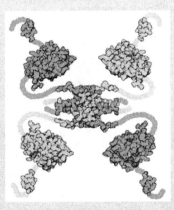

p53 molecule picture: Goodsell, D.S., The Scripps Institute, Featured Molecule: p53 Tumor Suppressor, *Bio.Com*, http://www.bio.com/ [accessed Sep 7, 2002].

Exhibit 2.3 Sickle Cell Anemia

Hemoglobin is a tetramer with four polypeptide chains: two identical α chains (141 residues) and two identical β chains (146 residues).

In people with sickle cell anemia, there is just one mutation in each of the β chains. The glutamic acid in position 6 is substituted by valine. This substitution, two residues out of a total of 474, is sufficient to cause the red blood cell to deform and constrict blood flow by blocking the capillaries.

SOURCE   Campbell, M.K., *Biochemistry*, 3rd edn., Harcourt Brace College Publishers, Orlando, FL, 1999.

Exhibit 2.4 Cystic Fibrosis

Cystic fibrosis (CF) is a hereditary disease of abnormal fluid secretion. It affects cells of the exocrine glands, such as intestine, sweat glands, pancreas, reproductive tract, and especially the respiratory tract. The disease affects about one in 2500 infants of the Caucasian population to varying degrees of seriousness. Patients produce thickened mucous that is difficult to get out of the airway. This leads to chronic lung infection, which progressively destroys pulmonary function.

CF is caused by the absence of a protein called cystic fibrosis transmembrane conductance regulator (CFTR). This protein is required for the transport of chloride ions across cell membranes. On the molecular level, there is a mutation in the gene that encodes for CFTR. As a result, CFTR cannot be processed properly by the cell and is unable to reach the exocrine glands to assume its transport function.

SOURCE   Karp, G., *Cell and Molecular Biology, Concepts and Experiments*, John Wiley & Sons, New York, 1996.

2.3.2   Targets

There are a number of techniques used for target identification. Radioligand binding was a common technique until recently. Now DNA microarrays, expressed sequence tags, and *in silico* methods are used.

Radioligand binding   The classical way to discover drug targets or receptors is to bind the potential receptors with radioligands (see Exhibit 2.5) so that targets can be picked out from a pool of other receptors. Bound receptors are then separated from the radioligands, cloned and their nucleotide sequence decoded. Potential drug molecules are then studied with these receptors or their nucleotide sequences to determine their interactions in terms of biochemical and functional properties.

Exhibit 2.5 Radioligands

Ligands are molecules that bind to a target. They may be endogenous (that is, produced by the body), such as hormones and neurotransmitters, or exogenous, such as drug molecules. Ligands (exogenous or endogenous) with high specificity for particular targets are labeled with radioisotopes. The tissue known to contain the target is mixed with a known quantity of the radioligands. Those targets bound with radioligands are separated by rapid filtration or centrifugation, followed by washing with cold buffers to remove unbound ligands. Scintillation counting techniques are used to reveal the amount of bound radioligands.

The target bound with radioligands can be isolated and its amino acid sequence determined. The sequence information enables classifications of the target based on previously known targets. Targets that do not appear to show homology to known ligands and that have no known endogenous ligand are called 'orphan' targets. Active research is ongoing to find molecules of compounds to interact with these orphan targets as possible sites for therapy.

Sequence information can be used to clone the target by using recombinant technology. In this way, biochemical pathways of the target can be studied in detail, rendering the development of a drug molecule with higher chances of success.

DNA microarray   DNA microarray, also known as DNA or gene chips, is a new technology to investigate how genes interact with one another and how they control biological mechanisms in the body. The gene expression profile is dynamic and responds to external stimuli rapidly. By measuring the expression profile, scientists can assess the clues for the regulatory mechanisms, biochemical pathways and cellular functions. In this way, microarrays enable scientists to find out the target genes that cause disease.

The heart of the technology is a glass slide or membrane that consists of a regular array of genes (Figure 2.2). Thousands of genes can be spotted on the array, using a photolithography method. Samples from healthy and diseased cells are mixed with the genes on the array. In this way, many genes can be studied and their expression levels in healthy and diseased states can be determined within a short time. The gene that is responsible for a particular disease can be identified. Exhibit 2.6 presents a more detailed explanation of microarrays.

Expressed sequence tags and in silico methods   Expressed Sequence Tags (ESTs) are short nucleotide sequences of complementary DNA with about 200–500 base pairs. They are parts of the DNA that code for the expression of particular proteins. EST sequencing provides a rapid method to scan for all the protein coding genes and to provide a tag for each gene on the genome.

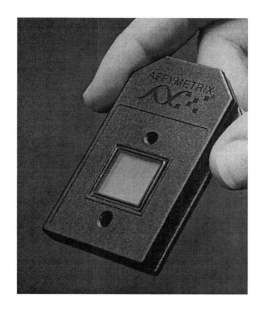 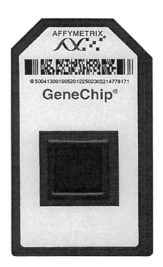

Figure 2.2 Microarray slides
Photo courtesy of Affymetrix, Inc., US.

Exhibit 2.6 Microarrays

To use the microarray, DNA is printed onto a solid support of membrane or glass slide. From healthy and diseased cells, mRNAs are isolated. The mRNAs are used to generate complementary DNAs (cDNAs). Fluorescent tags are attached to the cDNAs, and the cDNAs are then mixed and incubated with the microarray supports (slides).

Through a process called hybridization probing, the genes from the samples pair up with their complementary counterparts on the solid supports. When the hybridization step is completed, a scanner (laser beam and camera) is used to capture the fluorescence image of the array.

From comparison of the intensities and ratios of red and green fluorescence, the expression levels of genes from the healthy and diseased cells can be deciphered. For example, if the disease causes some types of genes to be expressed more, more of these genes will hybridize with the DNA on the solid support, providing a greater intensity of red fluorescence than of green. In this way, disease targets can be identified.

Continued

Exhibit 2.6 *Continued*

The flowchart shows a schematic representation of the use of a microarray for identification of disease genes.

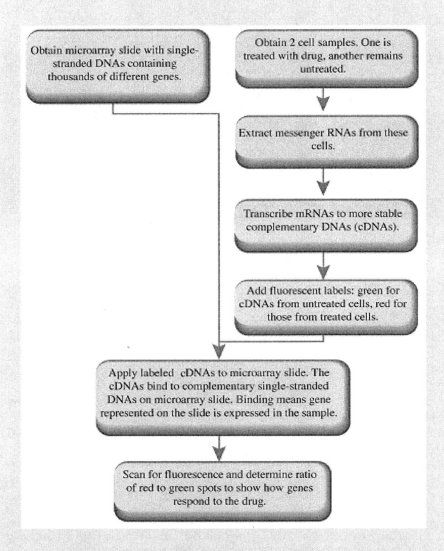

SOURCE   Friend, S.H. and Stoughton, R.B., The magic of microarrays, *Scientific American*, February, pp. 44–53 (2002).

The scanning of nucleotide sequences is achieved through *in silico* (computer) methods. The premise is that all proteins, even those with sequences that appear considerably different, can be members of families sharing essentially similar structures and functions.

Scientists carry out searches on databases. Each EST of interest can be compared with sequences in proteins, and the degree of match determined. A technique called threading is used. This involves using data on 3D protein structure, coupled with knowledge of the physicochemical properties of amino acids, to determine if the amino acid sequence is likely to fold in the same way as a sequence for which the structure is known. In this way, more information about the putative target protein can be assessed.

2.4 TARGET VALIDATION

Once a potential disease-causing target has been identified, a process of validation is carried out to confirm the functions and effects of the target. The ultimate target validation is a series of human clinical trials in which the effects of a drug on the target are evaluated. However, this kind of validation is at the other end of the drug discovery spectrum, when too much time and commitment have already been expended on the drug. What is required at this early stage is validation of the target identified, to lay the path for developing appropriate drugs aiming at this target. This will ensure that time, resources and investments can be optimized.

Some questions that target validation has to answer are:
- What is the function of the target?
- Which disease pathway does the target regulate?
- How important is this disease pathway?
- What is the expected therapeutic index if a drug is to interact with the target?

Validations can be divided into two groups: *in vitro* laboratory tests, and *in vivo* disease models using animals.

Typically, *in vitro* tests are cell- or tissue-based experiments. The aim is to study the biochemical functions of the target as a result of binding to potential drug ligands. Parameters such as ionic concentrations, enzyme activities and expression profiles are studied.

For *in vivo* studies, animal models are set up and how the target is involved in the disease is analyzed. One such model is the mouse knockout model (Exhibit 2.7). It should be borne in mind, however, that there are

Exhibit 2.7 Knockout Mice

Genetic research, such as by microarray, reveals the possible genes that may cause the disease under study. Transgenic mice are bred with the putative gene modified or inactivated, giving rise to the term 'knockout' mice models. The effects of gene knockouts are studied in relation to the progress of disease. It is also possible to study drug interactions by treating these mice with potential drug candidates.

SOURCE Harris, S., Transgenic knockouts as part of high-throughput, evidence-based target selection and validation strategies, *Drug Discovery Today*, 16, pp. 628–636 (2001).

differences between humans and animals in terms of gene expression, functional characteristics and biochemical reactions. Nevertheless, animal models are important for the evaluation of drug–target interactions in a living system.

More recently, *in silico* target validation has been used. This is similar to the method discussed for ESTs. The DNA sequence of the putative target is compared with those of known liganded receptors. Homology (similarity) of sequences and structures, if these are determined, can provide clues to ligands that are likely to interact with the target.

2.5 DRUG INTERACTIONS WITH TARGETS OR RECEPTORS

It should be clarified that targets identified using microarrays are mainly the genes that regulate or contribute to diseases. These gene targets give us the clues to the proteins that are affected. In most situations, it is the proteins or receptors that drug molecules are developed to interact with to provide the therapy. The exceptions are in cases such as antisense drugs and gene therapy, where the nucleotides and genes are targeted, respectively.

When presented to the target, drug molecules can elicit reactions to switch on or switch off certain biochemical reactions. The main drug targets in the human body can be classified into three categories:

- *Enzymes:* There are many different types of enzyme in the human body. They are required for a variety of functions. Drugs can interact with enzymes to modulate their enzymatic activities.
- *Intracellular receptors:* These receptors are in the cytoplasm or nucleus. Drugs or endogenous ligand molecules have to pass

through the cell membrane (a lipid bilayer) to interact with these receptors. The molecules must be hydrophobic or coupled to a hydrophobic carrier to cross the cell membrane.

- *Cell surface receptors:* These receptors are on cell surface and have an affinity for hydrophilic binding molecules. Signals are transduced from external stimuli to the cytoplasm, and affect cellular pathways via these surface receptors. There are three main superfamilies (groups) of cell surface receptors: G-protein coupled receptors, ion channel receptors, and catalytic receptors using enzymatic activities.

Hydrophilic, or water-soluble drugs do not cross membranes. They stay in the bloodstream for durations that are normally short, lasting of the order of seconds, and mediate responses of short duration. In contrast, hydrophobic drugs require carrier molecules for transport through the bloodstream. Hydrophobic drugs remain in the bloodstream and can persist for hours and days, providing much longer effects.

When the action of the drug is to activate or switch on a reaction, the drug is called an 'agonist'. On the other hand, if the drug switches off the reaction, or inhibits or blocks the binding of other agonist components onto the receptor, it is called an 'antagonist'. When the interaction is with an enzyme, the terms 'inducer' and 'inhibitor' are used to denote drugs that activate or deactivate the enzyme.

Appendix 3 lists some common drugs and their mechanisms of action, showing their roles as agonists or antagonists, and inducers or inhibitors. Figures 2.3 and 2.4 provide schematic lock and key representations of the agonist and antagonist actions. It should be noted that the drug molecule (agonist or antagonist), receptor and cell membrane are in fact complicated 3-dimensional structures. Only certain keys can be inserted into the lock and activate or deactivate the lock. Some facts about interactions between drug molecules and targets to bear in mind are:

- Binding is specific
- Binding occurs at particular sites in the target molecule
- Binding is reversible.

Allosteric binding occurs when two molecules bind to different sites on the target. When the two molecules are identical, it is called homotropic interaction. If the molecules differ from each other, it is called heterotropic interaction. Binding is competitive when two different ligand molecules compete for the same site. We discuss ligand binding further in Chapter 5. The specificity of ligand–receptor interaction is illustrated in Exhibit 2.8.

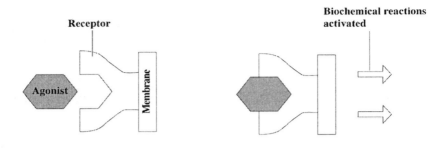

Figure 2.3 Agonist binding to receptor initiates biochemical reactions

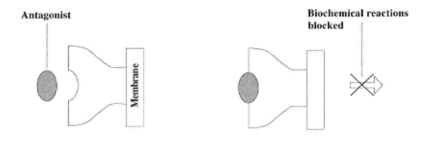

Figure 2.4 Antagonist binding to receptor blocks biochemical reactions

2.5.1   Types of interactions

Binding between drug molecule and receptor or enzyme is critically dependent on the shapes and sizes of the molecules. To deliver the therapeutic actions, drug molecules with the right shapes and sizes have to be designed to fit into the binding sites (pockets) of the receptor or enzyme. Another important factor is the nature of the coupling. Before a drug can fit into the binding site, it has to overcome thermal and vibrational motions at the cellular level. The attractive forces must be strong enough for the drug to dock with the binding site. When molecules couple together, the type of bonding can be divided into covalent bonding, and electrostatic interactions due to hydrogen bonding or van der Waals forces. The stronger the coupling between the drug and binding site, the more sustained is the interaction.

Exhibit 2.8 Aspirin (Acetylsalicylic Acid)

The enzyme prostaglandin H_2 synthase (PGHS) manufactures prostaglandin H_2, which causes fever and inflammation. PGHS contains two protein subunits with long channels.

The chemical arachidonic acid enters these channels and becomes converted to prostaglandin H_2. Aspirin, with the correct shape and size, enters these channels and blocks entry of arachidonic acid. As a result, the agent for causing fever and inflammation cannot be manufactured. Unfortunately, an undesirable effect of aspirin is that it blocks other types of PGHS, including the types that protect the stomach lining, giving rise to potential for stomach bleeding.

Recent advances with other anti-inflammatory drugs, ibuprofen and naproxen, which only work by physically blocking the channel to arachidonic acid, mean that the adverse effect of stomach bleeding can be avoided.

SOURCE Garavito, M., Aspirin, *Scientific American*, May, p. 108 (1999).

Covalent bonds are strong bonds. Actual bonds are formed between the interacting molecules via the sharing of electrons. Hence, this type of interaction is expected to provide long lasting effects although not many drug-receptor bonds are of this nature.

Electrostatic forces are due to the ionic charges residing on the molecules, which attract or repel each other. The macromolecular structures of the receptors and enzymes mean that there are a number of ionic charges to attract the oppositely charged drug molecules. The forces of electrostatic interactions are weaker than covalent bonding. Electrostatic interactions are more common in drug–receptor interactions. There are two types of electrostatic interactions:

- Hydrogen bonding
- Van der Waals forces.

Hydrogen bonds are due to the attractive forces between the distorted electron cloud of a hydrogen atom and other more electronegative atoms such as oxygen and nitrogen. The attractive forces are weaker than covalent bonds, but many hydrogen bonds can be formed in macromolecular protein molecules. Van der Waals forces are weaker attractive forces, due to the attraction between neutral atoms.

A third type of interaction is due to hydrophobic effects. These are the result of non-electrostatic domains interacting. This type of interaction occurs mainly with the highly lipid-soluble drugs in the lipid part within the cytoplasm of the cell.

2.6 ENZYMES

Enzymes are biological molecules that catalyze biochemical reactions. The thermodynamics of biochemical reactions are described in Exhibit 2.9.

Almost all enzymes are proteins. They provide templates whereby reactants (substrates) can bind and are favorably oriented to react and generate the products. The locations where the substrates bind are known as 'active sites'. Because of the specific 3D structures of the active sites, the functions of enzymes are specific, i.e. each particular type of enzymes catalyzes specific biochemical reactions. Enzymes speed up reactions, but

Exhibit 2.9 Thermodynamics of Enzymatic Reactions

In general, there are two types of biochemical reactions: exothermic and endothermic. Exothermic reactions are those where the energy states (free energy, labeled as G) of the reactants are higher than those of the products—they are energetically favorable. Endothermic reactions are those for which the products have higher energy states than the reactants—they are energetically unfavorable.

Regardless of whether the reaction is favorable, the reactants have to come together in close proximity to react. They have to overcome a potential energy barrier that may involve displacing solvating molecules around the reactants and reorientating the reactants. The energy needed to overcome this potential energy barrier is called the activation energy (see figure).

Enzymes bind to the reactants and provide an alternative mechanism of lower activation energy for the reaction to proceed. Hence, enzymes speed up biochemical reactions that are otherwise too sluggish to advance.

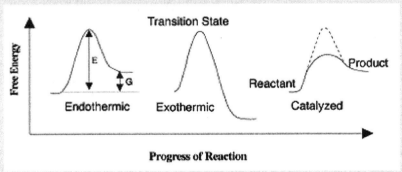

NOTE E is the potential energy barrier, known as the activation energy. G is the change in free energy. The catalyzed reaction provides an alternative reaction pathway with lower activation energy.

they are not consumed and do not become part of the products. Enzymes are grouped into six functional classes by the International Union of Biochemists (Table 2.2).

In some cases, enzymes require the assistance of coenzymes (cofactors) to ensure the reactions proceed. Coenzymes include vitamins, metal ions, acids and bases. They can act as transporters or electron acceptors or be involved in oxidation–reduction reactions. At the completion of the reaction, coenzymes are released, and they do not form part of the products. For some reactions that are energetically unfavorable, an energy source provided by the compound adenosine triphosphate (ATP) is needed to ensure the reactions proceed.

Enzymatic reactions can be impeded by the additions of exogenous molecules. This is how drugs are used to control biochemical reactions, and most drugs are used for inhibitory functions. Drugs may function as competitive inhibitors or as non-competitive inhibitors. Competitive inhibitors compete with the substrates for binding to the active sites, whereas non-competitive inhibitors bind to another location (allosteric site), but affect the active site and its consequential interactions with the substrates. Some drugs used as enzyme inhibitors are:

- Omeprazole (Losec, AstraZeneca): proton pump inhibitor for the prevention of relapse in reflux esophagitis
- Captopril (Capoten, Bristol-Myers Squibb): angiotensin-converting enzyme (ACE) inhibitor for the treatment of hypertension
- Imatinib mesylate (Gleevec, Novartis): tyrosine kinase inhibitor for the treatment of chronic myeloid leukemia (refer to Exhibit 7.3)

Table 2.2 Classification of enzymes

Number	Classification	Biochemical properties
1	Oxidoreductases	Remove or add hydrogen atoms in oxidation or reduction reactions.
2	Transferases	Transfer functional groups from one molecule to another. Kinases are specialized transferases that transfer phosphate from ATP to other molecules.
3	Hydrolases	Hydrolyze various functional groups.
4	Lyases	Add water, ammonia or carbon dioxide across double bonds, or remove these elements to produce double bonds.
5	Isomerases	Convert between different isomers.
6	Ligases	Form a bond between molecules.

- Sertraline (Zoloft, Pfizer): selective serotonin (5-hydroxytryptamine; 5HT) uptake inhibitor for treating major depression and obsessive compulsive disorder
- Atorvastatin (Lipitor, Pfizer) and simvastatin (Zocor, Merck): HMG-Coenzyme A inhibitors for the reduction of cholesterol level in blood (refer to Exhibit 1.3).

Exhibit 2.10 shows two new drugs, celecoxib (a COX-2 inhibitor) and orlistat (a lipase inhibitor) and their actions on disease targets.

Exhibit 2.10 Two New Drugs

COX-2 inhibitor

Celecoxib (Celebrex, Searle): This drug inhibits the enzyme COX-2, which is involved in pain and inflammation, but it has no effect on the COX-1 enzyme, which helps to maintain stomach lining. It is prescribed for the relief of pain and symptoms of osteoarthritis and rheumatoid arthritis. Previously, non-steroidal anti-inflammatory drugs (NSAIDs) were used. NSAIDs inhibit both COX-1 and COX-2 enzymes, and cause stomach bleeding.

Lipase inhibitor

Orlistat (Xenical, Roche): This drug inhibits the gastrointestinal lipase enzymes. It binds to the lipase through the serine site and inactivates the enzyme. Fat in the form of triglycerides cannot be hydrolyzed by the lipase and converted to free fatty acids and monoglycerides. Thus, there is no uptake of fat molecules into the cell tissue. This drug is prescribed for the treatment of obesity.

Drugs are also used to inhibit the enzymatic reactions of foreign pathogens that enter the human body. An example is the use of reverse transcriptase inhibitor and protease inhibitor for combating the human immunodeficiency virus (HIV), as shown in Exhibit 2.11.

2.7 RECEPTORS AND SIGNAL TRANSDUCTION

Cells communicate to coordinate the biochemical functions within the human body. If the communication system is interrupted or messages are not conveyed fully, our bodily functions can go haywire. An example of this is discussed in Exhibit 2.2: if the p53 protein is mutated, cell growth is unchecked and cancer can form.

Exhibit 2.11 Drugs against HIV

The diagram below shows the various stages of HIV infection of the CD4 cell (see also Exhibits 4.4 and 4.5).

Reverse transcriptase is an enzyme that makes a DNA copy of the virus RNA (Step 3). Once made, the DNA enters the cell nucleus and replicates into many copies. Another enzyme, the protease, is required to cut the HIV proteins into proper sizes and assemble into the viral particles (Step 7).

The drug zidovidine (AZT; Retrovir, GlaxoSmithKline) is a reverse transcriptase inhibitor. It is structurally similar to a nucleotide called thymidine except for an azido ($-N_3$) group in place of the $-OH$ group at the 3′ position of the thymidine nucleotide sugar. Thymidine is a building block for the viral DNA, and when AZT is incorporated into the DNA chain it blocks further chain linkages, as there is no $-OH$ group available.

At Step 6, large molecules of the viral proteins are made. Protease cleaves the large protein molecules into smaller pieces. Another drug, a protease inhibitor, is used to inhibit the protease, thus stopping the formation of new viruses.

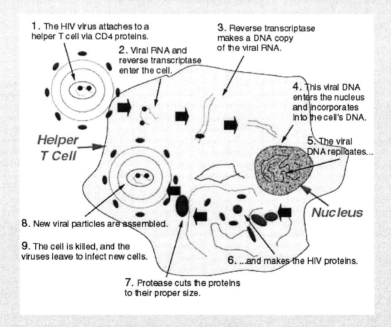

SOURCE   Casidy R. and Frey, R., *Drug Strategies to Target HIV: Enzyme Kinetics and Enzyme Inhibitors*, Washington University, http://wunmr.wustl.edu/EduDev/LabTutorials/HIV/DrugStrategies.html [accessed May 21, 2003].

There are hundreds of receptors on the cell surface. They act as antennas to receive signals from the extracellular environment. These signals may be from endogenous sources, such as neurotransmitters, cytokines and hormones, or exogenous sources, such as viruses and drugs. On receiving the signals, receptors transduce these signals to the cell interior. Within the cell, the signal may cause a cascade of reactions to proceed. Figure 2.5 illustrates this signal transduction process.

Signals may be relatively straightforward, as in the case of ion channels for opening and closing of channel gates for migration of ions. There are also signals that are more complex, involving the binding of ligand to the receptor. A consequence of the binding is a conformational (shape) change in the receptor, which leads to further amplifying processes.

We discuss below a number of receptor classes and analyze how signals are transduced. These receptors are G-protein coupled receptors (GPCRs), ion channel receptors, tyrosine kinases, and intracellular receptors. A list of selected drugs and target receptors is shown in Table 2.3.

2.7.1   G-protein coupled receptors

G-protein coupled receptors (GPCRs) represent possibly the most important class of target proteins for drug discovery. They are always involved in signaling from outside to inside the cell. The number of diseases that are caused by a GPCR malfunction is enormous, and therefore it is not surprising that most commonly prescribed medicines act on a GPCR. It is estimated that more than 30% of drugs target this receptor superfamily.

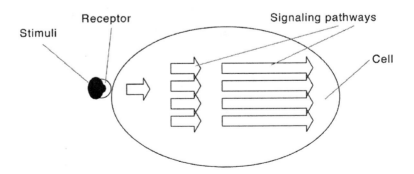

Figure 2.5 Signal transduction showing cascades of reaction occurring inside the cell

Table 2.3 Selected drugs and target receptors

Drug	Therapeutic category	Drug target
Omeprazole (Losec, AstraZeneca)	Gastrointestinal/metabolism	Ion channel
Simvastatin (Zocor, Pfizer)	Cardiovascular	Enzyme inhibitor
Atorvastatin (Lipitor, Pfizer)	Cardiovascular	Enzyme inhibitor
Amlodipine (Norvasc, Pfizer)	Cardiovascular	Ion channel
Lansoprazole (Takepron, Takeda)	Gastrointestinal/ metabolism	Ion channel
Loratadine (Claritin, Schering)	Respiratory	GPCR
Erythropoietin (Procrit, Ortho Biotech)	Hematology	Transmembrane agonist
Celecoxib (Celebrex, Pharmacia)	Musculoskeletal	Enzyme inhibitor
Fluoxetine (Prozac, Eli Lilly)	Central nervous system	GPCR
Olanzapine (Zyprexa, Eli Lilly)	Central nervous system	GPCR
Paroxetine (Seroxat, GlaxoSmithKline)	Central nervous system	GPCR
Rofecoxib (Vioxx, Merck)	Musculoskeletal	Enzyme inhibitor
Sertraline (Zoloft, Pfizer)	Central nervous system	GPCR
Erythropoietin (Epogen, Amgen)	Hematology	Transmembrane agonist
Augmentin/amoxillin plus clavulanic acid	Anti-infective	Enzyme inhibitor

CNS = central nervous system. GPCR = G-protein coupled receptor.
SOURCE Adapted from Renfrey, S. and Featherstone, J., From the analyst's couch: Structural proteomics, *Nature Reviews Drug Discovery*, 1, pp. 175–176 (2002).

The common feature of this superfamily (there are many different families and subtypes of receptors in this group) of receptors is that there are seven domains that cross the cell membrane (Figure 2.6). These seven transmembrane receptors are often referred to as serpentine receptors.

The serpentine receptors are coupled to the G-proteins (guanine nucleotide regulatory proteins) inside the cell. There are three subunits that make up the G-proteins: α, β, and γ. When a ligand, for example a drug or neurotransmitter, binds to the receptor on the cell surface, the shape of the receptor changes. This induces an activated change in the trimeric clusters of α, β, and γ subunits within the cell. A phosphorylation (the addition of a phosphate group, such as PO_3H_2, to a compound) reaction occurs, in which guanosine diphosphate (GDP) changes to guanosine triphosphate (GTP):

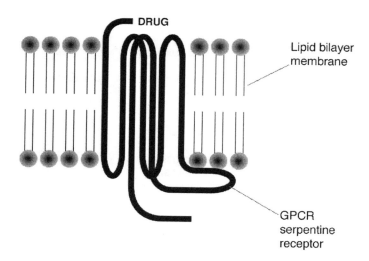

Figure 2.6   A G-protein coupled receptor

$$GDP + phosphate \rightarrow GTP$$

This reaction then switches on the effector molecule, and the signal is relayed along the pathway (see Figure 2.7). When the enzyme GTPase hydrolyzes GTP to GDP and removes the phosphate group, the trimeric subunits change back to the inactivated state. This receptor is once again ready to receive and transmit further signals.

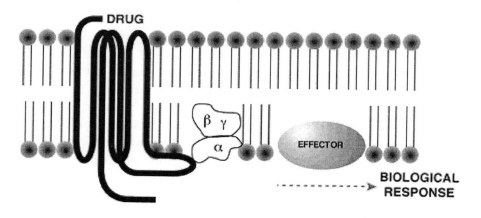

Figure 2.7 Signal cascade in GPCR

GPCRs are involved in a wide range of diseases, including asthma, hypertension, inflammation, cardiovascular disease, cancer, gastrointestinal and central nervous system diseases. From the Human Genome Project, it is estimated that there are about 1000 GPCRs. The current therapeutic drugs are only targeting about 50 of these GPCRs. There are many possibilities of developing new drugs to target this family of receptors.

2.7.2   Ion channel receptors

There are two main types of ion channel receptors: ligand-gated and voltage-gated. In addition, some ion channels are regulated through GPCRs or via activation by amino acids.

The ligand-gated family consists of receptors of the so-called cys-loop superfamily (nicotinic receptor, gamma-aminobutyric acid [GABA$_A$ and GABA$_C$] receptors, glycine receptors, 5-HT$_3$ receptors and some glutamate activated anionic channels). The common feature is that they are made up of five subunits (designated as two α, one β, one γ and one δ subunits - Figure 2.8). Natural ligands for this family of ion channels include acetylcholine, GABA, glycine and aspartic acid. They are, in general, synaptic transmitters.

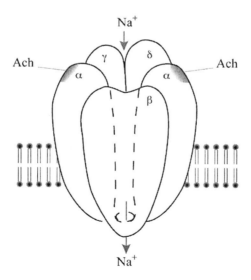

Figure 2.8   A ligand-gated ion channel receptor. ACh = acetylcholine. The binding of ACh to the α subunits opens the ion channel, allowing Na$^+$ ions to flow through the channel into the cell.

Normally, in the resting state, the channel is impermeable to ions. When a ligand binds to the receptor, it becomes activated, and opens a channel to a diameter of about 6.5 Å (6.5 × 10^{-10} m). This action allows the migration of, for example, extracellular sodium ions to the interior of the cell. A cascade of further changes then proceeds within the cell to amplify the signal.

Voltage-gated ion channels depend on changes of transmembrane voltage to regulate the opening and closing of channel gates. A common feature of this type of receptors is the presence of four domains, where each domain consists of six membrane-spanning regions. Some of these channels are the sodium, calcium and potassium channels, and they regulate the influx of these ions into the cell interior to propagate the signal.

Diseases mediated through ion channel receptors include cardiovascular disease, hypertension and central nervous system dysfunctions. A voltage-gated ion channel is a key to the treatment of cystic fibrosis (Exhibit 2.4).

2.7.3   Tyrosine kinases

This class of receptors transmits signals carried by hormones and growth factors. The structure consists of an extracellular domain for binding ligands and a cytoplasmic enzyme domain. The function of kinases is to enable phosphorylation. Phosphorylation regulates most aspects of cell life.

When a ligand binds to the receptors, the receptors dimerize and join together. This action activates the enzyme within the cell. As a result, protein molecules are phosphorylated (Figure 2.9).

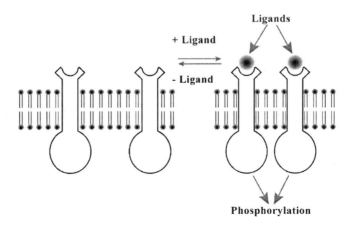

Figure 2.9   A tyrosine kinase receptor

Other kinase receptors are serine/threonine kinases, protein kinases, and mitogen-activated protein (MAP) kinases. Insulin, transforming growth factor-beta (TGF-β) and platelet-derived growth factor (PDGF) are the natural ligands that interact with kinase receptors.

2.7.4 Intracellular receptors

Intracellular (nuclear) receptors are located inside cells, in the cytoplasm or nucleus. Endogenous ligands such as hormones and drugs bind to these receptors to either activate or inhibit transcription messages from genes. There is a large superfamily of these intracellular receptors. The common feature is that they all have a single polypeptide chain consisting of three distinct domains:

- Amino terminus: this region in most instances is involved in activating or stimulating transcription
- DNA binding domain: amino acids in this region are responsible for binding of the receptor to specific sequences of DNA
- Carboxy terminus, or ligand-binding domain: this is the region that binds ligands.

2.8 ASSAY DEVELOPMENT

To study drug–receptor/enzyme interaction, it is not always convenient or appropriate to use a living system of the target receptor. Instead, biochemical assays can be devised to mimic the target. Very often, the assays use multicolor luminescence or fluorescence-based reagents. In this way, the reaction path can be followed in space and time to enable quantitative evaluation of the reaction.

Many parameters can be monitored, for example, free-ion concentrations, membrane potentials, activities of specific enzymes, rate of proton generation, transport of signaling molecules and gene expression.

Primary assays are devised to incorporate physiological or enzymatic targets for screening biological activity of potential drug compounds. The biological assays are then reconfirmed in specific biochemical and whole cell assays to characterize the target compound interaction.

Exhibit 2.12 shows some current assays used in ligand–receptor studies.

Exhibit 2.12 Reporter Assays and Bioluminescence

Assays can be prepared with a reporter system containing, for example, the firefly luciferase gene. The reporter cells are coupled to receptor genes. When a ligand binds to the receptor, luminescence glow can be observed. In this way, the effects of the signaling events are evaluated.

There are other reporter gene systems, such as β-galactosidase (a bacterial enzyme), chloramphenicol acetyltransferase (a bacterial enzyme) and aequorin (a jellyfish protein).

SOURCE Naylor, L.H., Reporter gene technology: The future looks bright, *Biochemical Pharmacology*, 58, pp. 749–757 (1999).

2.9 FURTHER READING

Cambridge Healthtech Institute, *Streamlining Drug Discovery with Breakthrough Technologies for Genomic Target Identification and Validation*, http://www.chireports.com/content/articles/targetart.asp [accessed May 7, 2002].

Campbell, M.K., *Biochemistry*, 3rd edn., Saunders College Publishing, Harcourt Brace College Publishers, Orlando, FL, 1999.

Campbell, N.A., Reece, J.B. and Mitchell, L.G., *Biology*, 5th edn., Benjamin/Cummings Publishing Company, Inc., Menlo Park, CA, 1999.

Cohen, J.S. and Hogan, M.E., The new genetic medicines, *Scientific American*, December, pp. 76–82 (1994).

Deller, M.C. and Jones, E.Y., Cell surface receptors, *Current Opinion in Structural Biology*, 10, pp. 213–219 (2000).

Dowell, S.J., Understanding GPCRs—from orphan receptors to novel drugs, *Drug Discovery Today*, 6, pp. 884–886 (2002).

Drug Discovery Process, http://www.arraybiopharma.com/discovery/index.cfm [accessed May 7, 2002].

Ezzell, C., Beyond the human genome, *Scientific American*, July, pp. 64–69 (2000).

Foreman, J.C. and Johansen, T. (eds.), *Textbook of Receptor Pharmacology*, CRC Press, FL, 2002.

Friend, S.H. and Stoughton, R.B., The magic of microarrays, *Scientific American*, February, pp. 44–53 (2002).

GPCRs,   http://www.cuebiotech.com/inside.php?section=technology&page=gpcr [accessed Jul 2, 2002].

Grahame-Smith, D.G. and Aronson, J.K., *Oxford Textbook of Clinical Pharmacology and Drug Therapy,* 2nd edn., Oxford University Press, Oxford, 1992.

Harris, S., Transgenic knockouts as part of high-throughput, Evidence-based target selection and validation strategies, *Drug Discovery Today,* 6, pp. 628–636 (2001).

Haseltine, W.A., Discovering genes for new medicines, *Scientific American,* March, pp. 92–97 (1997).

Kartzung, B.G. (ed.), *Basic & Clinical Pharmacology,* 6th edn., Appleton & Lange, Norwalk, Connecticut, 1995.

Kenakin, T.P., *Pharmacologic Analysis of Drug–Receptor Interaction,* Raven Press Books, New York, 1987.

Kirkpatrick, P., G-protein-coupled receptors: Putting the brake on inflammation, *Nature Reviews Drug Discovery,* 1, p. 99 (2002).

Leff, P. (ed.), *Receptor-Based Drug Design, Drugs and the Pharmaceutical Sciences,* Volume 89, Marcel Dekker, Inc., New York, 1998.

Persidis, A., Signal transduction as a drug-discovery platform, *Nature Biotechnology,* 16, pp. 1082–1083 (1998).

Pharmocodynamics, 'Drug–receptor interactions', in *The Merck Manual of Diagnosis and Therapy,* Section 22, Clinical Pharmacology, http://www.merck.com/pubs/mmanual/section22/chapter300/300b.htm [accessed May 7, 2002].

Pratt, W.B. and Taylor, P. (eds.), *Principles of Drug Action—The Basis of Pharmacology,* 3rd edn., Churchill Livingstone, New York, 1990.

Scott, J.D. and Pawson, T., Cell communication: The inside story, *Scientific American,* June, pp. 72–79 (2000).

Wise, A., Gearing, K. and Rees, S., Target validation of G-protein coupled receptors, *Drug Discovery Today,* 7, pp. 235–246 (2002).

CHAPTER 3

DRUG DISCOVERY: SMALL MOLECULE DRUGS

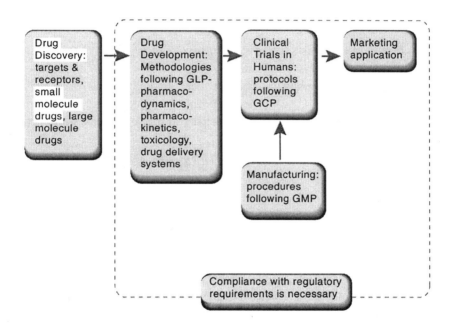

3.1   INTRODUCTION

The World Health Organization (WHO) in its May 2002 report estimated that currently up to 80% of the African people and a significant percentage of the worldwide population still practice some form of traditional medical treatment. Typically, these treatments are in the forms of decoctions, tinctures, syrups or ointments with plant or animal products (see Exhibit 3.1).

Exhibit 3.1 Forms of Traditional Medicines

Decoctions: Liquid extracts of active components and volatile oils from natural products.

Tinctures: These are made by steeping fresh or dried herbs in alcohol or vinegar.

Syrups: They are made by combining tinctures or medicinal liquors with honey or glycerin.

Ointments: Typically prepared by mixing floral or plant ingredients with essential oil and wax, such as beeswax.

However, for most readers of this book, the drugs that we are familiar with, such as analgesics (paracetamol), antibiotics (penicillin), hormones (insulin) and vaccines (hepatitis) are not part of the traditional medical armory. These drugs are either chemically synthesized (small molecule drugs with molecular weights of typically <500 Da) or produced using rDNA technology (protein-based large molecule drugs with molecular weights in excess of thousands of Daltons). We will describe the discovery methodologies for the small molecule drugs in this chapter and that for the protein-based large molecule drugs in Chapter 4.

There are two main approaches to discovering small molecule drugs: the irrational approach, or the more recent structured rational approach. Antisense and chiral drugs are two other drug discovery methodologies.

3.2   IRRATIONAL APPROACH

The basic steps of the irrational or random scanning approach are shown in Figure 3.1.

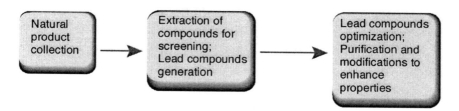

Figure 3.1 The basic steps of the irrational drug discovery process

3.2.1 Natural product collection

This approach of drug discovery commences with the collection of natural materials from their habitats. Such collections typically gather 1–5 kg of materials, which may consist of leaves, shoot, bark, and roots of plants. Marine life forms are collected as well. The locations are recorded, to facilitate further collection of materials should that be required.

An important aspect of natural product collection is to provide biodiversity, i.e. products with different and diverse chemical compositions so that potentially many variations of chemical compositions and structures can be extracted for testing.

Collections of natural products, or bioprospecting, used to be relatively straightforward, with little formality or encumbrances. Now, however, there are new rules (Exhibit 3.2) to protect the natural habitats.

3.2.2 Extraction of potential drug compounds

Compounds are extracted from natural materials using organic solvents such as alcohol. Tannins and chlorophylls from plant materials are normally removed using chromatographic columns, as they can interfere with the screening. In some cases, animal products, such as venoms from snakes, are gathered for screening. In other cases, collections of microorganisms are examined. Two examples are provided below:

- One of the first angiotensin-converting enzyme (ACE) inhibitors was teprotide. It is an antihypertensive drug for use after heart attacks. The active ingredient was isolated from the venom of a South American viper snake. Other well-known ACE inhibitors such as captopril and analopril were developed based on modifications to the venom chemical structures.
- Tetracyclines are a group of antibiotics derived from bacteria. Chlortetracycline was isolated from *Streptomyces aureofaciens* and

oxytetracycline from *S. rimosus*. Tetracyclines act by binding to receptors on the bacterial ribosome and inhibit bacterial protein synthesis.

Exhibit 3.3 shows the chemical formulas of some of the well-known drugs.

Exhibit 3.2   Regulations for Biodiversity Prospecting

Until recently, obtaining samples of plants, microorganisms, animals and marine life forms was straightforward. Normally a researcher would arrive at the collection site with permission from the local authority, and collect samples without much restriction.

There are now new rules for biodiversity prospecting regarding the collection of natural products. The 1993 Convention on Biological Diversity (CBD) established sovereign national rights over biological resources, and committed member countries to conserve them, develop them sustainably, and share the benefits resulting from their use.

CBD requires that permission must be obtained before biological samples can be taken. To comply with the CBD, an Access and Benefit-Sharing Agreement (ABA) has to be agreed between the researcher and the source country providing the natural products. The ABA sets out the clauses with respect to the observation, development and benefit sharing accruing from the use of natural products for medical applications.

With the ABA, the source country must know in advance how the natural products are to be exploited and the benefits that can be shared. If the CBD is not observed, the natural products can be treated as being poached and the patent based on these products may be invalidated.

SOURCE   Gollin, M.A., New rules for natural products research, *Nature Biotechnology*, 17, pp. 921–922 (1999).

Exhibit 3.3   Chemical Formulas of some Selected Drugs

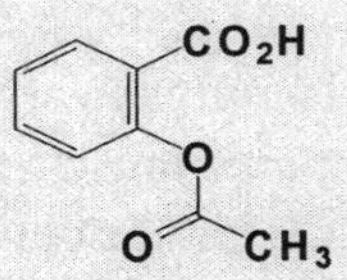

Aspirin 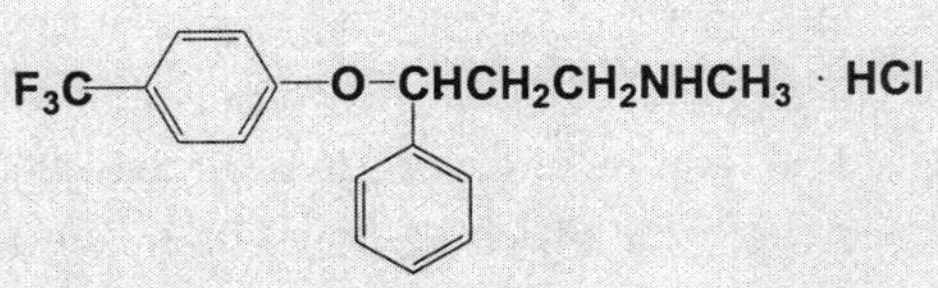   Prozac

Exhibit 3.3 *Continued*

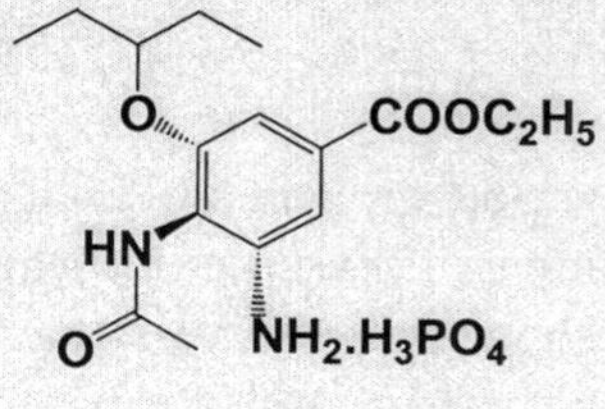

Tamiflu

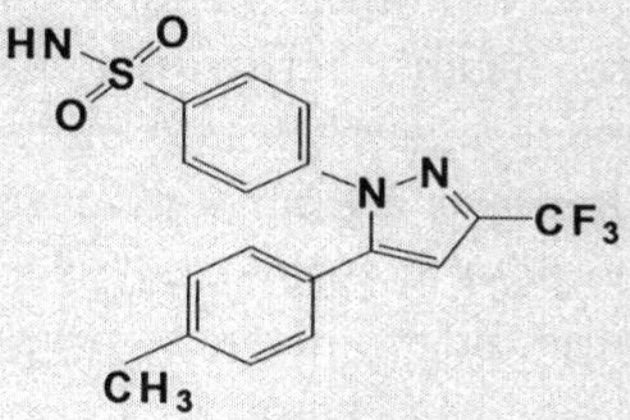

Celebrex

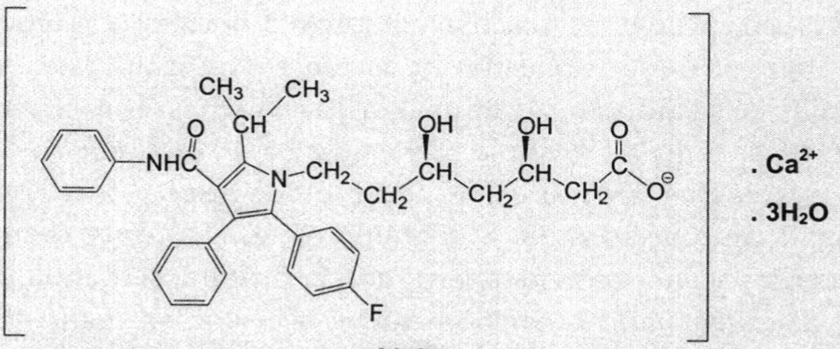

Lipitor

3.2.3 Screening compounds to find 'hits': lead compound generation

The next step is the screening of thousands of these compounds to find lead compounds or potential drug molecules that bind with receptors and modulate disease pathways. When an interaction happens, it is referred to as a 'hit'.

In some cases, compounds are purchased from laboratories or other suppliers. The collections of various compounds are called 'libraries', and libraries of large pharmaceutical organizations have from hundreds of thousands to millions of compounds. For example, the Developmental Therapeutics Program of the United States National Cancer Institute has a collection of more than 600 000 synthetic and natural compounds.

Lead compounds are those that have shown some desired biological activities when tested against the assays. However, these activities are not optimized. Modifications to the lead compounds are necessary to improve the physicochemical, pharmacokinetic and toxicological properties for clinical applications.

3.2.4   Purification and modifications to optimize lead compounds

Following 'hits', the lead compounds are purified using chromatographic techniques and their chemical compositions identified via spectroscopic and chemical means. Structures may be elucidated using X-ray or nuclear magnetic resonance (NMR) methods.

Further tests are carried out to evaluate the potency and specificity of the lead compounds isolated. This is usually followed up with modifications of the compounds to improve properties through synthesis of variations to the compounds via chemical processes in the laboratory and frequently with modifications to the functional groups. The optimized lead compounds go through many iterative processes to keep improving and optimizing the drug interaction properties to achieve improved potency and efficacy.

Only after all these exhaustive tests are a few candidates selected for preclinical *in vivo* studies using animal disease models. The current approach is to perform as much as possible of the tests based on tissue cultures or cell-based assays, as they are less costly and provide results more readily. At the end of this long process is the availability of selected drug candidates with sufficient efficacy and safety required for human clinical trial.

Drug discovery and development is a tortuous path—factors that constraint its development may sometimes arise from unexpected quarters, such as environmental groups (Exhibit 3.4).

Exhibit 3.4 Paclitaxel (Taxol)

Paclitaxel (Taxol, Bristol-Myers Squibb) is a chemotherapy drug for cancers of the ovaries, breasts and certain lung cancer. It was discovered by the US National Cancer Institute in the 1960s. Originally, it was extracted from the bark of the North American yew tree (*Taxus brevifolia*). Clinical tests had necessitated the harvesting of the bark, and this method damaged the trees irreversibly.

Environmental groups objected to this practice, and many demonstrations were staged. A solution was eventually found when the needles of the European yew tree (*Taxus baccata*) provided a source for the paclitaxel precursor without destroying the bark.

Paclitaxel was introduced by Bristol-Myers Squibb in 1993. Today paclitaxel or a precursor can be obtained from cell cultures of *Taxus* media formed by hybridizing *Taxus baccata* and *Taxus cuspidate*.

SOURCE   *The Taxol Story*, Taxolog Inc., 2000–2001, http://www.taxolog.com/taxol.html [accessed Aug 15, 2002].

3.2.5   High throughput screening

As we can imagine, the screening of thousands of natural products using wet laboratory chemistry process is extremely time-consuming. The latest technology in screening is based on laboratory automation and robotics systems. This is termed high throughput screening (HTS) or ultra-HTS (UHTS). These two systems can screen thousands and hundreds of thousands of samples per day, respectively.

The heart of the HTS system is a plate, or tray, which consists of tiny wells where assay reagents and samples are deposited, and their reactions monitored. The configuration of the plate has changed from 96 wells (in a matrix of 8 rows by 12 columns) to 384, and now to a high-density 1536-well format, which enables large-scale screening to be undertaken. Assay reagents may be coated onto the plates, or deposited in liquid form together with test samples into the wells. Both samples and assay reagents may be incubated, and those that interact show signals, which can be detected. A variety of detector systems is used, ranging from radioactive readouts to fluorescence and luminescence. These signals indicate 'hits', and the strengths of the signals show the quality of 'hits'. Lead compounds with good quality 'hits' warrant further evaluation as potential candidates for optimization or modification to become drug candidates. Exhibit 3.5 shows a schematic representation of HTS.

The aim of HTS and UHTS is cost-effectiveness and speed of compound scanning. Hence, the robotics system not only has to deliver fast and accurate liquid samples into the wells, it has to be miniaturized to conserve the volumes required of the valuable samples and expensive assay reagents. For the 1536 wells, the liquids being dispensed are in the nanoliter (10^{-9} L) to picoliter (10^{-12} L) range. The ink jet technology provided the technological basis for liquid dispensation in HTS.

The design of assay systems is another particularly important factor for testing the sample compounds. Assays have to be specific and sensitive. The assays used for HTS come in many forms. There are binding assays, or enzyme-based or cell-based assays. Cell-based assays have become an important test compared with other *in vitro* assays, as they can provide information about bioavailability, cytotoxicity and effects on biochemical pathway. Invariably, the enzyme-based and cell-based assay systems consist of receptors or mimetics of receptors (components that mimic active parts of receptors). Normally the assays are linked to an indicator that shows the ligand–receptor interaction as some forms of signal. Radioligand binding assays were used previously. However, because of the lengthy processing and limited data provided, radioligands binding assays have been superseded by other assays. Scintillation proximity assays (SPAs) and reporter systems such as luciferase (an enzyme in firefly that gives off light) are common forms of signal generation for assay systems (see Section 2.8). The advantage of cell-based assays over biochemical assays is that cell-based assays enable analysis of sample compound activity in an environment that is similar to the one in which a drug would act. It also provides a platform for toxicity studies.

Exhibit 3.5 High Throughput Screening

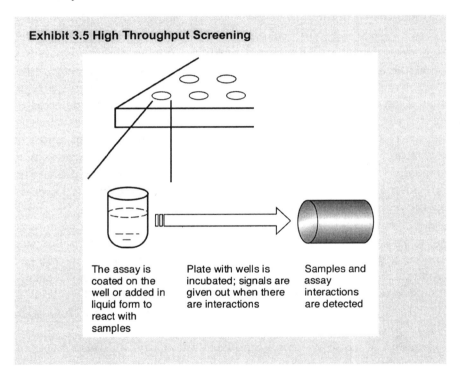

The assay is coated on the well or added in liquid form to react with samples

Plate with wells is incubated; signals are given out when there are interactions

Samples and assay interactions are detected

3.3   RATIONAL APPROACH

The premise for the rational approach is that drug discovery based on knowledge of the three-dimensional (3D) structure as well as the amino acid sequence of the chosen receptor molecule would reveal potential binding sites for drug molecules. Structural information and modeling simulations will help to design a drug that will fit precisely within the binding site, similar to the lock and key concepts discussed in Chapter 2. Such information about the receptor or protein structure will significantly improve the probability of obtaining a successful drug and eliminate unlikely drug candidates at a very early stage of drug discovery. The steps in rational drug discovery are summarized in Figure 3.2.

The standard techniques used for 3D structural determinations are X-ray crystallography and NMR spectroscopy. Modeling of drug–receptor interactions is studied using computational chemistry (*in silico*) methods and mining data using bioinformatics. The modeled drug is then synthesized using combinatorial chemistry, and screened against assays in HTS system. These enabling technologies are described below.

3.3.1 X-ray crystallography

To determine the structures of drug compounds or protein molecules using X-ray crystallography, it is necessary to have these compounds or molecules available in crystalline form. For example, when crystals of protein are formed, the protein molecules are arranged in orderly fashions like tiny imaginary 'cubes' stacked on top of each other. Each of these building blocks contains a molecule of protein, and is termed a unit cell (Figure 3.3).

For examining atomic structures with bond lengths of 1–2 Å, the interrogating beams ideally should have wavelengths of the same dimensions, to resolve atomic details. X-ray fulfils this criterion because its wavelength, for example, CuKα (X-ray using copper target) is 1.5418 Å ($1.5418 \times x10^{-10}$ m), which is similar to atomic dimensions.

When X-ray beams are focused on different orientations of these unit cells, the regular lattice arrangement scatters the X-ray and a 3D diffraction

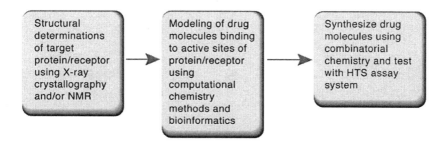

Figure 3.2 The basic steps of the rational drug discovery process

pattern consisting of thousands of diffraction spots is created. The intensity of each diffraction spot is the summation of constructive interference by the atoms (represented as electron density) in the molecule at a certain orientation, and the dimensions and pattern arrangement are due to the geometric positions of these atoms within the protein molecule. From the intensities and diffraction pattern, together with solving the phase angles of the diffracted beams, highly complex mathematical functions are used to determine the protein structure.   Figure 3.4 shows a diagrammatic representation of the structure determination process. A more detailed description of X-ray crystallography is presented in Exhibit 3.6.

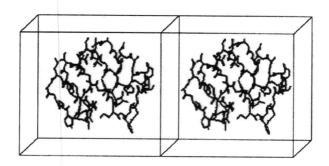

Figure 3.3 Crystalline molecules in 3D. Unit cells are imaginary blocks used to represent the regular arrangement of molecules in 3D space.

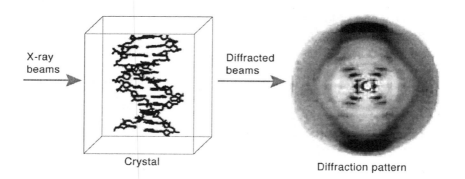

X-ray beams

Diffracted beams

Crystal

Diffraction pattern

Figure 3.4 Steps in X-ray structure determination. X-ray scattering by the crystal gives rise to a diffraction pattern. From the diffraction pattern, the molecular structure can be determined using Fourier transformation mathematical calculations. SOURCE for diffraction photograph   Nicholls, H., Double helix photo not taken by Franklin, *BioMedNet News and Comments*,   2003,   http://news.bmn.com/news/story?day=030425&story   =1#caption_name [Accessed 28 April 2003].

Exhibit 3.6 X-ray Crystallography

Electrons are the components in atoms that scatter X-rays. The magnitude of scattering is measured in terms of the atomic scattering factor, f, which is proportional to the number of electrons in the atom. Hence, heavier atoms have higher atomic scattering factors. For a molecule composed of many atoms, the combined scattering of X-rays by a group of atoms is known as the structure factor, which is the summation of all the atomic scattering factors in space from the unit cell. This is given by the equation:

$$F(hkl) = \sum f_j \cos 2\pi(hx_j + ky_j + lz_j) + \sum f_j \sin 2\pi(hx_j + ky_j + lz_j)$$

where F is the structure factor, f is the atomic scattering factor, h, k, l are the indices for imaginary diffracting planes and x, y, z the position of the scattering atom.

It should be noted that F is a vector quantity with magnitude and direction (phase angle).

The diffraction pattern provides us with intensity and geometric information. The equation for intensity of each diffracting plane, I_{hkl}, is given by:

$$I(hkl) = |F(hkl)|^2.LP.A$$

where LP is a combined geometry and polarization factor and A is the absorption correction factor.

To determine the structure, we have to locate the atoms, which are given by the electron density equation:

$$\rho(xyz) = \frac{1}{V} \sum_h \sum_k \sum_l F(hkl) \exp(-2\pi i(hx + ky + lz))$$

where V is the volume of the unit cell.

Notice that we need F, a complex quantity, to find the electron density. However, from the intensity we can only derive the amplitude of F. The lack of phase information requires specific methods for solution, beyond the scope of this book.

From the intensity, the value for the observed F is obtained. This is substituted into the electron density equation for locating the atoms that determine the structure of the protein. Through an iterative process, the observed and calculated F values are compared to determine the 'goodness of fit' and hence the quality of the structure.

The quality function is given by the crystallographic reliability factor, R_f:

$$R_f = \sum |F_o - F_c| / F_o$$

where F_o is the observed structure amplitude from the real molecule, and F_c is the structure factor calculated from the derived structure.

A perfect match has $R_f = 0$. Most protein structures have R_f values of 0.05–0.10, and a completely random structure gives an R_f of 0.59.

A major drawback with X-ray crystallography is the requirement to obtain crystals of proteins, which is a difficult process. However, techniques are being improved and many structures of proteins have been solved, more than 13 000 at the time of this writing. The very nature of crystallization also means that the protein molecules are 'frozen' in space, rather than in the natural liquid state as found in the human body.

When a ligand is co-crystallized with protein, the active binding site is easily discernable from the structure determined. In situations where it is not possible to insert the ligand, the active site on the protein, which is normally in the form of a clef or pocket on the surface, can be inferred from comparison with other known structures. Once the structure of the active site is known, potential drug molecules can be designed using computational chemistry methods (Exhibit 3.7). Examples of some of the well-known drugs discovered using X-ray crystallography are the human immunodeficiency virus (HIV) drugs, such as amprenavir (Agenerase) and nelfinavir (Viracept). They were designed by studying the interactions of potential drug

---

Exhibit 3.7 Development of Zanamivir (Relenza) and Oseltamivir (Tamiflu)

Flu virus has two types of spikes on the surface: neuraminidase and hemagglutinin. The neuraminidase and hemagglutinin undergo mutations, and these mutations account for the different types of flu viruses (Exhibit 4.2).

The virus uses its hemagglutinin to bind to human cells by interacting with the sialic acid on the human cell surface. The cell then takes up the virus. The virus eventually enters the nucleus, where it replicates to produce many new genes. The genes combine to become multiple copies of viruses, which are released from the cell. When viruses are released, there is a coating of sialic acid on the hemagglutinin, rendering it unable to bind to new cell surface. But the neuraminidase of the virus is able to cleave the sialic acid, thereby letting the hemagglutinin loose to attach and infect other cells.

There is a conserved part on neuraminidase, and this does not mutate or bind to sialic acid. X-ray crystallography revealed that this conserved part is a cleft with four parts. Drug molecules were designed to fit into this cleft and jam the neuraminidase, so that it is not available to cleave the sialic acid. When the sialic acid remains intact on the hemagglutinin, the virus is unable to attach to new cells and propagate the infection.

Two drugs were designed: zanamivir (Relenza) by Glaxo Wellcome and oseltamivir (Tamiflu) by Roche. Zanamivir is a powder that has to be inhaled, and oseltamivir is an oral drug.

SOURCE   Laver, W.G., Bischofberger, N. and Webster, R.G., Disarming flu viruses, *Scientific American*, January, pp. 78–87 (1999).

compounds using the crystal structure of HIV protease. The flu drugs zanamivir (Relenza) and oseltamivir (Tamiflu) were developed with extensive modeling of the crystal structure of neuraminidase, as described in Exhibit 3.7. compounds using the crystal structure of HIV protease. The flu drugs zanamivir (Relenza) and oseltamivir (Tamiflu) were developed with extensive modeling of the crystal structure of neuraminidase, as described in Exhibit 3.7.

3.3.2 Nuclear magnetic resonance spectroscopy

NMR is another powerful tool for determining the 3D structures of compounds. In contrast to X-ray crystallography, NMR requires that the compound be in solution, rather than crystalline. It provides information about the number and types of atoms in the molecule and the electronic environment around these atoms.

The principle behind NMR is that, when a molecule is placed in a strong external magnetic field, certain nuclei of atoms within the molecule, such as ^{1}H, ^{13}C, ^{15}N, ^{19}F and ^{31}P, will resonate as they absorb energy at specific frequencies that are characteristics of their electronic environment. Because most drug and protein molecules are composed of hydrogen, carbon, nitrogen, fluorine and phosphorus, NMR is ideally suited to unravel structural information of drugs and proteins.

An NMR spectrum shows the types of environment around the nuclei (atoms) and the ratios of these nuclei. Compared with X-ray crystallography, NMR has the advantage of being carried out in concentrated solutions rather than requiring crystal samples. The solution states are more representative of the native environment of receptor proteins. NMR can be used to study ligand–receptor interactions. A receptor protein is labeled with isotopes such as ^{13}C or ^{15}N, and changes in their spectra when bound with ligands can be monitored.

However, NMR is limited to molecules with molecular weights of less than 35 kDa. Both techniques, X-ray crystallography and NMR, when combined can provide invaluable information for drug design. With the precise binding site topologies derived from X-ray crystallography and dynamic properties obtained from NMR, tailor-made drug molecules can be designed to fit in the binding sites.

Exhibit 3.8 presents a more detailed description on NMR, and Exhibit 3.9 illustrates the use of NMR in drug discovery.

Exhibit 3.8 Principles of NMR

It is a fundamental property of atomic particles, such as electrons, protons and neutrons, to have spins. Spins can be classified as +½ or –½ spin. For example, a deuterium atom, ^2H, has one unpaired electron, one unpaired proton and one unpaired neutron. The total nuclear spin = ½ (from the proton) + ½ (from the neutron) = 1. Hence, the nuclear spins are paired and result in no net spin for the nucleus. For atoms such as ^1H, ^{13}C, ^{15}N, ^{19}F and ^{31}P, the nuclei consist of protons with unpaired spins.

In the presence of an external magnetic field, the spin of the nucleus can align in two energy states: with or against the field. When energy is applied at the right frequency, resonance occurs and the spin flips from one energy state to another according to the formula:

$$\nu = \gamma B$$

where ν is the frequency, γ is the gyromagnetic ratio and B is the external field strength.

Nuclei are affected by the microenvironment around them. Electrons around the nuclei shield the magnetic field experienced by the nuclei. If the electrons are withdrawn, the nuclei will experience a stronger magnetic field and require more energy (higher resonance frequency) to flip the spins, and vice versa. For ^1H NMR, the hydrogen nuclei of a compound can resonate downfield (higher frequency) or upfield (lower frequency) relative to a standard called tetramethylsilane (TMS).

The NMR spectrum also provides information about the number of nuclei under each distinct environment. This is given by the area under each resonant peak representing the relative number of nuclei of each type. Furthermore, the surrounding nuclei also cause a splitting pattern. For example, a H surrounded by 'n' other H neighbors will have its resonance peak split into 'n+1' peaks.

SOURCE Hornak, J.P., *The basics of NMR*, http://www.cis.rit.edu/htbooks/nmr/ [accessed Oct 31, 2002].

Exhibit 3.9 NMR in Drug Discovery

In addition to being used for structural determinations of protein targets, NMR is increasingly being used to examine the dynamic interactions of ligand–receptor binding. Two NMR properties are particularly important: chemical shift and nuclear spin relaxation.

When a ligand binds to a protein receptor, it perturbs the microchemical environment of the protein nuclei through bond formation, hydrogen bonding and/or van der Waals forces. The shifting of the resonance frequency reflects the strengths of the interaction.

Exhibit 3.9 *Continued*

The nucleus absorbs the magnetic energy and flips to another spin state. After a finite time, the spin state reverts to the original state through an equilibrium process. Generally, small molecules with fast rotational motions have slow relaxation rates. When a ligand binds to a target, the interaction slows the rotational motions. The relaxation time thus changes. This is observed via the nuclear overhauser effects (NOEs), which are a measure of Brownian motions (rotational motions of molecules). A negative NOE for a small molecule is indicative of binding to the protein target.

An example of the use of NMR to design inhibitors of the protein kinase p38 is shown below. The first NMR spectrum shows the resonance peaks of nicotinic acid (a) and 2-phenoxy benzoic acid (b) in the absence of a target enzyme. When a target enzyme is added, in this case the p38 MAP kinase, binding of the ligand and the enzyme causes line broadening and attenuation of the resonance peaks. This is shown by the second NMR spectrum, in which the affected peaks are those of the 2-phenoxy benzoic acid (from 7.2 ppm to 6.6 ppm), indicating the interactions between p38 MAP kinase and 2-phenoxy benzoic acid.

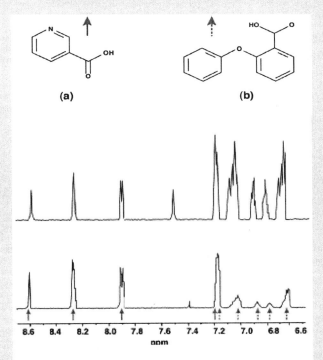

SOURCE Reprinted with permission from Pellecchia, M., Sem, D.S. and Wuthrich, K., NMR in drug discovery, *Nature Reviews Drug Discovery*, 1, pp. 211–219 (2002).

3.3.3   Bioinformatics

Bioinformatics is the use of information technology for the collation and analysis of biological data. This field of study started in the 1980s; it was initially set up by the US Department of Energy for the storage and retrieval of short sequences of DNA. The database is called GenBank. Now GenBank has been transferred to the National Institutes of Health's National Center for Biotechnology Information (NCBI). Many more databases, both public and private, have been set up to enable scientists to deposit, revise, retrieve and analyze biological information. The Human Genome Project is a prime example of bioinformatics. Terabytes (2^{40} bytes) of capacity are used to store the sequence information of billions of DNA base pairs.

As bioinformatics evolves and matures, more and more information beyond sequences of DNAs and amino acids is added to the database. The amount of data that can be generated is phenomenal. It is reported that the growth in bioinformatics data exceeded even the well-known Moore's Law for electronics, which states that the number of transistors on a chip doubles every 18 months. The Internet has played a central role in the growth of bioinformatics. It provides a comprehensive and easily accessible means for information storage, retrieval and analysis.

A process called data mining is used to extract the ever-expanding valuable information from the databases. Data mining consists of complex computer algorithms and mathematical functions with testable hypotheses for a range of analyses. The analyses include homology comparison, gene identification, RNA transcription and protein translation. Some of these are discussed in Chapter 2 under microarrays and expressed sequence tags for target identification. Newly sequenced DNA can be compared with previously sequenced DNA segments of model organisms. Sequences that match or closely resemble model systems enable scientists to predict the likely proteins being produced. Bioinformatics also assists scientists to assess the probable 3D structures of proteins. Bioinformatics, in conjunction with structural data from X-ray crystallography and NMR, helps scientists to focus on the likely target and the binding sites for drugs to be designed.

In addition, bioinformatics databases have been expanded to integrate data on absorption, distribution, metabolism, excretion and toxicity of drugs. Through these comprehensive sets of data, scientists have at their disposal powerful means to relate disease targets and their cellular functions to physiological and pathological processes.

Another application of bioinformatics is the use of pharmocogenomics.

There are some diseases, such as sickle cell anemia (Exhibit 2.3), in which the difference of one amino acid group can have drastic consequences. These differences in nucleotides are termed single nucleotide polymorphisms (SNPs). SNPs, whether due to genetic origins or environmental factors, translate to individual differences. By understanding these SNPs using bioinformatics, more individualized medicines with better efficacy and less adverse effects can be prescribed.

In essence, bioinformatics is applied as below:

- Scan the DNA sequences to determine locations of genes
- Analyze transcription and translations of genetic codes to proteins (see Appendix 2.2.3)
- Determine possible functions and structures for proteins
- Predict binding sites for drug interactions and modulations of causative effects of disease pathway
- Provide information for drugs to be designed to fit the binding sites
- Analyze SNPs for tailored prescriptions to individuals.

A simplified bioinformatics process for provision of information is shown in Figure 3.5.

3.3.4 Computational chemistry

Computational chemistry is an *in silico* method (computational approach) that is used to determine the structure–activity relationships (SARs) of ligand–protein receptor binding. It encompasses a number of techniques, such as computer assisted drug design, computer aided molecular design and computer assisted molecular modeling. There are many software algorithms written for computational chemistry, with different emphasis on modeling and SAR functions.

When a ligand (drug molecule) interacts with a protein, the protein bonds with the drug and undergoes varying degrees of conformational change to accommodate the drug. As a result, the biological activity regulated by the protein is modified, as shown by the equation below, relating SAR as a function of the interaction:

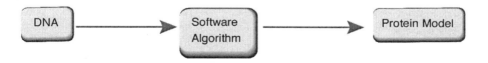

Figure 3.5 Bioinformatics flow of information

SAR = f (ligand–protein bonds and conformational change)

The aim of computational chemistry is to perform virtual screening using computer-generated ligands via a *de novo* drug design method—the design of drug compounds by incremental construction of a ligand model within a model of the receptor or enzyme active site. Libraries of virtual ligands are generated on computer based on certain building blocks or framework (scaffolds) of chemical compounds. The method uses a genetic algorithm, which simulates the genetic evolutionary process to produce 'generations' of virtual compounds with new structures that have improved ability to bind to the receptor protein, similar to the concept of 'survival for the fittest' in the biological process.

To maximize the chances of success, it is necessary to build in 'drug-like' properties. One of the 'drug-like' criteria adopted is the 'Lipinski Rule of 5'— so named because of its emphasis on the number 5 and multiples of 5. The rule states that potential drug candidates are likely to have poor absorption and permeability if they have:

- >5 hydrogen bond donors (the sum of –OH and NH_2 groups)
- Molecular weight >500
- Log P (the octanol/water partition coefficient, which indicates lipophilicity) >5, or
- >10 hydrogen bond acceptors (the sum of nitrogen and oxygen atoms).

Using information about the 3D shape of a protein receptor active site, which is derived from X-ray crystallography or NMR, ligands from the virtual library can be selected and fitted into the site. This is a modeling process known as docking simulation (Figure 3.6).

Ligands are selected based on their 'drug-like' properties, shapes, and the orientations and distributions of chemical functional groups complementary to those of the protein. For example, a hydrogen bond donor of the ligand matches with a hydrogen bond acceptor of the protein, where positive electrostatic charge aligns with negative electrostatic charge and so on. Constituent side chains or functional groups of the ligands are varied to provide many different configurations for the docking analysis, with a view to optimize the best ligands that can be used as potential drug candidates.

Docking simulation is distinct from wet laboratory chemistry, where chemical reactions are performed using real rather than virtual compounds.

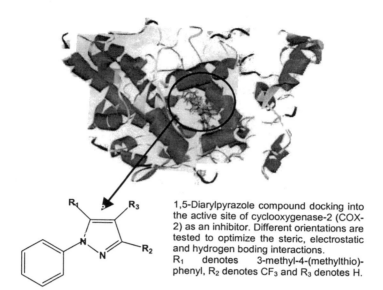

1,5-Diarylpyrazole compound docking into the active site of cyclooxygenase-2 (COX-2) as an inhibitor. Different orientations are tested to optimize the steric, electrostatic and hydrogen boding interactions. R_1 denotes 3-methyl-4-(methylthio)-phenyl, R_2 denotes CF_3 and R_3 denotes H.

Figure 3.6 Docking simulations. SOURCE Reprinted with permission from Liu, H., Huang, X., Shen, J., et al., Inhibitory mode of 1,5-diarylpyrazole derivatives against cyclooxygenase-2 and cyclooxygenase-1: Molecular docking and 3D QSAR analyses, *Journal of Medicinal Chemistry*, 45, pp. 4816–4827 (2002).

The docking approach is more cost effective and efficient than the conventional chemical synthesis route. It allows a large database of virtual compounds to be screened and matched up with the binding site of the targeted protein.

Scoring systems are set up to quantitatively calculate how well the ligand docks with the active site in terms of alignment, hydrogen bonding, van der Waals forces, and electrostatic and hydrophobic interactions. In addition, flexibilities of both the ligands and protein in the binding process as they accommodate each other have to be considered.

The affinity of interactions can be calculated in a number of ways. One example is the force field method to calculate the free energy of binding for the ligand–protein system before and after the docking, as given by the equation:

$$\Delta G = T\Delta S_{rt} + n_r E_r + \Sigma n_x E_x$$

where ΔG is the free energy of binding, $T\Delta S_{rt}$ is the loss of overall rotational and translational entropy upon binding, n_r is the number of internal degrees of conformational freedom lost on binding, E_r is the energy equivalent of the entropy loss, n_x is the number of functional groups in the ligand, and E_x is the binding energy associated with each ligand functional group (Andrews, 2000).

The energy calculations include the rotational and translational changes and torsional angular effects of the ligands and protein, as well as solvation and de-solvation energies because ligands have to displace water molecules normally residing in the active site. An analogy is fitting a hand into a rubber glove. The fingers have to be extended and the glove stretched to accommodate the fit similar to the rotational, translational and torsional changes required for a good fit. Entrapped air inside the glove has to be expelled, much like the ligand replacing the water molecules at the active site. A schematic view is shown in Figure 3.7.

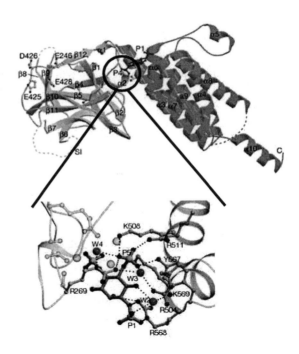

Figure 3.7 A ligand fitting into a binding site. Binding of inositol 1,4,5-trisphosphate (InsP₃) with its receptor. The InsP₃ receptor plays a key role in cellular and physiological processes. SOURCE Reprinted with permission from Bosanac, I., Alattia, J.R., Mal, T.K., et al. Structure of the inositol 1,4,5-trisphosphate receptor binding core in complex with its ligand, *Nature*, 420, pp. 696–700 (2002).

There are other scoring functions for rating the docking of ligands to the protein binding site. These functions include *ab initio* (from first principle) quantum mechanical calculations, which take into account the electronic populations of the entire ligand–protein system and the bonding scheme, and molecular Monte Carlo iterative processes, which consider thermodynamic properties, minimum energy structures and kinetic coefficients.

The result of computational chemistry is some potential drug candidates. These can be synthesized using combinatorial or wet-laboratory techniques, and then tested with assays. The advantage is to screen an array of ligands virtually in a cost effective manner and compress the discovery timeline. Exhibit 3.10 shows a typical workflow process for virtual screening.

Exhibit 3.10 Virtual Screening Process

Presented below is a pictorial description of the workflow of a virtual screening run against a specific target. The typical workflow consists of a preparation of the virtual library database and the target. Docking simulations are next taken, and various scoring functions are used to rate the 'goodness' of fit for the potential candidate to the target.

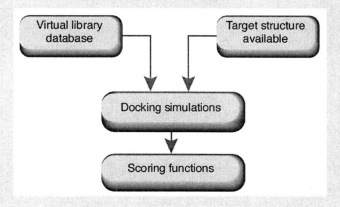

3.3.5 Combinatorial chemistry

Combinatorial chemistry is a laboratory chemistry technique to synthesize a diverse range of compounds through methodical combinations of building block components. These building blocks (reagents) are added to reaction vessels, and the reactions proceed simultaneously to generate an almost infinite array of compounds, limited only by the imaginations of the scientists. This technique is in contrast to traditional methods, in which compounds are synthesized sequentially by mixing one reagent with another and with further reagents to build up the compound. By using combinatorial chemistry techniques, large libraries of many thousands of compounds can be prepared very quickly, unlike the laborious task needed to collect natural compounds from the field. However, there is a debate as to which method, combinatorial chemistry or natural collection, would provide more diverse range of compounds and biodiversity to be tested.

The selection of building blocks is based on information derived from, for example, computational chemistry, where potential virtual ligand molecules are modeled to fit the receptor protein binding site. Combinatorial chemistry commences with a scaffold or framework to which additional groups are added to improve the binding affinity. Compounds are prepared and later screened using HTS. In this way, many compounds are tested within a short timeframe to speed up drug discovery.

There are two basic combinatorial chemistry techniques: (a) parallel synthesis and (b) split and mix methods. They are illustrated below.

Parallel synthesis: We start the reaction by using two sets of building blocks, amines (A) and carboxylic acids (B). The amines are first attached to solid supports, normally polystyrene beads coated with linking groups, in separate reaction vessels for each amine. After the amines have been attached, excess unreacted amines are washed off. Next, the carboxylic acids are added to the amines to form the desired amides. We illustrate these steps in Figure 3.8. Assuming there are eight amines to react with 12 carboxylic acids in a 96-well plate with eight rows and 12 columns of tiny wells, the amines, A1 to A8, are added across the rows to each well containing the polystyrene beads. Different types of carboxylic acids, B1 to B12, are added to the wells in each column.

After the reactions, the compounds are separated from the beads, for instance by using UV light, which severs the linking groups. Purification steps are applied to separate the enantiomeric compounds (see Section 3.5). From a mere 20 reagents, eight amines plus 12 carboxylic acids, we end up with 96 different compounds. By using different types of reagents, for example X, Y and Z, we generate XxYxZ compounds. Hence, very large libraries are obtained through such combinations.

Split and mix: Here we use eight amines and eight carboxylic acids as our example. The amines are added to eight different reaction vessels and attached to polystyrene beads. Next, all the amines bound to polystyrene are

A1	A1	A1	A1	A1	A1	A1	A1	A1	A1	A1	A1
B1	B2	B3	B4	B5	B6	B7	B8	B9	B10	B11	B12
A2	A2	A2	A2	A2	A2	A2	A2	A2	A2	A2	A2
B1	B2	B3	B4	B5	B6	B7	B8	B9	B10	B11	B12
A3	A3	A3	A3	A3	A3	A3	A3	A3	A3	A3	A3
B1	B2	B3	B4	B5	B6	B7	B8	B9	B10	B11	B12
A4	A4	A4	A4	A4	A4	A4	A4	A4	A4	A4	A4
B1	B2	B3	B4	B5	B6	B7	B8	B9	B10	B11	B12
A5	A5	A5	A5	A5	A5	A5	A5	A5	A5	A5	A5
B1	B2	B3	B4	B5	B6	B7	B8	B9	B10	B11	B12
A6	A6	A6	A6	A6	A6	A6	A6	A6	A6	A6	A6
B1	B2	B3	B4	B5	B6	B7	B8	B9	B10	B11	B12
A7	A7	A7	A7	A7	A7	A7	A7	A7	A7	A7	A7
B1	B2	B3	B4	B5	B6	B7	B8	B9	B10	B11	B12
A8	A8	A8	A8	A8	A8	A8	A8	A8	A8	A8	A8
B1	B2	B3	B4	B5	B6	B7	B8	B9	B10	B11	B12

Figure 3.8 Additions of amines (A) and carboxylic acids (B) in a 96-well plate

taken and mixed in one reaction vessel. The mixed amines are then split into eight vessels of equal portions. Each of these vessels contains amines of A1 to A8 bound to the beads. Carboxylic acids are separately added to each vessel: B1 to vessel 1, B2 to vessel 2, and so on. The compounds prepared would be as follow:

Vessel 1: A1B1, A2B1, A3B1,...A8B1
Vessel 2: A1B2, A2B2, A3B2,...A8B2
.
.
Vessel 8: A1B8, A2B8, A3B8,...A8B8.

Compounds can be tagged via 'coding' groups on the polystyrene beads. The coding can be performed for each reaction step. At the completion of the reactions, each compound can be uniquely identified through a decoding process. All the compounds are screened, tested against target assays and the potent ones ('hits') are selected for analysis, which may include further synthesis to refine the 'hits' and optimization to yield lead compounds.

Exhibit 3.11 gives a synopsis of the development of Gleevec using the rational approach.

Exhibit 3.11 A Rational Approach to the Development of Imatinib Mesylate (Gleevec)

Imatinib mesylate (Gleevec, Novartis; Glivec in countries other than the US) is a drug for the treatment of chronic myeloid leukemia (CML). CML is a result of a chromosomal problem, and gives rise to high levels of white blood cells. An enzyme called *BCR-ABL* is involved. The *BCR-ABL* gene encodes a protein with elevated tyrosine kinase activity (See Exhibit 7.3).

The lead compound for Gleevec was identified in screening of a combinatorial library. This compound is a phenylaminopyrimidine derivative that inhibits protein kinase C (PKC). It is a signal transduction inhibitor. Using docking studies and X-ray crystallography, different groups were introduced into the basic phenylaminopyrimidine template. Stronger PKC inhibition was obtained with a 3'-pyridyl group, compound (a). An amide group provided an inhibitory effect on *BCR-ABL* tyrosine kinase, compound (b). Compound (c) lost PKC activity, but improved tyrosine kinase inhibition. Solubility and bioavailability were studied, and finally a methylpiperazine compound (d), code name ST1571, was selected for clinical trial.

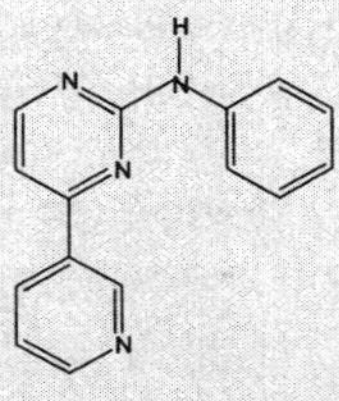

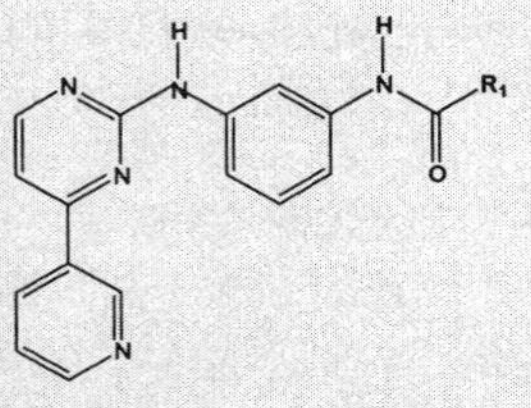

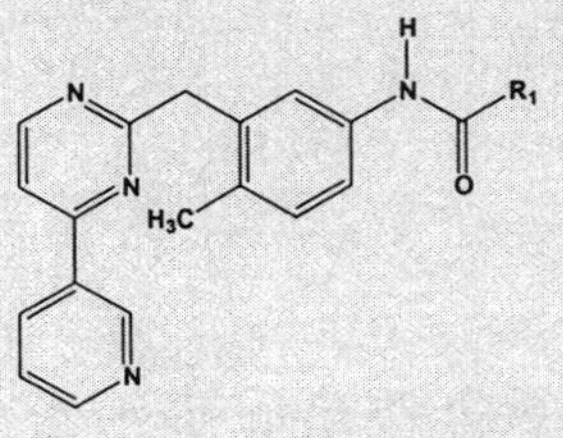

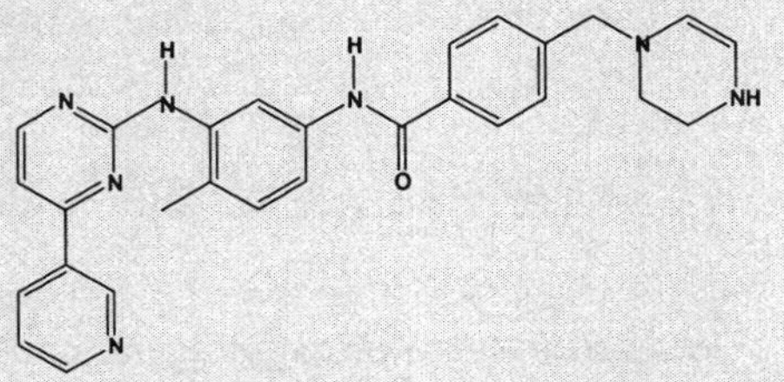

SOURCE   Reprinted with permission from Capdeville, R., Buchdunger, E., Zimmermann, J. and Matter A., Glivec (ST1571, Imatinib), a rationally developed, targeted anticancer drug, *Nature Reviews Drug Discovery*, 1, pp. 493–502 (2002).

3.4   ANTISENSE APPROACH

Genetic information is transcribed from the genes in the DNA to mRNA. The information is then translated from the mRNA to synthesize the protein (refer to Appendix 2). This process is depicted below:

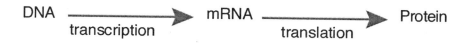

The aim of antisense therapy is to identify the genes that are involved in disease pathogenesis. Short lengths of oligonucleotides of complementary sense (hence 'antisense') are bound to DNA or mRNA (Figure 3.8). These antisense drugs are therefore used to block expression activity of the gene. Information (the sense) from either the gene (DNA) or the mRNA is blocked from being processed (transcribed or translated), and the manufacture of protein is thus terminated.

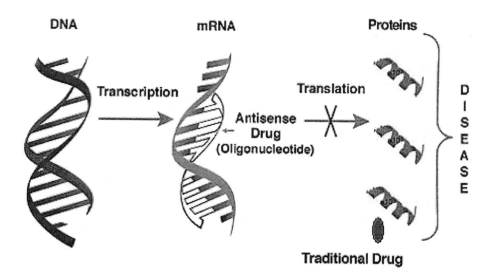

Figure 3.8   Mode of action for antisense drugs. An example is Fomivirsen (Vitravene, Isis Pharmaceuticals), which is a 21-nucleotide phosphorothioate that binds to the complementary mRNA of cytomegalovirus and blocks the translation process. Cytomegalovirus is a virus that belongs to the herpes group. SOURCE Chang, Y.T., *Keyword of the Post Genomic Era—Library*, New York University, 2002, http://www.nyu.edu/classes/ytchang/book/e003.html [accessed Sep 10, 2002].

A strategy for antisense therapy is based on the binding of oligodeoxyribonucleotides to the double helix DNA. This stops gene expression either by restricting the unwinding of the DNA or by preventing the binding of transcription factor complexes to the gene promoter. Another strategy centers on the mRNA. Oligoribonucleotides form a hybrid with the mRNA. Such a duplex formation ties up the mRNA, preventing the encoded translation message from being processed to form the protein.

Although all these seem like elegant ways to stop the disease at the source, at the DNA or mRNA level, there are practical problems. First, the antisense drug has to be delivered to the cell interior, and the polar groups of oligonucleotides have problems crossing the cell membrane to enter the cytoplasm and nucleus; secondly, the oligonucleotides have to bind to the intended gene sequence through hydrogen bonding; and, thirdly, the drug should not exert toxicities or side effects as a result of the interaction. For these reasons, there have been difficulties in bringing antisense drugs to the market. Currently, there is only one antisense drug in the market—Vitravene (active ingredient: fomivirsen) for the treatment of cytomegalovirus-induced retinitis (inflammation of the retina) in AIDS patients. However, the sales of this drug were well under US$1 million in 2001. Listed in Table 3.1 are some of the antisense drugs undergoing clinical trials. Two examples of experimental antisense drugs are provided in Exhibit 3.12.

3.5   CHIRAL DRUGS

Most drugs and biological molecules are chiral. 'Chirality' means 'handedness', i.e. left and right hand mirror images. This is because of the

Table 3.1 Antisense drugs currently undergoing trials

Antisense drugs	Treatment focus
Resten-NG, Phase II	Cancer, re-stenosis
HGTV43, Phase II	Antiviral (HIV)
EPI2010, Phase II	Respiratory diseases
Genasense, Phase III	Various cancer
GTI2040, Phase II	Cancer
ORI1001, Phase I	Antiviral

SOURCE Dove, A., Antisense and sensibility, *Nature Biotechnology*, 20, pp. 121–124 (2002).

Exhibit 3.12 Antisense Drugs

Bcl-2

B cell lymphoma protein 2 (Bcl-2) is a family of proteins that regulate apoptosis (programmed cell death). Apoptosis is a necessary process whereby aged or damaged cells are replaced by new cells. Dysfunction of the apoptosis process results in disease: inhibition of apoptosis results in cancer, autoimmune disorder and viral infection, whereas increased apoptosis gives rise to neurodegenerative disorders, myelodysplastic syndromes, ischemic injury, and toxin-induced liver disease.

Some lymphomas, for example, are related to over-expression of Bcl-2. Antisense oligonucleotides are specially designed to target the over-expression of Bcl-2. Oblimersen (Genasense) is an antisense drug by Genta to block Bcl-2 production and enhance the efficacy of other standard chemotherapy drugs such as paclitaxel, fludarabine, irinotecan and cyclophosphamide.

ICAM-1

Intracellular adhesion molecule 1 (ICAM-1), an immunoglobulin, plays an important role in the transport and activation of leukocytes. In Crohn's disease (inflammation of the alimentary tract), there is an over-expression of ICAM-1, which causes inflammation. Laboratory studies show that antisense oligonucleotides can reduce the expression of ICAM-1 and hence inflammation.

SOURCE Opalinska, J.B. and Gewirtz, A.M., Nucleic-acid therapeutics: Basic principles and recent applications, *Nature Reviews Drug Discovery*, 1, pp. 503–514 (2002).

existence within the molecules of chiral centers. For example, a carbon atom attached to four different groups can be oriented in such a way that two different molecules that are mirror images are obtained (Figure 3.9).

The two forms of mirror images are called enantiomers, or stereoisomers. All amino acids in proteins are 'left-handed', and all sugars in DNA and RNA are 'right-handed'. Drug molecules with chiral centers when synthesized without special separation steps in the reaction process result in 50/50 mixtures of both the left- and right-handed forms. The mixture is often referred to as a racemic mixture.

As we can imagine, putting the right hand into a left-handed glove is not going to give a good fit. Similarly, the presentation of a racemic mixture of drug to a chiral binding site in a protein will not result in effective therapeutic treatment. One drug isomer is the actual effective component, while the other isomer may have varying degree of activity. The other isomer may have little or no net effect, or it may nullify the activity of the active isomer. Worse still, it may cause an adverse reaction.

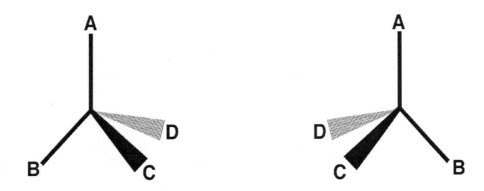

Figure 3.9 Chiral molecules   Black triangular bond projects out of the page, gray triangular bond projects into the page.

Before the 1980s, most drugs were manufactured in racemic mixtures. These drugs are being 'rediscovered' so that only the active isomers are synthesized. The reason is that the active isomer is more effective in the absence of its mirror image, or it can be prescribed in higher dose without the adverse reaction due to the inactive isomer. Another reason is that pharmaceutical companies are rediscovering the active isomer to extend the life cycle of blockbuster drugs. This is illustrated in Exhibit 3.13.

3.6 CLOSING REMARKS

Drug discovery is extremely challenging and demanding. The attrition rate for failures is very high. Although the above approaches for drug discovery afford a higher probability of success, the astute observations and inventiveness of the scientists are critical ingredients for success. Exhibit 3.14 shows how the careful observation by Fleming gave rise to one of the most effective drugs.

Very often drugs are discovered through persistent work and continual optimization and many tests and trials. This is exemplified by the history behind the discovery of sildenafil (Viagra, Pfizer), a drug for the treatment of erectile dysfunction, and the AIDS vaccine, zidovidine (Retovir, GlaxoSmithKline) (Exhibits 3.15 and 3.16).

Exhibit 3.13 Omeprazole and Esomeprazole

AstraZeneca launched omeprazole in 1988. It is a safe and effective drug for acid reflux, functioning as a proton pump inhibitor. However, the patent has expired and AstraZeneca has to compete against generics. The company developed the active isomer and called it esomeprazole. It was approved by the Mutual Recognition process in Europe in July 2000, and by the US Food and Drug Administration in February 2001. The chemical formulas for omeprazole and esomeprazole are shown below.

It was reported that healing of reflux esophagitis with 40mg per day of Esomeprazole is effective in 78% of patients after 4 weeks of treatment and in 93% of patients after 8 weeks, compared to 65% and 87% of patients treated with 20mg per day of Omeprazole.

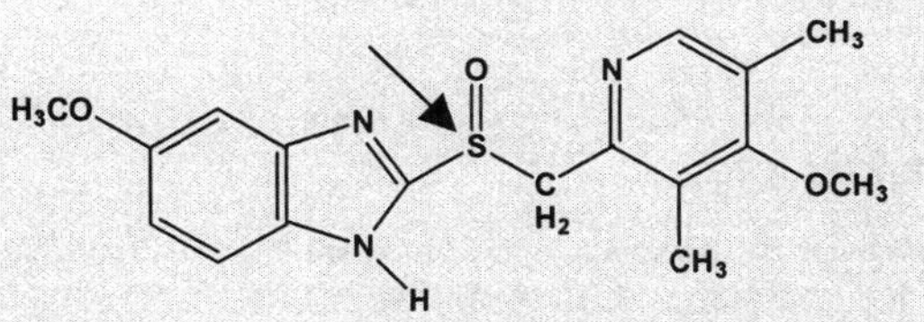

Omeprazole
Launched 1988

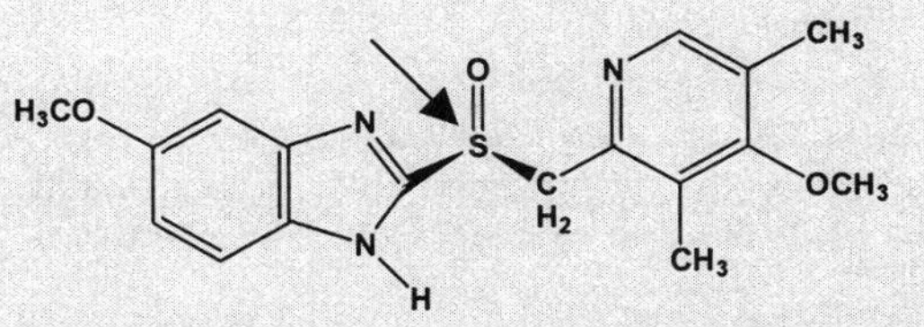

Esomeprazole
Launched 2000

NOTE The arrows point to the chiral centers.

SOURCE Reprinted with permission from Agranat, I., Caner, H. and Caldwell, J., Putting chirality to work: The strategy of chiral switches of drug molecules, *Nature Reviews Drug Discovery*, 1, pp. 753–768 (2002).

Exhibit 3.14 Importance of Observation in Drug Discovery

Alexander Fleming was studying bacteria. In 1928, he noticed that the bacterial cultures that he was growing were ruined when there was a mould present in the culture. The mould turned out to be *Penicillium*, which produces a substance called penicillin. This was found to be very effective in killing a variety of bacteria.

Exhibit 3.15 Discovery of Viagra

The long, tortuous path from drug discovery to commercialization is amply demonstrated by the sildenafil (Viagra) story.

Scientists at the Pfizer laboratory set out to discover an anti-hypertensive drug. The mechanism to lower blood pressure is:

- Atrial natriuretic peptide binds to the GPCR receptor

- This binding activates the enzyme guanylate cyclase

- Guanylate cyclase converts guanosine triphosphate (GTP) to cyclic guanosine monophosphate (cyclicGMP)

- CyclicGMP lowers intracellular calcium, leading to (i) release of sodium in kidney cells or (ii) relaxation of smooth muscle in blood vessels.

The enzyme phosphodiesterase (PDE) converts cyclicGMP to GMP. The Pfizer scientists wanted to develop a drug to inhibit PDE so that the level of cyclicGMP remains high, so that point 4 can proceed.

Sildenafil was developed. However, there are different types of PDEs (nine are known today). As discussed previously, a potent drug has to be specific. Sildenafil inhibits PDE-5, which is absent in the kidney, although sildenafil's effect on smooth muscle relaxation was confirmed. The direction of the drug changed to treating angina instead, as sildenafil relaxes the vascular muscle of the heart.

At clinical trials, sildenafil did not work well as a treatment for angina. Instead, it was observed that it overcomes erectile dysfunction. Later, it was found that cyclicGMP also increases the level of nitric oxide, which is needed in penile erections.

Hence, we can see how the focus of treatment for sildenafil changed from anti-hypertensive to angina treatment to overcoming erectile dysfunction, giving rise to the drug called Viagra.

Exhibit 3.16 Retovir, an AIDS Vaccine

Zidovudine (Retrovir, also known as AZT), was the first drug approved for the treatment of AIDS. The drug was first studied in 1964 as an anti-cancer drug, but it showed little promise. It was not until the 1980s, when desperate searches began for a way to treat victims of HIV, that scientists at Burroughs Wellcome Co., of Research Triangle Park, NC, took another look at zidovudine. After it showed very positive results in human testing, it was approved by the FDA in March 1987 for AIDS treatment.

3.7 FURTHER READING

Agranat, I., Caner, H. and Caldwell, J., Putting chirality to work: The strategy of chiral switches, *Nature Reviews Drug Discovery*, 1, pp. 753–768 (2002).

Andrews, P. R., 'Drug-receptor interactions' in Kubinyi, H. (ed.), *3D QSAR in Drug Design: Theory, Methods and Applications*, Kluwer/Escom, The Netherlands, 2000.

Bioinformatics, University of Texas at Austin, http://biotech.icmb.utexas.edu /pages/bioinfo.html [accessed Oct 22, 2002].

Blundell, T.L., Jhoti, H. and Abell, C., High-throughput crystallography for lead discovery in drug design, *Nature Reviews Drug Discovery*, 1, pp. 45–54 (2002).

Bohm, H.J. and Schneider, G. (eds.), *Virtual Screening for Bioactive Molecules*, Wiley-VCH, Weinheim, Germany, 2000.

Bolger, R., High-throughput screening: New frontiers for the 21st century, *Drug Discovery Today*, 4, pp. 251–253 (1999).

Brazil, M., High throughput screening—molecular beacons for DNA binding, *Nature Reviews Drug Discovery*, 1, pp. 98–99 (2002).

Cohen, J.S. and Hogan, M.E., Antisense—the new genetic medicines, *Scientific American*, December, pp. 76–82 (1994).

Cohen, N.C. (ed.), *Guidebook on Molecular Modeling in Drug Design*, Academic Press, San Diego, California, 1996.

Devlin, J.P. (ed.), *High Throughput Screening*, Marcel Dekker, New York, 1997.

Dobson, C.M. and Fersht, A.R. (eds.), *Protein Folding*, Cambridge University Press, Cambridge, UK, 1995.

Dove, A., Antisense and sensibility, *Nature Biotechnology*, 20, pp. 121–124 (2002).

Dunn, D., The broader applications of uHTS, *Drug Discovery Today*, 6, p. 828 (2001).

Food and Drug Administration, *From Test Tube to Patient: New Drug Development in the United States*, 2nd edn., FDA, Rockville, MD, 1995, http://www.fda.gov/fdac/special/newdrug/ndd_toc.html [accessed Sep 22, 2002].

Ganellin, C.R. and Roberts, S.M., *Medicinal Chemistry—The Role of Organic Chemistry in Drug Discovery*, 2nd edn., Academic Press, London, 1993.

Glusker, J.P. and Trueblood, K.N., *Crystal Structure Analysis, A Primer*, 2nd edn., Oxford University Press, Oxford, 1985.

Harvey, A.L. (ed.), *Advances in Drug Discovery Techniques*, John Wiley & Sons, New York, 1998.

Howard, K., The bioinformatics gold rush, *Scientific American*, July, pp. 58–63 (2000).

Kourounakis, P.N. and Rekka, E. (eds.), *Advanced Drug Design and Development, A Medicinal Chemistry Approach*, Ellis Horwood Limited, Chichester, UK, 1994.

Larvol, B.L. and Wilkerson, L.J., In silico drug discovery: Tools for bridging the NCE gap, *Nature Biochemistry*, 16, Supplement, pp. 33–34 (1998).

Liebman M.N., Biomedical informatics: The future for drug development, *Drug Discovery Today*, 7, pp. s197–s203 (2002).

Lyne, P.D., Structure-based virtual screening: An overview, *Drug Discovery Today*, 7, pp. 1047–1055 (2002).

Opalinska, J.B. and Gewirtz, A.M., Nucleic-acid therapeutics: Basic principles and recent applications', *Nature Reviews Drug Discovery*, 1, pp. 503–514 (2002).

Parrill, A.L. and Reddy, M.R., *Rational Drug Design—Novel Methodology and Practical Applications*, American Chemical Society, Washington, DC, 1999.

Reid, D.G. (ed.), *Protein NMR Techniques*, Humana Press, New Jersey, 1997.

Rupp, B., *X-ray 101—An Interactive Web Tutorial*, http://www-structure. llnl.gov/Xray/101index.html [accessed Aug 25, 2002].

Sittampalam, S.S., Kahl, S.D. and Janzen, W.P., High-throughput screening: Advances in assay technologies, *Current Opinion in Chemical Biology*, 1, pp. 384–391 (1997).

Terrett, N.K., *Combinatorial Chemistry*, Oxford University Press, Oxford, 1998.

Walters, W.P., Stahl, M.T. and Murcko, M.A., Virtual screening—an overview, *Drug Discovery Today*, 3, pp. 160–178 (1998).

Watt, A. and Morrison, D., Strategic and technical challenges for drug discovery, *Drug Discovery Today*, 6, pp. 290–292 (2001).

Weiner, D.B. and Williams, W.V. (eds.), *Chemical and Structural Approaches to Rational Drug Design*, CRC Press, FL, 1994.

Welling, P.G., Lasagna, L. and Banakar, U.V. (eds.), *The Drug Development Process: Increasing Efficiency and Cost Effectiveness*, Marcel Dekker, New York, 1996.

Wermuth, C.G., Koga, N., Konig, H. and Metcalf, B.W. (eds.), *Medicinal Chemistry for the 21st Century*, Blackwell Scientific Publications, Oxford, 1992.

Wolke, J. and Ullmann D., Miniaturized HTS technologies—uHTS, *Drug Discovery Today*, 6, pp. 637–646 (2001).

CHAPTER 4

DRUG DISCOVERY: LARGE MOLECULE DRUGS

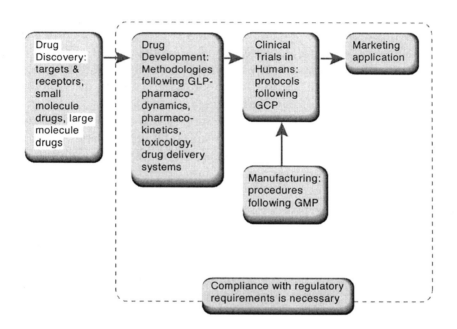

4.1   INTRODUCTION

Unlike the small molecule drugs (pharmaceuticals) described in Chapter 3, large molecule drugs (biopharmaceuticals) are mainly protein-based. Another distinction is that these protein-based drugs are, in the main, similar to natural biological compounds found in the human body or they are fragments that mimic the active part of the natural compounds.

The discovery of pharmaceuticals commences with the scanning of hundreds of compounds, whether with actual materials (irrational approach) or virtual simulations (rational approach). To discover biopharmaceuticals, we have to examine the compounds within us, for example, hormones or other biological response modifiers, and how they affect the biological processes. In some cases, we study the pathogens such as the influenza virus or bacteria to derive the vaccines. In other cases, we copy these biological response modifiers and use them as replacement therapy.

Pharmaceuticals are new chemical entities (NCEs) and they are produced (synthesized) in manufacturing plants using techniques based on chemical reactions of reactants. Biopharmaceuticals are made using totally different methods. These protein-based drugs are 'manufactured' in biological systems such as living cells, producing the desired protein molecules in large reaction vessels or by extraction from animal serum.

Biopharmaceuticals are becoming increasingly important. The reason is that they are more potent and specific, as they are similar to the proteins within the body, and hence are more effective in treating our diseases. There are three major areas in which biopharmaceuticals are used: as prophylactic (preventive, as in the case of vaccines), therapeutic (antibodies) and replacement (hormones, growth factors) therapy. Exhibit 4.1 presents selected statistics for biopharmaceuticals.

Another term that is used for protein-based drugs is biologics. The FDA definition for biologics is:

"A biological product subject to licensure under the Public Health Service Act is any virus, therapeutic serum, toxin, antitoxin, vaccine, blood, blood component or derivative, allergenic product, or analogous product, applicable to the prevention, treatment or cure of diseases or injuries to humans. Biological products include, but are not limited to, bacterial and viral vaccines, human blood and plasma and their derivatives, and certain products produced by biotechnology, such as interferons and erythropoietins.   Biologics encompass many different protein-based drugs, and include blood products such as clotting factors extracted from blood".

Exhibit 4.1 Biopharmaceuticals

There are at present about 150 biopharmaceutical drugs approved for marketing in USA and EU. This market is worth more than US$ 30billion.

Around 500 biopharmaceuticals are now in clinical trials, for diseases ranging from cancer to cardiovascular and infectious diseases.

SOURCE   Walsh, G., Biopharmaceutical benchmarks - 2003, *Nature Biotechnology*, 21, pp. 865–870 (2003).

Biopharmaceutical drugs are becoming increasingly important. Over 30% of the 37 new drugs launched in 2001 are biopharmaceuticals, according to the IMS HEALTH LifeCycle service.

SOURCE   *LifeCycle*, http://www.ims-global.com/insight/news_story/0204/news_story_020412.htm [accessed Jun 10, 2002].

In this chapter, we discuss the following topics, but exclude blood products:

- Vaccines
- Antibodies
- Cytokines
- Hormones
- Gene therapy
- Stem cells.

We have included gene therapy and stem cells to present a more comprehensive perspective on medical treatments, although they are not drugs by our conventional definitions.

4.2 VACCINES

Most of us were vaccinated soon after we were born. As we grow up and go through different stages of life, we are further vaccinated against other diseases. The basis of vaccination is that administering a small quantity of a vaccine (antigen that has been treated) stimulates our immune system and causes antibodies to be secreted to react against the foreign antigen. Later in life, when we encounter another exposure to the same antigen, our immune system will evoke a 'memory' response and activate the defense mechanisms by generating antibodies to combat the invading antigen.

A vaccine formulation contains antigenic components that are obtained from or derived from the pathogen. These pathogens include mainly viruses, bacteria, parasites and fungi. Research has shown that the part of the pathogen, which causes disease, termed virulence, can be decoupled from the protective part, so-called immunity. Vaccine development focuses on means to reduce the virulence factor while retaining the immunity stimulation. Administration of vaccines may be oral or parenteral. After the initial vaccination, booster doses may be needed to maximize the immunological effects.

4.2.1   Traditional vaccines

Traditionally vaccines are prepared in a number of ways:
- Attenuated vaccines
- Killed or inactivated vaccines
- Toxoids.

Attenuated vaccines   The virulence of a pathogen can be reduced in a number of ways: by chemical treatment, by temperature adaptation, or by growing the pathogen in species other than the natural host (a process called 'passaging').

The advantages of attenuated vaccines are (a) the low cost of preparation, (b) they elicit the desired immunological response and (c) normally a single dose is sufficient. The disadvantages are (a) a potential to revert to virulence and (b) a limited shelf life.

Examples of attenuated vaccines are *Bacillus Calmette-Guerin* (BCG) for immunization against tuberculosis, Sabin vaccine for poliomyelitis, attenuated *Paramyxovirus parotitidus* against mumps, and attenuated measles virus against measles.

Killed or inactivated vaccines   Chemical and temperature treatment are normally used to kill or inactivate the pathogen. Formaldehyde treatment is one of the more common methods. Other chemicals used are phenol and acetone. Another method is to irradiate the pathogen to render it inactive.

The advantages are (a) non-reversal to virulence and (b) relatively stable shelf life. The disadvantages are (a) higher cost of production, (b) more control is required for production to ensure reliable processes for complete inactivation and (c) there is a possibility of reduced immunological response due to the treatment processes, so multiple booster vaccinations may be required.

Examples of killed or inactivated vaccines are cholera vaccine containing dead strains of *Vibrio cholerae,* hepatitis A vaccine with inactivated hepatitis A virus, pertussis vaccine with killed strains of *Bordetella pertussis,* typhoid vaccine with killed *Salmonella typhi,* and influenza vaccine with various strains of inactivated influenza viruses (see Exhibit 4.2 for a discussion on influenza viruses and vaccines).

Toxoids Toxoids are derived from the toxins secreted by a pathogen. The advantages and disadvantages are similar to those for killed or inactivated vaccines.

Examples are diphtheria and tetanus vaccines. Diphtheria vaccine is produced by formaldehyde treatment of the toxin secreted by *Corynebacterium diptheriae.* Similarly, tetanus vaccine is obtained from toxins of cultured *Clostridium tetani* that has been treated with formaldehyde.

Exhibit 4.2 Influenza Viruses and Vaccines

Influenza is caused by the influenza (Orthomyxoviruses) viruses. There are three types of influenza viruses, Influenza A, B and C (based on their protein matrix, influenza A and B have 8 RNA fragments, C has 7). Influenza A can infect humans and other animals, while influenza B and C mainly infect humans only. Unlike influenza A and B, influenza C virus causes very mild illness and does not cause epidemics. Influenza A is categorized into subtypes based on its surface antigens: hemagglutinin and neuraminidase (see Exhibit 3.7). There are no subtype classifications for influenza B. Influenza virus undergoes frequent mutations as it replicates, with Influenza A changing more rapidly than B, causing antigenic shifts in the hemagglutinin and neuraminidase.

The nomenclature for classifying influenza virus is:
Type/Site Isolated/Isolate No./Year, e.g.
A/New Caledonia/20/99(H3N2), B/Hong Kong/330/2001.

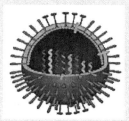 source Reprinted with permission from Dr Cann, A. J., *Influenza Virus Haemagglutination,* http://www-micro.msb.le.ac.uk/ LabWork/haem/haem1.htm [accessed May 2, 2003].

There have been three influenza pandemics in the 20th century: in 1918 (Spanish Flu, H5N1), 1957 (Asian Flu, H2N2) and 1968 (Hong Kong Flu, H3N2). The pandemic in 1918 killed more than 20 million people worldwide, and the other two took the lives of 1.5 million people combined. In 1997, the first avian (chicken) flu was transmitted to humans in Hong Kong. It was caused by Influenza A H5N1.

Continued

Exhibit 4.2 *Continued*

Antibodies responsive to influenza antigens are specific to the subtype and strain. To have an effective influenza vaccine, it is a requirement that there is an accurate prediction of the subtype and strain that are expected to circulate in the influenza season months before the season begins. When the antigenic match between vaccine and circulating viruses is close, influenza vaccine is 70%–90% effective.

The World Health Organization (WHO) has a network of 110 centers worldwide that monitor influenza activity and ensure virus isolates and information are sent to WHO for strain identification and action. Each February (for the Northern Hemisphere winter) and September (for the Southern hemisphere winter) the WHO provides advanced recommendations for the composition of the influenza vaccine to be manufactured. For the November 2002 – April 2003 season, the February 2002 recommendation was:
 A/New Caledonia/20/99(H3N2)-like
 A/Moscow/10/99(H3N2)-like
 B/Hong Kong/330/2001-like.

Similarly, the FDA CBER recommended similar trivalent influenza vaccine to be prepared for the 2002–2003 US winter season:
 A/New Caledonia/20/99 (H1N1)-like
 A/Panama/2007/99 (H3N2), an A/Moscow/10/99-like virus
 B/Hong Kong/330/2001-like.

4.2.2   New vaccines

Advances in genomics, molecular biology and recombinant technology have provided new directions for the discovery, development and manufacture of vaccines. One of the current approaches is a minimalist strategy to decouple the virulence and immunity functions. The aim is to use only the immunity part to confer protection, so that the vaccine is safe to be administered. The approach can be divided into subunit, vector-based, DNA and peptide vaccines.

Subunit vaccines Subunit vaccines use only a part of the bacteria or virus instead of the entire pathogen. Normally, the part is derived from the outside envelope protein of the pathogen. Discovery of the relevant envelope protein requires knowledge of the genome sequence of the pathogen by identifying open reading frames (ORFs, see Exhibit 4.3) that potentially encode novel antigenic surface proteins known as epitopes (Exhibit 4.3), which bind to antibodies. When identified, the ORFs are cloned to express protein epitopes using self-replicating plasmids (see Exhibit 10.8). The binding properties of the epitopes can be studied using enzyme-linked immunosorbent assay (ELISA, Exhibit 4.3) or a fluorescent activated cell sorter (FACS, Exhibit 4.3). After laboratory testing, the leading candidates of epitopes are injected into animals to determine whether they elicit any antibody response. Those that work are selected and optimized to become vaccine candidates with further tests before human clinical trials. Researchers are also working on multiple epitope subunit vaccines, which can provide different antigenic binding sites.

Exhibit 4.3 Important Concepts Related to Subunit Vaccines

An **open reading frame (ORF)** is a sequence of nucleotide in the RNA or DNA that has the potential to encode protein. The start triplet is ATG. It is followed by a string of triplets that code for amino acids. The stop triplet is TAA, TAG or TGA (see Exhibit A2.3).

An **epitope** is an antigenic determinant of the pathogen. It consists of certain chemical groups that are antigenic, which means that it will elicit a specific immune response by binding to antibodies.

The **enzyme linked immunosorbent assay (ELISA)** is a method for determining the presence of specific antibodies. Antigens are first solubilized and coated onto solid support, such as 96-well plates. Test samples with antibodies are added, and the antibodies bind to the antigens on the plate. Excess unbound sample is washed off, and the antigen–antibody complex is incubated. The antigen–antibody complex is linked to an enzyme (e.g. alkaline phosphatase, horseradish peroxidase). The labeling with the enzyme catalyzes certain biochemical reactions and provides a readout (color) to show the presence or absence of the specific antibodies. The process can also be used for detecting antigens. In this case, the antibodies are coated onto the substrate, followed by antigen attachment and conjugation to an enzyme.

A **fluorescence-activated cell sorter (FACS)** is a flow cytometry instrument used to separate and identify cells in a heterogeneous population. Cell mixtures to be sorted are first bound to fluorescent dyes such as fluorescein or phycoerythrin. The labeled cells are then pumped through the instrument and are excited by a laser beam. Cells that fluoresce are detected, and an electrostatic charge is applied. The charged cells are separated using voltage deflection.

Vector-based vaccines   Viruses and bacteria are detoxified and used as vehicles to carry vaccines. Subunit vaccines are being delivered by carrier vehicles to elicit the immune response. An example is the use of canarypox (a virus that infects birds, but not humans) to carry envelope proteins for HIV treatment. Multiple types of envelope proteins can be delivered with this method. Clinical trials with this type of vector-based vaccines are being investigated.

DNA vaccines   DNA vaccines are sometimes called nucleic vaccines or genetic immunization. The host (patient) is directly injected with selected viral genes, which contain engineered DNA sequences that code for antigens. The host's own cells take up these genes and express the antigens, which are then presented to the immune cells and activate the immune response.

Peptide vaccines   Peptide vaccines are chemically synthesized and normally consist of 8–24 amino acids. In comparison with protein molecules, peptide vaccines are relatively small. They are also known as peptidomimetic vaccines, as they mimic the epitopes. Complex structures of cyclic components, branched chains or other configurations can be built into the peptide chain. In this way, they possess conformations similar to the epitopes and can be recognized by immune cells. An *in silico* vaccine design approach has been used to find potential epitopes. A critical aspect of peptide vaccines is to produce 3D structures similar to the native epitopes of the pathogen.

4.2.3   Adjuvants

Very often vaccines are formulated with certain substances to enhance the immune response. These substances are called adjuvants (from the Latin *adjuvare,* which means 'to help'). The most common adjuvants for human use are aluminum hydroxide, aluminum phosphate and calcium phosphate. Other adjuvants being used include bacteria and cholesterol. Mineral oil emulsions are normally the adjuvants used in animal studies. The adjuvant known as Freund's Complete Adjuvant consists of killed *tubercle bacilli* in water-in-mineral oil emulsion, and Freund's Incomplete Adjuvant is a water-in-oil emulsion. Both these adjuvants are effective in stimulating an immune response, but they cause unacceptable side effects in humans.

There are three basic mechanisms by which adjuvants assist in improving immune response. First, adjuvants help the immune response by forming reservoirs of antigens and providing sustained release of antigens over a long period. Secondly, adjuvants act as non-specific mediators of immune cell function by stimulating or modulating immune cells. Thirdly, adjuvants can serve as vehicles to deliver the antigen to the spleen and/or lymph nodes, where immune response is initiated.

Edible food sources have been tested to deliver vaccines orally; for example, transgenic potato tuber-based vaccines have been developed. Other food sources, such as bananas, tomatoes and corn, are being tested in laboratories (see Section 11.12). Mucosal vaccines utilizing genetically modified enterotoxins are a method to deliver vaccines intranasally. Research in this area has to ensure the safety aspect of using enterotoxins.

4.2.4 Recent vaccine research and clinical activities

The field of vaccine research is very active. Exhibit 4.4 summarizes examples of some recent work and clinical results for selected vaccines.

Exhibit 4.4 Recent Work on Vaccines

Alzheimer's disease

The vaccine being tested contains a small protein called β amyloid (Aβ). This protein forms abnormal deposits, or 'plaques', in the brains of people with Alzheimer's disease. Researchers believe that Aβ deposition causes loss of mental function by killing the brain neurons. The strategy of Aβ vaccination is to stimulate the immune system to clean up plaques and prevent further Aβ deposits. Although preclinical and Phase I studies showed the potential of the vaccine, the Phase II clinical trial was halted because 15 of 360 patients developed severe brain inflammation. Further studies showed that the Aβ did generate the desired antibody response. An acceptable vaccine may still be possible by modifying the epitope to reduce the inflammation effect.

SOURCE Frantz, S., Alzheimer's disease vaccine revisited, *Nature Reviews Drug Discovery*, 1, p. 933 (2002).

Pneumococcal

In October 2002, the FDA approved the use of Prevnar for immunization of infants and toddlers against otitis media—middle ear infection. Prevnar is a pneumococcal seven-valent conjugate vaccine. It is formulated with a sterile solution of saccharides conjugated to the antigen, *Streptococcus pneumoniae*.

SOURCE Center for Biologics Evaluation and Research, *Product Approval Information*, FDA, Rockville, MD, http://www.fda.gov/cber/approvltr/ pneuled100102L.htm [accessed Oct 10, 2002].

Cancer

In cancer, the immune system does not recognize the changes in cancer cells. Cancer vaccines seek to mimic cancer-specific changes by using synthetic peptides to challenge the immune system. When these peptides are taken up by T cells, the immune system is activated. The T cells search for cancer cells with specific markers and proceed to kill them. Some vaccines being tested are (a) a peptide called β-defensin 2, which activates the immune system against tumor activity, and (b) an outer coat protein of the human papillomavirus to act as a vaccine against cervical cancer.

SOURCE National Institutes of Health, *Cancer Vaccine*, http://www.nih.gov [accessed Oct 28, 2002].   *Continued*

Exhibit 4.4 *Continued*

AIDS (see Exhibit 2.11)

AIDS is caused by HIV infection. HIV belongs to a large family of retroviruses, the Lentiviridae. The HIV genome is within the RNA. Following infection in humans, the RNA genome of HIV is reverse-transcribed into DNA and integrated within the human cell. HIV undergoes frequent mutation and therefore is highly variable. One technique for producing an AIDS vaccine is to reproduce, using recombinant technology, the surface proteins on the HIV. There are two particular envelope proteins being investigated: gp120 and gp41. gp120 is a trimeric protein, and is held together by three transmembrane gp41 proteins. Laboratory studies have shown that vaccines based on these proteins can induce antibody responses to different strains of HIV. Other AIDS treatments are the use of (a) antiviral (AZT, a reverse transcriptase inhibitor) drugs, (b) drugs (indinavir) that target and inhibit the production of HIV protease, an enzyme required to assemble new virus particles, and (c) gene therapy—control of viral genome expression through the use of synthetic oligonucleotides.

Malaria

Malaria is a major disease in tropical countries. According to the WHO, 300–500 million individuals are infected with malaria. The death tolls are 1.5–3.5 million yearly. There are four species of malaria parasites that infect humans: *Plasmodium falciparum*, *P. vivax*, *P. ovale*, and *P. malariae*. Of these, *P. falciparum*, the predominant malarial parasite found in Africa, is the most virulent. There are four stages in the *P. falciparum* life cycle: (a) sporozoite (3–5 minutes when it is injected into the blood stream by mosquito), (b) liver stage (1–2 weeks after the parasite enters the liver, during which it matures; no symptoms are shown in stages a and b), (c) blood stage (2 or more days/cycle during which red blood cells are invaded and parasites rupture out of red blood cells; fevers and chills are manifested) and (d) sexual stage (10–14 days during which parasites mature into the sexual form, ready to be picked up by a mosquito to infect the next person). Vaccine strategies are of three types: pre-erythrocytic (stages a and b), blood stage (stage c) and transmission-blocking (stage d).

SOURCE Dubovsky, F., *Creating a Vaccine against Malaria*, Malaria Vaccine Initiative, Rockville, MD, 2001, http://www.malariavaccine.org/files/ Creating_a_Vaccine_ against_Malaria.pdf, [accessed Nov 22, 2002].

Chicken pox

Chicken pox is a highly contagious viral infection that causes rash-like blisters on the skin surface and mucous membranes. It is generally mild and not normally life-threatening. For adults, the symptoms are more serious and uncomfortable than for children. The disease can also be deadly for some people, such as pregnant women, people with leukemia, or immunosuppressed patients. Varivax (varicella virus vaccine live) from Merck & Co. was tested on about 11 000 children and adults, and was approved by the FDA in March 1995 as a chicken pox vaccine.

4.3 ANTIBODIES

Antibodies are produced by the B cells of the immune system (Exhibit 4.5). They are like weapons of our defense system and can be described as 'homing devices' that target antigens and destroy them. Antibodies are immunoglobulins (proteins with immune functions) and are categorized into five different classes: immunoglobulin G and D (IgG and IgD, ~75%), immunoglobulin A (IgA ~15%), immunoglobulin M (IgM ~15%) and immunoglobulin E (IgE <1%). They differ from each other in size, charge, carbohydrate content and amino acid composition. Within each class, there are subclasses that show slight differences in structure and function from other members of the class.

Exhibit 4.5 Human Immune System

The human immune system is a remarkable system for combating against foreign substances that invade the body. It protects us from infections by pathogens such as viruses, bacteria, parasite and fungi. An important aspect of the immune system is the self–non-self recognition function, by means of markers present on a protein called the major histocompatibility complex (MHC). Substances without such markers are discerned and targeted for destruction. Although in most cases the immune system functions properly, at times it breaks down. For some people, the immune system lacks the normal discrimination capability and reverts to attack and destroy their own body cells as if they are foreign. This gives rise to autoimmune diseases such as rheumatoid arthritis, diabetes, multiple sclerosis and systemic lupus erythematosus. There are also occasions when the immune system responds with undue sensitivities to innocuous substances such as airborne pollen, leading to allergies, as in the case of asthma and hay fever.

Immune responses are mediated through the lymphocytes called B cells and T cells. Lymphocytes are a particular type of white blood cells. White blood cells (leukocytes) are divided into granulocytes (neutrophils, 55%–70%; eosinophils, 1%–3%; and basophils, 0.5%–1%) and agranulocytes (lymphocytes [B and T cells], 20%–40%; and monocytes, 1%–6%). There are 5000 to 10 000 white blood cells per milliliter of blood, compared with five million red blood cells in the same volume.

When pathogens enter the human body, cells called macrophages (meaning 'big eaters') engulf and ingest the pathogens (antigens). The antigens are processed by the macrophages, and parts of the antigens are displayed on the surface in the form of short peptide chains bound to the MHC protein. These antigen-presenting cells (APCs) of macrophages and dendritic cells activate the immune response by sensitizing the B and T cells.

Continued

Exhibit 4.5 *Continued*

B cells are produced by the bone marrow. In response to activation of CD4+ T helper cells (see below), B cells proliferate and produce antibodies (The term CD stands for 'cluster of differentiation'. They are proteins coating cell surfaces. Altogether there are more than 160 different types of CDs). The antibodies produced by B cells circulate in the bloodstream and bind to antigens. Once bound, other cells are in turn activated to destroy the antigens.

T cells are lymphocytes produced by the thymus gland. There are two types of T cells involved in immune response: CD4+ (CD positive, helper cells) and CD8+ (CD positive, also called T killer, or suppressor cells). When the APCs present the antigens to CD4+ helper T cells, the secretory function is activated and growth factors such as cytokines are secreted to signal the proliferation of CD8+ killer cells and B cells. When the CD8+ cells are activated by the APCs, the CD8+ killer T cells directly kill those cells expressing the antigens. Activated B cells produce antibodies, as described above.

It is estimated that every B and T cell has about 100 000 protein molecules on the surface. There are many variations to these surface molecules, which act as receptors for antigens. As many as 10^{18} different surface receptors can be produced, thus giving rise to a vast probability for the B and T cells to recognize and bind to a vast array of antigens.

NOTE   CD4 is a receptor for HIV. Hence, people infected with HIV have suppressed immune response and develop AIDS because the CD4 cannot function normally.

4.3.1   Antibody structure

The structure of an antibody is normally depicted as a capital letter 'Y' configuration. IgG is the most predominant antibody. It is a tetrameric molecule consisting of two identical heavy (H) polypeptide chains of about 440 amino acids and two identical light (L) polypeptide chains of about 220 amino acids (Figure 4.1). The four chains are held together by disulfide bonds and non-covalent interactions.

Within the light and heavy chains are domains, which consist of about 110 amino acids. The domains that have similar polypeptide sequence are termed constant domains. These are the C_H1, C_H2 and C_H3 domains of the heavy chain and the C_L domain of the light chain. Where the sequence is variable, the domains are called variable domains, one each on the heavy and light chain: V_H and V_L. The variability is confined to particular regions of the variable domain, called the complementarity-determining regions. These regions have the appropriate 3D structure to bind to antigens.

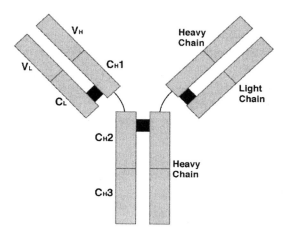

Figure 4.1 IgG antibody molecule

An antibody can be cleaved by enzymes such as papain and pepsin into different fragments (Figure 4.2).

These different fragments are:

- *Variable fragment (Fv):* The tips of the two 'Y' arms vary greatly from one antibody to another. They are the regions that bind to epitopes of antigens and bring them to the natural killer cells and macrophages for destruction.
- *Antigen-binding fragments (Fab), Fab´ and F(ab´)₂:* various parts that contain the variable fragment.
- *Constant fragment (Fc):* This is the stem of the letter 'Y'. It is the part that is identical for all antibodies of the same class; for example, all IgGs have the same Fc. The Fc fragment is the part that links the antibody to other receptors and trigger immune response and antigen destruction.

4.3.2 Traditional antibodies

Several decades ago, antibodies were obtained by extraction from blood samples of immunized animals or human donors. These are polyclonal antibodies, because several different types of antibodies are obtained through this method, although IgG is normally the predominant component. The steps for obtaining polyclonal antibodies are illustrated in Figure 4.3.

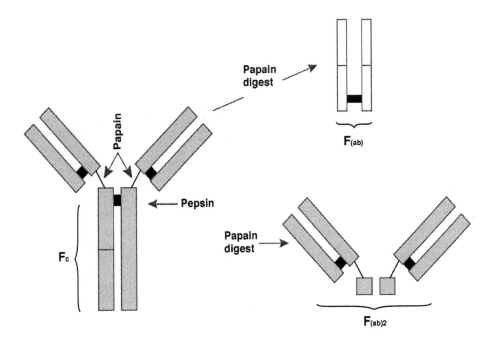

Figure 4.2 Different fragments of the antibody molecule

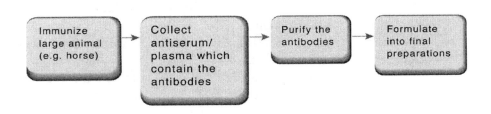

Figure 4.3 Production of polyclonal antibodies from horse antisera. SOURCE Walsh, G., *Biopharmaceuticals: Biochemistry and Biotechnology*, John Wiley & Sons, New York, 1998.

Examples of some of polyclonal antibodies are:

- *Antibodies derived from horse antisera:* botulism antitoxin, diphtheria antitoxin, scorpion venom antisera, snake venom antisera, spider antivenins and tetanus antitoxin
- *Antibodies derived from human donors:* hepatitis A and B

immunoglobulins,   measles   immunoglobulins,   rabies immunoglobulin and tetanus immunoglobulin.

Although polyclonal antibodies have been used for passive immunization and therapeutic treatments, there are cases when hypersensitivities are induced. The reason is that polyclonal antibodies contain not only the specific antibody that binds to the desired antigen, but also other antibodies, which our immune system will treat as foreign substances and act against.

4.3.3   Monoclonal antibodies

The next development was the production of monoclonal antibodies (MAbs) in the mid 1970s. This uses hybridoma technology, which involves the fusion of antibody-producing B cells to immortal myeloma cells. Figure 4.4 shows the preparation of MAbs using hybridoma techniques. A more detailed discussion of biopharmaceuticals production is presented in Section 10.5.

MAbs are specific in binding to epitopes of antigens. Because MAbs are produced using murine (mouse) spleen cells, human immune system can react against these murine MAbs. The allergic reaction is called human anti-mouse antibodies (HAMA) and it can neutralize the effect of the MAbs, or even induce rashes, swelling, kidney problems; it may even be life threatening. In other cases, the murine MAbs may not be as effective as human antibodies because of their murine origin.

4.3.4   Humanization of antibodies

As discussed above, murine antibodies have limitations. The next phase of development is to make these murine MAbs more like human antibodies, by using genetic engineering techniques. A recent approach is to 'humanize' the antibodies to reduce HAMA and improve the avidity of the MAbs (avidity is a measure of the affinity or interaction of the binding of an antibody to an antigen). Several strategies have been adopted. They include replacing certain fragments of the antibodies.

Chimeric antibodies   The first generation is the chimeric antibodies (chimeric comes from the word Chimera, a Greek mythology beast made of three animals: lion, snake and goat). This type of antibody consists of both murine and human parts. The murine Fv fragments are retained and linked to the Fc fragment of human IgG. An example of the chimeric antibody is ReoPro, which prevents blood clots by binding to a receptor on platelets.

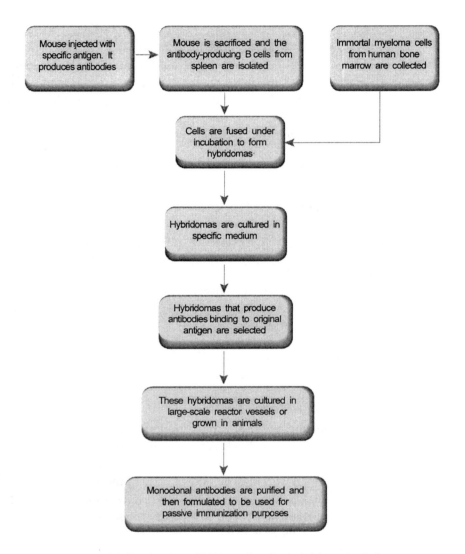

Figure 4.4 Production of MAbs using the hybridoma technique

Humanized antibodies   To further improve the avidity and reduce antigenicity, only the specific antigen-binding region is derived from mouse, while the remainder of the antibody is constructed using human proteins. These are the humanized antibodies, and include the breast cancer targeting MAb called Herceptin.

Full human antibody Full human antibodies are the current engineered antibodies. Several techniques are used to construct these antibodies. One method is to fuse human B cells to myeloma cells. These hybridomas will produce fully human MAbs. Another method is to genetically alter mice in the laboratory to contain human antibody producing genes. In response to antigens, antibodies resembling the human antibodies are produced. A third method is the use of phage display. A type of filamentous bacteriophage (virus) is used. Genes that code for the antibodies are isolated from human B cells. These genes are inserted into the virus, and *E. coli* is infected with the virus. As the virus reproduces within *E. coli*, antibodies are also produced. In this way, many copies of the human antibodies are 'photocopied' and become available.

4.3.5 Conjugate antibodies

Antibodies are also prepared to carry 'payloads'. Materials such as toxins, enzymes or even radioisotopes can be fused to the antibodies (Figure 4.5). The strategy here is to use antibodies as vehicles to deliver more effective treatment to specific target cells. Immunotoxins are fusion proteins consisting of a toxin connected to a MAb. Immunocytokines consist of a fusion of rDNA encoding the heavy chain of a MAb with the DNA encoding a cytokine. The aim is to obtain a high local concentration of cytokine to generate an anti-tumor response. Zevalin and Bexxar are two new conjugate antibody drugs, which carry radioisotope yttrium (^{90}Y) and iodine (^{131}I) for the treatment of non-Hodgkin's lymphoma.

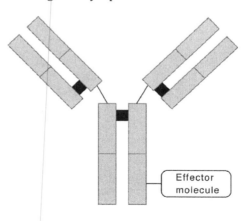

Effector molecule

Figure 4.5 Conjugate antibodies

Another variation to conjugate antibodies is to use bispecific antibodies. These are produced using chemical means and recombinant techniques to fuse separate hybridomas into a hybrid hybridoma (Figure 4.6). Bispecific antibodies use one arm of the Fv to target the antigen or tumor cell and the other arm carries the effector molecule of toxins, radioisotopes or other drugs.

4.4 CYTOKINES

Cytokines are produced mainly by the leukocytes (white blood cells). They are potent polypeptide molecules that regulate the immune and inflammation functions, as well as hemopoiesis (production of blood cells) and wound healing. There are two major classes of cytokines: (a) lymphokines and monokines, and (b) growth factors.

4.4.1   Lymphokines and monokines

Cytokines produced by lymphocytes are called lymphokines, and those produced by monocytes are termed monokines. Lymphocytes and monocytes are different types of white blood cells. The major lymphokines are interferons (IFNs) and some interleukins (ILs). Monokines include other interleukins and tumor necrosis factor (TNF).

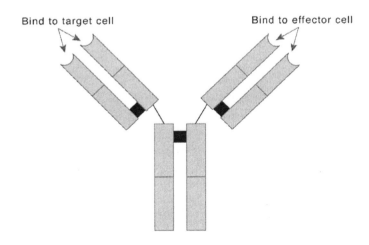

Figure 4.6 Bispecific antibody

Interferons There are two types of interferons: Type I, which includes IFN-α and IFN-β and Type II consisting of IFN-γ. IFN-α and β have about 30% homology in amino acid sequence. There are two more recently discovered Type I interferons; they are called IFN-ω and IFN-τ. IFN-α and IFN-β each have 166 amino acids, and IFN-γ has 143. Both IFN-α and IFN-β are of single chain structure and bind to the same type of cell surface receptors, whereas IFN-γ is a dimer of two identical chains and interacts with another type of receptors. All our cells can produce Type I interferons when infected by viruses, bacteria and fungi. However, only T cells and natural killer cells can produce Type II interferon. Type I interferon binds to receptor, which in turn activates tyrosine kinase phosphorylation and the subsequent transcription pathway that induces viral resistance. Similarly, Type II interferon binds to another receptor and activates the immune response.

Because of its antiviral and anticancer effects, IFN-α is used in the treatment of hepatitis and various forms of cancer, such as Kaposi's sarcoma, non-Hodgkin's lymphoma and hairy cell leukemia. Exhibit 4.6 describes the treatment of hepatitis C with IFN-α. IFN-β is used for treating multiple sclerosis, a chronic disease of the nervous system. The medical application of IFN-γ is for cancer, AIDS and leprosy.

Exhibit 4.6 Hepatitis C and Interferon

Hepatitis C is caused by a virus contracted through contaminated blood. Most infected patients show no sign of hepatitis for a long time. Of those infected, about 15% will clear the virus, and 85% develop chronic hepatitis. Up to 30% of patients with chronic hepatitis C will develop cirrhosis within 20 years, and 5% will develop liver cancer. The WHO estimates that more than 170 million people worldwide are infected with hepatitis C.

Interferon is the approved treatment for hepatitis C. In general, there are four different treatments: (a) IFN-*a*, (b) combination therapy of IFN-*a* and another drug called ribavirin, (c) pegylated IFN-*a* and (d) pegylated IFN-*a* with ribavirin. Pegylated interferon contains polyethylene glycol, which slows down the body's absorption of interferon. In this way, a more controlled release of interferon is achieved to prolong absorption. Interferons were extracted and purified from human blood supplies up until the 1980s. The amount produced was very low. Since then, interferons have been produced using recombinant technology from a variety of cells: *E. coli*, fungus, yeast and mammalian.

Patients receiving IFN experience side effects similar to influenza symptoms: headache, nausea and tiredness. IFN also decreases red blood cells, white blood cells and platelet counts. A measure of the effectiveness of IFN treatment is the marker called alanine aminotransferase in blood. The normal range is 10–70 U/L.

Interleukins   Interleukins are proteins produced mainly by leukocytes. There are many interleukins within this family (Table 4.1). Interleukins have a number of functions, but principally in mediating and directing immune cells to proliferate and differentiate. Each interleukin binds to specific receptor and produces its response.

IL-2 is possibly the most-studied interleukin. It is also called T cell growth factor. IL-2 is a 15 kDa glycoprotein produced by CD4+ T helper cells. It has 133 amino acids. There are four helical regions and a short β-sheet section (Figure 4.7).

Table 4.1 Selected interleukins

Cytokine	Origin	Target cell	Effect on immune response
IL-2	T cell	T cell, NK cell	Proliferation of antigen-specific cells and other immune cells
IL-3	T cell	Bone marrow cells	Growth/differentiation of all cell types
IL-4	T cell	B cell	Stimulation of Immunoglobulin (Ig) heavy chain switching to IgE
IL-5	T cell	B cell, Eosinophil	Growth /differentiation of eosinophils
IL-7	Bone marrow stroma cell	Lymphocyte	Growth factor
IL-10	Macrophage, T cell	Macrophage, T cell	Inhibit macrophage function, control of immune response
IL-15	Macrophage	NK cell, T cell	Proliferation

SOURCE   Adapted with permission from Zane, H.D., *Immunology—Theoretical and Practical Concepts in Laboratory Medicine*, W. B. Saunders Company, Pennsylvania, 2001.

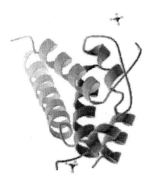

Figure 4.7 Interleukin 2 (IL-2) molecule.   SOURCE Reprinted with permission from Protein Date Bank, PDB ID: 1M47, http://www.rcsb.org/pdb/cgi/explore.cgi?job=summary&pdbId=1M47&page=, Arkin, M. M., Randal, M., Delano, W. L. et. al., Binding of Small Molecules to an Adaptive Protein-Protein Interface, *Proc.Nat.Acad.Sci.USA* 100 pp. 1603 (2003).

IL-2 promotes the growth of B cells for antibody production and induces the release of IFN-γ and TNF (see below). It has been approved by the FDA for the treatment of different types of cancer, including metastatic melanoma and metastatic renal carcinoma. Although IL-2 has not been approved to treat HIV/AIDS, many clinical trials using IL-2 are being conducted. The strategy is to complement the anti-HIV therapy by boosting the immune system with IL-2. The replacement therapy of IL-2 administered to AIDS patients increases production of CD4+ T cells and the activities of natural killer cells to combat HIV. Therapeutic IL-2 is manufactured using recombinant technology.

Tumor necrosis factor There are two types of tumor necrosis factor: TNF-α and TNF-β. Of the two, TNF-α has been studied in more detail. TNF-α is a 157 amino acid polypeptide. It is a mediator of immune regulation, including the activation of macrophages and induction of the proliferation of T cells. Another TNF-α function is its cytotoxic effects on a number of tumor cells. Recent research, however, concentrates on its property in the stimulation of inflammation, particularly in the case of rheumatoid arthritis. Clinical trials are being conducted with drugs to block TNF-α with anti-TNF-α monoclonal antibodies. These antibodies target the excessive levels of TNF-α in synovial fluids of joints and provide relief to sufferers of rheumatoid arthritis (Exhibit 4.7).

Exhibit 4.7 Rheumatoid Arthritis and TNF-*α*

Rheumatoid arthritis is an autoimmune disease of the synovial lining of joints. Typically, the joints affected are those in the extremities: fingers, wrist, toes and ankles. It is a debilitating disease in which ligaments may be damaged and joints deformed.

In the late 1980s, scientists found that TNF-*α* is involved in causing arthritis. Standard drug treatment for rheumatoid arthritis used to be methotrexate, steroids and non-steroidal anti-inflammatory drugs (NSAIDs). These drugs are non-specific and their effectiveness is variable. The new set of drugs in the late 1990s was designed to specifically target TNF-*α*. Two drugs are especially effective; they are infliximab (Remicade, Centocor) (a chimeric antibody that targets the TNF-*α*) and etanercept (Enbrel, Wyeth) (a soluble protein receptor for TNF-*α* that neutralizes its effect).

The success of these two drugs provides impetus for the development of other anti-inflammatory drugs aiming at specific inflammatory agents.

4.4.2   Growth factors

As the name implies, growth factors stimulate cell growth and maintenance. We will discuss the following growth factors:

- Erythropoietin
- Colony stimulating growth factors.

Erythropoietin   Erythropoietin (EPO) is a glycoprotein produced by specialized cells in the kidneys. It has 166 amino acids and a molecular weight of approximately 36 kDa. EPO stimulates the stem cells of bone marrow to produce red blood cells. It is used to treat anemia and chronic infections such as HIV and cancer treatment with chemotherapy where anemia is induced. Patients feel tired and breathless owing to the low level of red blood cells. EPO can be prescribed instead of blood transfusion.

Biopharmaceutical quantities of EPO are produced with recombinant cells. This is achieved through the isolation of the human gene that codes for EPO and transfection of the gene into cell lines such as Chinese hamster ovary cells (see Section 10.5). The product is called rhEPO—recombinant human EPO. EPO is normally administered subcutaneously and is generally well tolerated by patients.

EPO is considered a banned performance-enhancing drug in the sports arena, where athletes use EPO to boost their red blood cells with the expectation of boosting performance (see Exhibit 4.8 for a brief review of performance enhancing drugs).

Colony stimulating growth factors   Growth factors such as granulocyte macrophage colony stimulating factor (GM-CSF) and macrophage colony stimulating factor (M-CSF) are involved in the regulation of the immune and inflammatory responses. GM-CSF is a glycoprotein with 127 amino acids and a molecular weight of about 22 kDa. It is produced by macrophages and T cells.

Clinically, GM-CSF is used to stimulate production of blood cells, in particular patients who have received chemotherapy. M-CSF is a glycoprotein that can exist in different forms. The number of amino acids ranges from just over 200 to about 500, and molecular weight varies between 45 and 90 kDa. M-CSF is being evaluated clinically for its anti-tumor activity.

Exhibit 4.8 Performance-enhancing Drugs

To help them excel in sports, some athletes use drugs to boost their performance. There are several areas where drugs are used by athletes:

To increase oxygen delivery
To build muscle and bone
To mask pain
To mask use of other drugs
As stimulants

EPO is used in blood doping to generate more red blood cells for carrying oxygen. It is particularly favored by endurance athletes to enhance their performance. Human growth hormone (hGH, see description in Section 4.5.2) is used to build up muscle and bone strength. Both EPO and hGH are banned in sport.

The recombinant EPO and hGH produced are almost replicas of those that occur naturally in our body. Hence, it is very difficult to detect these banned substances if taken by athletes. Another difficulty is the need to develop reliable and sensitive test methods that take into account differences of these substances in athletes of different racial groups.

SOURCE Zorpette, G., All doped up—and going for gold, *Scientific American*, May, pp. 20–22 (2000); Freudenrich, C., *How Performance-Enhancing Drugs Work*, http://entertainment.howstuffworks.com/athletic-drug-test1.htm [accessed Sep 24, 2002].

4.5 HORMONES

Hormones are intercellular messengers. They are typically (a) steroids (e.g. estrogens, androgens and mineral corticoids, which control the level of water and salts excreted by the kidney), (b) polypeptides (e.g. insulin and endorphins) and (c) amino acid derivatives (e.g. epinephrine, or adrenaline, and norepinephrine, or noradrenaline). Hormones maintain homeostasis—the balance of biological activities in the body; for example, insulin controls blood glucose level, epinephrine and norepinephrine mediate response to external environment, and growth hormone promotes normal healthy growth and development.

4.5.1 Insulin

Insulin is produced in the pancreas by β cells in the region called the islets of Langerhans. It is a polypeptide hormone consisting of two chains: an A chain with 21 amino acids with an internal disulfide bond, and a B chain with 30 amino acids. There are two disulfide bonds joining these two chains together

(Figure 4.8). The molecular weight is around 6.8 kDa. Insulin regulates the blood glucose level to within a narrow range of 3.5–8.0 mmol/L of blood.

Insulin was originally (since the 1930s) obtained from porcine and bovine extracts. Bovine insulin differs from human insulin by three amino acids, and it can elicit an antibody response that reduces its effectiveness. Porcine insulin, however, differs in only one amino acid. An enzymatic process can yield insulin identical to the human form. Currently, insulin is produced via the rDNA process; it was the first recombinant biopharmaceutical approved by the FDA (in the early 1980s). The recombinant insulin removes the reliance on animal sources of insulin and ensures that reliable and consistent insulin is manufactured under controlled manufacturing processes. A description of diabetes mellitus and insulin is presented in Exhibit 4.9.

4.5.2   Human growth hormone

Human growth hormone (hGH) is a polypeptide with 191 amino acids. It is secreted by the pituitary gland. This hormone stimulates the production of insulin-like growth factor-1 (IGF-1) from the liver. Most of the positive effects of hGH are mediated by the IGF-1 system, which also includes specific binding proteins.

A major function of hGH is the promotion of anabolic activity, i.e. bone and tissue growth due to increase in metabolic processes. Other biological effects of hGH are stimulation of protein synthesis, elevation of blood glucose level and improvement of liver function.

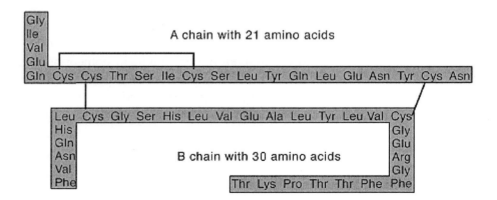

Figure 4.8 Human insulin molecule. Refer to Table A2.1 for the names of amino acids.

Exhibit 4.9 Diabetes Mellitus and Insulin

Diabetes mellitus occurs when the human body does not produce enough insulin. This form of diabetes is called insulin-dependent diabetes mellitus (IDDM, or juvenile diabetes, or Type I diabetes). IDDM is an autoimmune disease (see Exhibit 4.5) in which the β cells are targeted by the body's own immune system and progressively destroyed. Once destroyed, they are unable to produce insulin.

Production of insulin is triggered when there is a rise in blood sugar, for example after a meal. Most of our body cells have insulin receptors, which bind to the insulin secreted. When the insulin binds to the receptor, other receptors on the cell are activated to absorb sugar (glucose) from the bloodstream into the cell.

When there is insufficient insulin to bind to receptors, the cells are starved because sugar cannot reach the interior to provide energy for vital biological processes. Patients with IDDM become unwell when this happens. They depend on insulin injection for survival.

Another form of diabetes is non-insulin dependent diabetes mellitus (NIDDM, or adult diabetes, or Type II diabetes). In this case, insulin is produced and a normal insulin level is detected in blood. But for various reasons its effect is reduced. This may be caused by a reduced number of insulin receptors on cells, or reduced effectiveness in binding to these receptors. The cause is complex and may involve genetic make-up, changes in lifestyle, nutritional habits and environmental factors.

Overproduction of hGH during puberty leads to gigantism, and deficiency during this period results in dwarfism. The current main therapeutic use of hGH is for the treatment of short stature. As discussed in Exhibit 4.8, hGH is used by athletes illegally to enhance their performance. This hormone is also sold without prescription with claims of improvement to body composition (lean body mass, fat mass, fluid volume), bone strength, immune function, youthful vigor and general well being.

4.6 GENE THERAPY

In essence, gene therapy can be described as 'good genes for bad genes'. The technology involves the transfer of normal functional genes to replace genetically faulty ones so that proper control of protein expression and biochemical processes can take place. Although this seems straightforward, the major question is 'How do we get the normal genes to the intended location?'.

This question revolves around the delivery tools for the genes. The transport system or vehicles used are called vectors (gene carriers). There are two basic gene therapy techniques: *in vitro* and *in situ* methods.

For the *in vitro* method, some of the patient's tissues, which have the genetic fault, are removed. Cells are selected from these tissues and normal genes are loaded into the cells with vectors. The modified cells are then returned to the patient to correct the genetic fault. With the *in situ* method, genes encapsulated by the vectors are injected directly into the tissues to be treated. Figure 4.9 shows the basis for gene therapy.

Whether using the *in vitro* or *in situ* method, genes are first loaded onto the vectors. A number of vectors are used (Table 4.2).

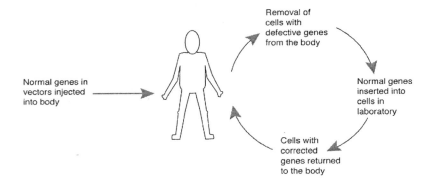

Figure 4.9 Basis of gene therapy

Table 4.2 Vectors for gene therapy

Retrovirus	Adenovirus	Adeno-associated virus	Liposomes	Naked DNA
Advantages Integrates genes to host chromosomes, chance of long term stability	Large capacity for carrying foreign genes	Integrates genes to host chromosomes	Do not have viral genes, so do not cause disease	Do not have viral genes, so do not cause disease
Disadvantages Integration is random, mostly on dividing cells	Transient function of genes	Small capacity for foreign genes	Less efficient than viruses	Inefficient gene transfer

SOURCE   Friedman, T., Overcoming the obstacles to gene therapy, *Scientific American*, June, pp. 96–101 (1997).

The most common vectors used today are viruses, with retroviruses being the preferred candidates, as they are efficient vectors for entering humans and replicating their genes within human cells. Scientists take advantage of this biological function. Disease-causing genes from the viruses are removed, and the therapeutic genes are inserted. Retroviruses carrying the desired therapeutic genes are placed in the patient's body. When the viruses invade the cells, they 'infect' these host cells and the therapeutic genes are added to the host DNA. In this way, the new genes function and take over from the original faulty genes.

Theoretically, this appears to be a fitting solution to gene problems. However, there are problems, such as immune and inflammation responses, toxicity, and means to target the intended cells. Non-viral vectors may overcome the problems with viral delivery agents. Lipids, in the form of liposomes and other lipid complexes, are being studied. Injection of DNA directly into a patient's muscle cells is another avenue being researched.

Another hurdle surrounding gene therapy is the identification of genes causing the disease. Effective cures can only arise when there is a good understanding of the roles of particular genes in diseases. Some of the diseases to which gene therapy may be applicable are cancer, hemophilia, sickle cell anemia, cystic fibrosis, insulin-dependent diabetes mellitus (see Exhibit 4.9), emphysema, Alzheimer's disease, Huntington's disease and severe combined immune deficiency (SCID). To date, the FDA has not approved any gene therapy product. Numerous clinical trials are in progress (Exhibit 4.10). Another question on gene therapy is the ethical considerations. This issue is discussed in Section 11.6.

Exhibit 4.10 Gene Therapy Trials

The first gene therapy trial was conducted in September 1990. A four-year-old girl with SCID (an inherited immune disorder disease, otherwise known as the 'Bubble Boy' syndrome) was treated in Cleveland, US. She is doing well some 10 years after the treatment. A second girl with the same disorder underwent gene therapy and she too continues to do well.

These are the successes; there are many failures as well. More than 400 gene therapy clinical trials have been conducted, mainly on cancer, but not many cases worked. In 1999, an 18-year old boy in Pennsylvania, US, unexpectedly died from a reaction to gene therapy when he was treated for a metabolic disease. This trial raised many issues, and many trials with discrepancies and unreported adverse events were suspended by the FDA. The FDA has since introduced tighter controls for gene therapy trials.

SOURCE Thompson, L., Human gene therapy—harsh lessons, high hopes, *FDA Consumer Magazine*, September–October (2000).

4.7   STEM CELLS

Stem cells are divided into three different categories: totipotent, pluripotent and multipotent. A description of the genesis of stem cells is shown in Figure 4.10.

Totipotent stem cells are obtained from embryos that are less than five days old. These cells have the full potential to develop into another individual and every cell type.

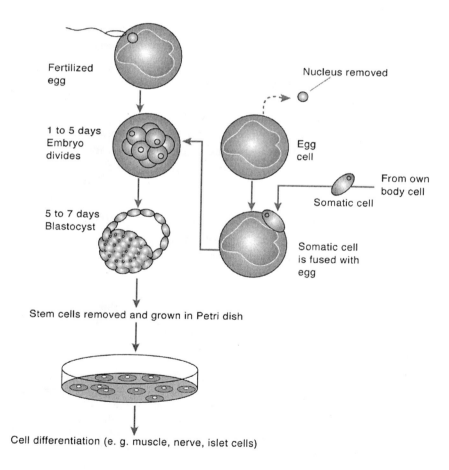

Figure 4.10 Genesis of different stem cells

After about five days and several cycles of cell division, the totipotent cells form a hollow sphere of cells called a blastocyst. The blastocyst has an outer layer of cells surrounding clusters of cells. Those cells on the outside continue to divide and grow into the placenta and supporting tissues. The clusters of cells on the inside divide and form virtually all the cell types, except the placenta and supporting tissues, which give rise to a human being. These are the pluripotent stem cells, and they give rise to many different types of cells, but not a new individual.

Pluripotent cells continue to develop, differentiate and specialize into different cells. They become the specialized stem cells, such as blood, skin and nerve stem cells. These differentiated stem cells are multipotent, i.e. they have the potential to produce specialized cells. For example, blood stem cells in bone marrow produce red blood cells, white blood cells and platelets, but not other types of cells.

There are two general avenues for stem cell research: pluripotent and multipotent stem cells. Pluripotent stem cells are obtained by two methods. One method is to harvest the clusters of cells from the blastocysts of human embryos. Another method is the isolation of pluripotent cells from fetuses in terminated pregnancies. Multipotent stem cells are derived from umbilical cords or adult stem cells. However, because of the specialization of these cells, their potential to develop into a myriad of different cells is limited.

A burning issue is the ethics of obtaining pluripotent stem cells from embryos and fetuses. The US government has acted on this issue and declared that federal funds for stem cell research have to meet certain criteria. It requires that funding will only be provided to research with stem cells obtained before 9 August 2001, as a cut-off date to limit research to pre-existing stem cells. Refer to Section 11.7 for an ethical debate on stem cells.

The potential contribution of stem cells to medical treatment lies in their capability to differentiate and grow into normal, healthy cells. Using pluripotent stem cells, scientists are devising means to culture them in the laboratories and coax them to grow into various specialized cells. Rather than gene therapy, with stem cells we have the potential of cell therapy to repair our diseased tissues and organs. This will circumvent the problem of lack of donor organs. Stem cells can also provide the possibility for healthy cells to cure disabilities such as strokes, Parkinson's disease and diabetes.

A drawback for stem cell therapy is the problem of cell rejection due to the host's immune system recognizing the cells as foreign. This rejection issue has to be overcome to ensure stem cell therapy as a viable treatment.

Recently, French scientists reported on research progress of stem cell transplants for curing children with sickle cell anemia. A mix of anti-rejection drugs was used to suppress rejection of the new stem cells.

Although research into stem cells is new, the use of stem cells for therapy has been with us for some time. Most of us are familiar with bone marrow transplant for patients with leukemia. This procedure involves finding a matching donor to harvest bone marrow stem cells and transfuse them to the patient with leukemia (see Exhibit 4.11 for details).

Exhibit 4.11 Bone Marrow Transplant

Bone marrow is the spongy tissue inside the cavities of our bones. Bone marrow stem cells grow and divide into the various types of blood cells: white blood cells (leukocytes) that fight infection, red blood cells (erythrocytes) that transport oxygen, and platelets that are the agents for clotting.

Patients with leukemia have a condition in which the stem cells in the bone marrow malfunction and produce an excessive number of immature white blood cells, which interfere with normal blood cell production.

The aim of a bone marrow transplant is to replace the abnormal bone marrow stem cells with healthy stem cells from a donor. Healthy stem cells are normally harvested using a syringe to withdraw bone marrow from the rear hip bone of the donor. They are then infused into the patient via a catheter in the chest area. Before the infusion, the patient receives chemotherapy or radiotherapy to destroy the diseased bone marrow stem cells so that the infused stem cells have a chance to grow free of complications from diseased cells.

There are a number of terms used in the transplant procedure:

Allogeneic transplant: The person giving the bone marrow or stem cells is a genetically matched family member (usually a brother or sister).

Unrelated allogeneic transplant: The person donating marrow is unrelated to the patient.

Syngeneic transplant: The person donating the bone marrow or stem cell is an identical twin.

Autologous transplant: The patient donates his or her own bone marrow or stem cells before treatment, for re-infusion later. This happens when a patient is receiving radiotherapy or chemotherapy in such a high dose that the bone marrow is destroyed. The bone marrow stem cells collected previously are re-injected into the patient to reinforce the immune system.

SOURCE   Bone Marrow and Stem Cells Transplant Support, *Bone Marrow Transplant Overview,* http://www.bmtsupport.ie/bmtoverview.html [accessed Sep 2, 2002].

4.8 FURTHER READING

Austen, F.A., Burakoff, S.J., Rosen, F.S. and Strom, T.B., *Therapeutic Immunology*, 2nd edn., Blackwell Science, Inc., Malden, US, 2001.

Baxter, A.M. and Gwadz, R.W., *Malaria: Prevention and Therapy (Emphasis on Africa)*, National Library of Medicine, 1997, http://www.nlm.nih.gov/pubs/resources.html.A [Accessed Sep 28, 2002].

De Groot, A.S. and Rothman, F.G., In silico predictions: In vivo veritas, *Nature Biotechnology*, 17, pp. 533–534 (1999).

DeWitt, N., *In silico* vaccine design?, *Nature Biotechnology*, 17, p. 523 (1999).

Di Bisceglie, A. and Bacon, B.R., The unmet challenges of hepatitis C, *Scientific American*, October, pp. 80–85 (1999).

Dubel, S., *The Recombinant Antibody Pages*, http://www.tu-bs.de/institute/ibb/biotech/SD/SDscFvSite.html [accessed Mar 26, 2002].

Ezzell, C., Magic bullets fly again, *Scientific American*, October, pp. 34–41 (2001).

Felgner, P.L., Nonviral strategies for gene therapy, *Scientific American*, June, pp. 103–106 (1997).

Friedmann, T., Overcoming the obstacles to gene therapy, *Scientific American*, June, pp. 96–101 (1997).

Funaro, A., Horenstein, A.L., Santoro, P. et al., Monoclonal antibodies and therapy of human cancers, *Biotechnology Advances*, 18, pp. 385–401 (2000).

George, A.J.T. and Urch, C.E. (eds.), *Diagnostic and Therapeutic Antibodies*, Humana Press, New Jersey, 2000.

Gibbs, W.W., Try, try again, *Scientific American*, July, pp. 101–103 (1993).

Green, B.A. and Baker, S.M., Recent advances and novel strategies in vaccine development, *Current Opinion in Microbiology*, 5, pp. 483–488 (2002).

Hanly, W.C., Bennett, B.T. and Artwohl, J.E., *Overview of Adjuvants*, Biologic Resources Laboratory, University of Illinois, Chicago, http://www.nal.usda.gov/awic/pubs/antibody/overview.htm [accessed Nov 21, 2002].

Haseltine, W.A., Beyond chicken soup, *Scientific American*, November, pp. 56–63 (2001).

Hudson, P.J., Recombinant antibody constructs in cancer therapy, *Current Opinion in Immunology*, 11, pp. 548–557 (1999).

Johnson, H.M., Bazer, F.W., Szente, B.E. and Jarpe, M.A., How interferons fight disease, *Scientific American*, May, pp. 68–75 (1994).

Klegerman, M.E. and Groves, M.J., *Pharmaceutical Biotechnology, Fundamentals and Essentials*, Interpharm Press, Inc., Buffalo Grove, US, 1992.

Laver, W.G., Bischofberger, N. and Webster, R.G., Disarming flu viruses, *Scientific American*, January, pp. 78–87 (1999).

Lee, C.K., Human vaccine development and approval process in the USA, *Journal of Biomedical Research* 1, pp. 46–51 (1991).

Lubiniecki, A.S., Monoclonal antibody products: Achievement and prospects, *Bioprocessing Journal*, 2, Mar/Apr, pp. 21–26 (2003).

Mandavilli, A., Gene-therapy trials for hemophilia make comeback, *BioMedNet*, October 1, 2002, http://news.bmn.com/news/story?day=021001&story=1 [accessed Nov 27, 2002].

McKay, D., Alzheimer's vaccine?, *Trends in Biotechnology*, 19, pp. 379–380 (2001).

National Institutes of Health, *Research for Malaria Vaccine Development*, NIH, Bethesda, MD, http://www.niaid.nih.gov/dmid/malaria/malvacdv/support.htm, [accessed Feb 6, 2002].

National Institutes of Health, *Stem Cell Research*, NIH, Bethesda, MD, 2000, http://www.nih.gov/ [accessed Nov 25, 2002].

National Institutes of Health, *Stem Cells: A Primer*, NIH, Bethesda, MD, 2002, http://www.nih.gov/ [accessed Nov 25, 2002].

Pizzi, R.A., The science and politics of stem cells, *Modern Drug Discovery*, 5, pp. 32–34, 36–37 (2002).

Sayers, J.R. Acres of antibodies: The future of recombinant biomolecule production?, *Trends in Biotechnology*, 19, pp. 429–430 (2001).

Scheibner, V., Adjuvants, preservatives and tissue fixatives in vaccines, *Nexus*, 8, Dec & Feb (2000–2001) http://www.whale.to/vaccine/adjuvants.html [accessed Nov 21, 2002].

Sinclair, M., Surface vaccine combo, *Nature Biotechnology*, 18, p. 586 (2000).

Singh, M. and O'Hagan, D., Advances in vaccine adjuvants, *Nature Biotechnology*, 17, pp. 1075–1081 (1999).

Walsh, G., *Biopharmaceuticals: Biochemistry and Biotechnology*, John Wiley & Sons, Chichester, UK, 1998.

Wigzell, H., The immune system as a therapeutic agent, *Scientific American*, September, pp. 126–134 (1993).

CHAPTER 5

DRUG DEVELOPMENT AND PRECLINICAL STUDIES

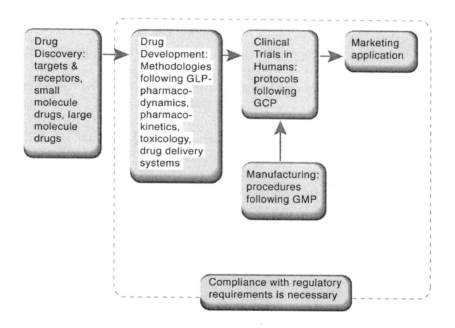

5.1 INTRODUCTION

In earlier chapters, we discussed the discovery of new drugs. After a lead compound has been identified, it is subjected to a development process to optimize its properties. The development process includes pharmacological studies of the lead compound and its effects on toxicity, carcinogenicity, mutagenicity and reproductive development. These data are important for determining the safety and effectiveness of the lead compound as a potential drug.

An ideal drug is potent, efficacious and specific, that is, it must have strong effects on a specific targeted biological pathway and minimal effects on all other pathways, to reduce side effects. In reality, no drugs are perfectly effective and absolutely safe. The aim of pharmacological studies is to obtain data on the safety and effectiveness of the lead compound. Many iterations of optimization of the lead compound may be necessary to yield a potential drug for clinical trial.

The potency, efficacy and safety of a drug depend on the chemical and structural specificity of drug–target interaction. In pharmacology, we are concerned with pharmacodynamics, pharmacokinetics and toxicity. In simplified terms, pharmacodynamics deals with the actions of the drug on the target, whereas pharmacokinetics is about the actions of the body on the drug. Toxicity information in preclinical studies provides us with confidence in the safety aspect of the potential drug. These data for pharmacodynamics, pharmacokinetics and toxicity enable the dose and dosing regimen to be set for the clinical trials.

Although pharmaceutical firms are increasingly using *in vitro* methods to evaluate pharmacological responses, some aspects of pharmacological developments have no alternatives but to use *in vivo* tests in animals to study the effects of a potential drug in living systems. Pharmacological and toxicity studies using animals are regulated under Good Laboratory Practice with strict guidelines, requiring scientists to follow established protocols. Readers are referred to FDA 21 CFR Part 58 'Good laboratory practice for nonclinical laboratory studies'. This regulation details the requirements for the conduct of nonclinical laboratory studies intended to support applications for clinical trials and marketing approvals (Investigational New Drug [IND] and New Drug Application [NDA]; see Chapter 8). The contents list for this guideline is presented in Exhibit 5.1.

Examples of some of these requirements are:
- Personnel must have the education, training and experience to

conduct the nonclinical studies

- A quality assurance unit should be set up
- Materials for the studies must be appropriately tested for identity, strength, purity, stability, and uniformity
- Appropriate personnel, resources, facilities, equipment, materials, and methodologies must be available
- The studies must be conducted under specifically designed protocols with an appropriate quality system established to handle data, deviations and reporting
- Animals must be isolated, their health status checked, and they must be given the appropriate welfare
- Nonclinical laboratory studies must be conducted in accordance with the protocols.

Exhibit 5.1 FDA 21 CFR Part 58 *Good Laboratory Practice for Nonclinical Laboratory Studies*: Table of Contents

Scope
Definitions
Applicability to studies performed under grants and contracts
Inspection of a testing facility
Personnel
Testing facility management
Study director
Quality assurance unit
General
Animal care facilities
Facilities for handling test and control articles
Laboratory operation areas
Specimen and data storage facilities
Equipment design
Maintenance and calibration of equipment
Standard operating procedures
Reagents and solutions
Animal care
Test and control article characterization
Test and control article handling
Mixtures of articles with carriers
Protocol

Continued

Exhibit 5.1 *Continued*

Conduct of a nonclinical laboratory study
Reporting of nonclinical laboratory study results
Storage and retrieval of records and data
Retention of records
Purpose
Grounds for disqualification
Notice of and opportunity for hearing on proposed disqualification
Final order on disqualification
Actions upon disqualification
Public disclosure of information regarding disqualification
Alternative or additional actions to disqualification
Suspension or termination of a testing facility by a sponsor
Reinstatement of a disqualified testing facility

Drug development also extends to formulation and delivery. Most drugs that are administered to patients contain more than just the active pharmaceutical ingredients (the drug molecules that interact with the receptors or enzymes). Other chemical components are often added to improve manufacturing processing, or the stability and bioavailability of drugs. Effective delivery of drugs to target sites is an important factor to optimize efficacy and reduce side effects. The development process also includes the design and development of new manufacturing and testing methodologies for cost-effective production of drugs in compliance with regulatory requirements. Drugs are manufactured under Good Manufacturing Practice, which is discussed in Chapters 9 and 10.

5.2   PHARMACODYNAMICS

The chemical and structural aspects of pharmacodynamics are discussed in Chapters 2, 3 and 4, where we considered drug–target interactions. When a drug binds to a target, it may regulate the receptor as an agonist or antagonist, or act as an inducer or inhibitor in the case of an enzyme. The lock and key chemical and structural interaction is *a priori* to achieving a potent and safe drug. In this chapter, we focus on the quantitative mathematical relationships of drug–target interactions, in addition to the chemical and structural aspects covered in Chapters 2, 3 and 4.

Pharmacodynamics is the study to determine dose–response effects. We are interested in finding out the effects of a drug on some particular response, such as heart rate, enzyme levels or muscle relaxation or contraction. When a drug binds to a receptor, the ensuing response is complex. The following example is an idealized case, which illustrates the drug–receptor interaction:

$$D + R \underset{k_{-1}}{\overset{k_1}{\rightleftarrows}} D*R \Longrightarrow Response$$

where D is the drug, R is the receptor, and D*R is the drug–receptor complex.

The response may be local or via a signal transduction process. The rate for the forward reaction of drug binding to receptor is proportional to the concentrations of both the drug and target. Conversely, the rate for the reverse reaction, i.e. dissociation of the drug–receptor complex, is proportional to concentration of the drug–receptor complex. At equilibrium, both forward and reverse reactions are equal. Mathematically we have:

$$k_1[D][R] = k_{-1} [D*R] \tag{1}$$

where k_1 is the forward reaction rate constant, k_{-1} is the reverse reaction rate constant, and [D], [R] and [D*R] are the concentrations of the drug, receptor and drug–receptor complex, respectively.

Rearranging Equation (1), we obtain:

$$\frac{[D][R]}{[D*R]} = \frac{k_{-1}}{k_1} = K_D \tag{2}$$

where K_D is the equilibrium dissociation constant.

When half the receptors are bound, we have [R] = [D*R]. Substituting into Equation (2), K_D is equal to [D]. This means that K_D is the concentration of the drug that, at equilibrium, will bind to half the number of receptors.

If we consider all the available receptors as 100% and [D*R] are the occupied receptors with drug at the binding sites, then [R], which is the percentage of free, unoccupied receptors, can be substituted with 100 − [D*R]. Equation (2) can be re-written as:

$$[D] = \frac{K_D[D*R]}{100 - [D*R]} \qquad (3)$$

Equation (3) is a hyperbolic function showing the relationship between dose of drug, [D], and its effects resulting from drug–receptor interaction, [D*R]. A graphical representation of this dose–effect, or dose–response curve, is shown in Figure 5.1. The graph shows that, at low doses, the effects are approximately linear in proportion to the doses. However, as the dose increases, there is gradually a diminishing return in effects. A maximum is reached and at this point all available receptors are bound with drug molecules. Further increase in dose does not generate any increase in effects. The point E_{max} is the maximum effect, and EC_{50} is the concentration of the drug that produces 50% of the maximum effect.

Very often, the dose–effect curve is redrawn using a logarithmic scale for the dose. This gives rise to a sigmoid curve, as shown in Figure 5.2. It is a mathematical transformation, which shows an approximate linear portion for the 20% to 80% maximal effect scale, which is usually the dose level for a therapeutic drug. Doses above 80% provide very little increase in therapeutic effects but with a concomitant rise in the risk of adverse reactions.

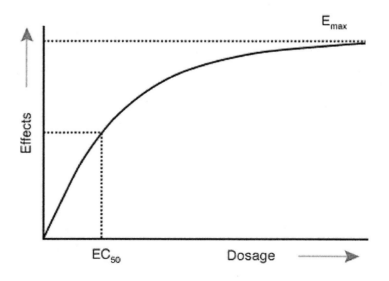

Figure 5.1 Dose–effect curve

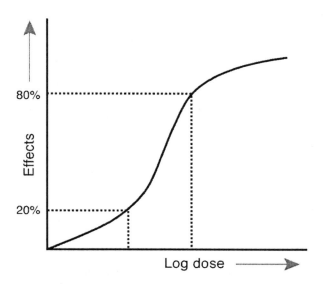

Figure 5.2 Dose–effect curve with logarithmic scale for dose

Scientists also study the potency, effectiveness, safety margin and therapeutic index of a drug. These terms are described below with reference to Figures 5.3 and 5.4.

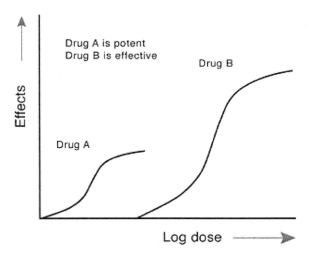

Figure 5.3 Potency and effectiveness

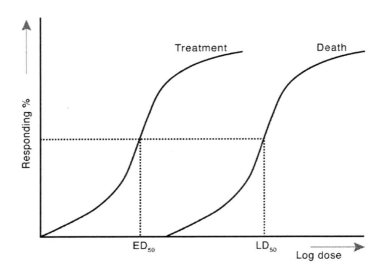

Figure 5.4 Therapeutic index

Potency: This is the dose required to generate an effect. A potent drug elicits an effect at a low dose.

Effectiveness: This is the intensity of the effect or response. It is a measure of the affinity of the drug for the receptor. An effective drug is one that can achieve effects in the vicinity of E_{max}.

Therapeutic Index: The index is given by the ratio:

$$\frac{LD_{50}}{ED_{50}}$$

where LD_{50} is the lethal dose for 50% of the population, and ED_{50} is the effective dose for 50% of the population.

When there is a large difference in dose between ED_{50} and LD_{50} the therapeutic index of the drug is high.

Safety Margin: This is the separation of two doses: one that produces therapeutic effects and one that elicits adverse reaction. The standard safety margin (SSM) is given by:

$$SSM = \frac{LD_1 - ED_{99}}{ED_{99}} \times 100$$

where LD_1 is the lethal dose for 1% of the population, and ED_{99} is the effective dose for 99% of the population.

A large safety margin is achieved when there is a significant difference between the ED_{99} and LD_1 doses.

5.3 PHARMACOKINETICS

For a drug to interact with a target, it has to be present in sufficient concentration in the fluid medium surrounding the cells with receptors. Pharmacokinetics is the study of the kinetics of absorption, distribution, metabolism and excretion (ADME) of drugs. It analyzes the way the human body deals with a drug after it has been administered, and the transportation of the drug to the specific site for drug–receptor interaction. For example, a person has a headache and takes an aspirin to abate the pain. How does the aspirin travel from our mouth to reach the site in the brain where the headache is and act to reduce the pain?

There are several ways to administer a drug. They include:

- Intravenous
- Oral
- Buccal
- Sublingual
- Rectal
- Subcutaneous
- Intramuscular
- Transdermal
- Topical
- Inhalational.

With the exception of intravenous administration, where a drug is injected directly into the bloodstream, all the routes of administration require the drug to be absorbed before it can enter the bloodstream for distribution to target sites. Metabolism may precede distribution to the site of action, for example, in the case of oral administration. The human body also has a clearance process to eliminate drugs through excretion. We will consider absorption, distribution, metabolism and excretion in the sections below, with reference to Figure 5.5.

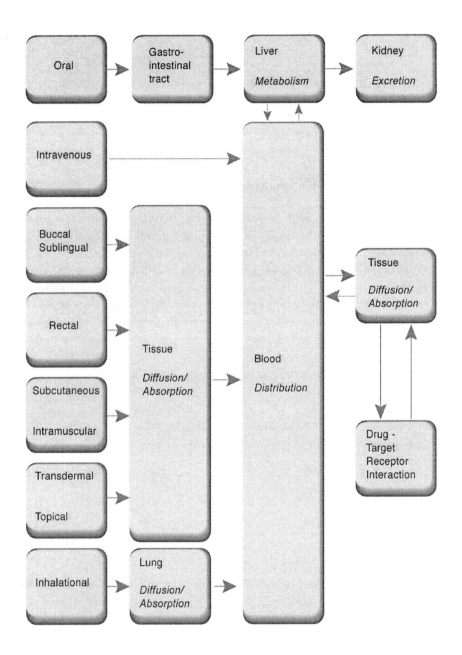

Figure 5.5   Schematic representation of drug absorption, distribution, metabolism and excretion

5.3.1 Transport mechanism

Except for intravenous injection, drug molecules have to cross cell membranes to reach target sites. There are four basic transport mechanisms:

- Passive diffusion
- Facilitated diffusion
- Active transport
- Pinocytosis.

Passive diffusion Diffusion is the random movement of molecules in fluid. If a fluid is separated by a semi-permeable membrane, more dissolved molecules will diffuse across the membrane from the higher concentration side to the lower concentration side than in the reverse direction. This process will continue until equilibrium is achieved, whereby both sides have the same concentration. When equilibrium is reached, there are equal numbers of molecules crossing the membrane in both directions.

Drug molecules are transported across cell membranes. Because of the lipid bilayer construction of the membrane (Appendix 2), non-polar (lipid-soluble) molecules are able to diffuse and penetrate the cell membrane. Polar molecules, however, cannot penetrate cell membrane readily via passive diffusion and rely on other transport mechanisms.

Lipid solubility determines the readiness of drug molecules to cross the gastrointestinal tract, blood–brain barrier and other tissues. Molecular size is another factor that determines the diffusion of drugs across membrane, with the smaller molecules able to diffuse more readily. Exhibit 5.2 describes the kinetics for diffusion of drug molecules across cell membrane.

Facilitated diffusion Polar drug molecules have been observed to cross cell membranes. The transport mechanism is via carrier systems. Transmembrane carriers, such as proteins, are similar to receptors and bind to polar and non-polar drug molecules. They facilitate the diffusion of drugs across the cell membrane. The facilitated diffusion rate is faster than passive diffusion, and may be controlled by enzymes or hormones. Facilitated diffusion is from a region of high concentration to low concentration. However, these carriers, or transporters, may become saturated at high drug concentration. In this case, the transportation rate plateaus until the carriers are cleared of the drugs in preparation for another cycle of transportation.

Active transport The active transport mechanism requires energy to drive the transportation of drugs against the concentration gradient, from low to high. The transportation rate is dependent on the availability of carriers and energy supply via a number of biological pathways.

Exhibit 5.2 Diffusion of Drugs

Most drugs are weak acids or bases. Under different pH conditions, they become ionized and cannot diffuse through the cell membrane. This ionization process is illustrated below:

Weak Acid: $AH \leftrightarrow A^- + H^+$

$$pK_a = pH + \log_{10} \frac{[AH]}{[A^-]} \qquad (4)$$

Weak Base: $BH^+ \leftrightarrow B + H^+$

$$pK_a = pH + \log_{10} \frac{[BH^+]}{[B]} \qquad (5)$$

AH and B are the unionized acid and base, respectively, and A^- and BH^+ are the ionized forms. The lipid solubility of AH and B are dependent on the chemical structure of the drugs. In most instances, they are of sufficient solubility to diffuse across the cell membranes. However, as the equations show, the pH environment affects the ionization of a drug. We illustrate this with aspirin (a weak acid drug, $pK_a = 3.5$) as an example and apply Equation (4):

Blood: high pH (7.4) environment

$$3.5 = 7.4 + \log_{10} \frac{[AH]}{[A^-]}$$

$$\log_{10} \frac{[AH]}{[A^-]} = -3.9$$

$$\frac{[AH]}{[A^-]} = 0.00126$$

The ionized form is dominant. Therefore, less lipid soluble.

Stomach: low pH (3.0) environment

$$3.5 = 3.0 + \log_{10} \frac{[AH]}{[A^-]}$$

$$\log_{10} \frac{[AH]}{[A^-]} = 0.5$$

$$\frac{[AH]}{[A^-]} = 3.16$$

There is more of the unionized form. Therefore, more lipid soluble.

A similar method is used to calculate the unionized to ionized forms for basic drugs using Equation (5).

SOURCE Adapted with permission from Rang, H.P., Dale, M.M., Ritter, J.M. and Gardner, R., *Pharmacology*, 3rd edn., Churchill Livingstone, New York, 1995, p. 70.

Pinocytosis   Pinocytosis involves the engulfing of fluids by a cell. The process commences with the infolding of cell membrane around fluids containing the drug. The membrane then fuses and forms a vesicle with fluid core. In this way, the drug is taken into the cell interior within the vesicle.

5.3.2   Absorption

Oral administration   The oral route is the most common way of administering a drug. For a drug to be absorbed into the bloodstream, it has to be soluble in the fluids of our gastrointestinal tract. Drugs are often formulated with excipients (components other than the active drug) to improve manufacturing and dissolution processes (see Section 5.5).

Our gastrointestinal tract is lined with epithelial cells, and drugs have to cross the cell membrane (see Exhibit 5.2). In the stomach, where pH is low, drugs that are weak acids are absorbed faster. In the intestine, where pH is high, weak basic drugs are absorbed preferentially. Figure 5.6 shows the absorption of drugs under different pH environment.

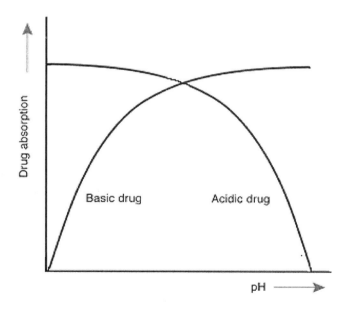

Figure 5.6 Absorption of drugs in different pH environments

In reality, there is more than just passive diffusion at work for drugs to traverse the cell membrane. Most drugs are absorbed in the intestine. Often, if an oral drug is taken and a fast response is desired, the drug is taken on an empty stomach to ensure a quick passage through the stomach for absorption in the intestine to take place.

Drugs absorbed through the gastrointestinal tract pass into the hepatic portal vein, which drains into the liver. The liver metabolizes the drug, which leads to reduction in the availability of the drug for interaction with receptors. This is called first pass metabolism.

A plot of the drug concentration in the bloodstream over time for a single dose is shown in Figure 5.7. At a certain time after administration, the rate of drug absorption equals the rate of clearance. This is an equilibrium condition called 'steady state'.

The area under the curve represents the total amount of drug in the blood. It is a measurement of the bioavailability of the drug. Comparison of drug concentrations in the bloodstream administered via intravenous injection and oral route provides information for the bioavailability of the oral drug. This is because the oral drug is metabolized in the liver before reaching the general blood circulation (see Section 5.3.4), whereas the total amount of drug is injected into the bloodstream intravenously. In general, oral doses are higher than intravenous doses to take into account the effects of first pass metabolism.

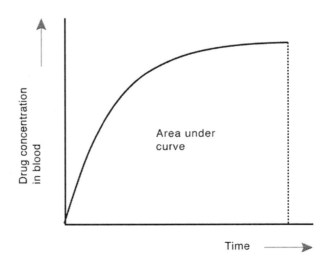

Figure 5.7 Drug concentration in bloodstream vs time for a single dose

Buccal and sublingual administration   Drugs can be absorbed through the oral cavity. Buccal (between the gums and cheek) and sublingual (underneath the tongue) can be effective means of drug administration. In both cases, drugs can enter the blood circulation without first pass metabolism in the liver.

Rectal administration   Rectal administration of drugs may be applied when the patient is unable to take drug orally and some other routes are impractical. The drug administered via the rectum is absorbed and partially bypasses the liver. However, the absorption of drugs may be unreliable in certain cases.

Subcutaneous and intramuscular administration   Subcutaneous and intramuscular administration can be used to deliver protein-based drugs. The absorption of drug is faster than with the oral route. The rate of absorption is determined by the blood flow pattern and diffusion of drug molecules in tissues.

Transdermal and topical administration   Transdermal administration is to apply the drug on the skin surface. The drug is absorbed and transported by blood to receptors, which may be remote from the part of the skin where the transdermal patch is. The first pass metabolism is circumvented. Topical administration is to apply the drug for local effects. The typical areas for topical applications are the skin, eyes, throat, nose and vagina.

Inhalation administration   Aerosol particles of drug can be inhaled into the lungs. Because of the large surface area of the alveoli, absorption is rapid and effective. As the lungs are richly supplied with capillaries, distribution of inhalational drugs is very quick.

Intravenous administration   When a drug is injected, the entire dose can be considered as being available in the bloodstream to be distributed to the target site. Hence, the dosage can be controlled, unlike with other routes of administration where the bioavailability of the drug may be unpredictable because of diffusion processes. Intravenous injection is the normal route for administration of protein-based drugs, as they are likely to be destroyed when taken orally because of the pH conditions in the gastrointestinal tract.

The onset of drug action with intravenous injection is quick, and this method is especially useful for emergency cases. However, intravenous injection is potentially the most dangerous. Once a drug is injected, there is no means to stop it from circulating throughout the body. The complete circulation of blood in the body takes about a minute, and hence an adverse reaction can occur almost instantaneously.

5.3.3   Distribution

When a drug is in the bloodstream, it is distributed to various tissues. The distribution pattern depends on a number of factors:

- Vascularity nature of the tissue
- Binding of the drug to protein molecules in blood plasma
- Diffusion of the drug.

When a tissue is perfused with blood supply, drug molecules in the blood are transported to the tissue rapidly until equilibrium is reached. On the other hand, the drug may bind to albumin and proteins in the blood, rendering less of it available for distribution to tissues. In general, acid drugs bind to albumins and basic drugs to glycoproteins. The third factor for drug distribution is passive diffusion. Lipid-soluble drugs can cross the cell membrane more readily than polar drugs and move into the tissues to interact with receptors.

The volume of distribution (Vd) is an important parameter. It is represented by the following equation:

$$Vd = \frac{\text{Amount of drug in the body}}{\text{Concentration of drug in blood}}$$

Vd is a hypothetical volume. When the concentration of drug in blood is low, Vd may turn out to be a large value, many times more than the volume of a person of around 60–70 liters. Highly lipid-soluble drugs have a very high volume of distribution. Lipid insoluble drugs, which remain in the blood, have a low Vd.

For example, obesity affects Vd because lipid-soluble drugs diffuse into the adipose tissues of the obese person. Vd is a useful parameter for determining the loading dose for a drug to attain equilibrium after the drug is administered.

Distribution of drugs is restricted in two areas: the brain and the placenta. Refer to Exhibit 5.3 for a brief description.

Exhibit 5.3 Barriers to Drug Distribution

Blood–brain barrier
Distribution of drugs to the brain tissue is restricted for some types of drugs. The reason is that the brain has a sheath of connective tissue cells, the astrocytes, surrounding it, forming a barrier to passive diffusion for polar drugs. In addition, the endothelial cells of the brain capillaries are joined more tightly together, curtailing further the diffusion of polar drugs to the brain. Lipid-soluble drugs, however, can diffuse into the brain more readily and bring forth their effects.

Placental barrier
The placental barrier consists of several layers of cells between the maternal and fetal circulatory systems. Diffusion of polar drugs is limited. However, lipid-soluble drugs can pass through the barrier. Fetuses are rich in lipids and may form a reservoir for sequestering lipid soluble drugs.

5.3.4 Metabolism

Many drugs are metabolized in the body; their chemical structures are altered and pharmacological activity reduced. The liver is the major organ for metabolizing drugs, a secondary role is played by the kidneys. Some drugs are metabolized in tissue systems.

Two types of biochemical metabolism reactions take place in the liver: Phase I and Phase II reactions. Phase I reactions include oxidation, reduction and hydrolysis, which transform the drugs into metabolites. A family of enzymes called cytochrome P-450 is responsible for these reactions. They convert lipid-soluble drugs to more water-soluble metabolites. Phase II reactions involve the addition or conjugation of subgroups, such as –OH, –NH and –SH to the drug molecules. Enzymes other than P-450 are responsible for these reactions. These reactions give rise to more polar molecules, which are less lipid-soluble and are excreted from the body. Exhibit 5.4 describes some of the drug metabolism studies recommended by the Food and Drug Administration (FDA).

5.3.5 Excretion

Drugs are excreted from the body by the following routes:
- Kidneys
- Lungs
- Intestine and colon
- Skin.

Exhibit 5.4 Metabolism Studies

The aim of metabolism studies is to (i) identify metabolic pathways, and (ii) investigate the possibility of drug–drug interactions.

Pharmacogenetics influences the therapeutic effects of drugs. A drug that is normally metabolized by the P-450 2D6 enzyme will not be metabolized in about 7% of the Caucasian population. Co-administration of drugs may have different effects which are either (i) additive, or synergistic, or (ii) antagonistic.

Some drugs are administered in a pro-drug form. They are metabolized, and the metabolites elicit the interactions with receptors.

P-450 enzymes have been cloned and *in vitro* studies can be performed using these enzyme systems. Metabolic pathways can be studied by incubating the drug with the P-450 enzymes. Similarly, drug–drug interactions can be studied.

SOURCE Center for Drug Evaluation and Research, *Guidance for Industry, Drug Metabolism/Drug Interaction Studies in the Drug Development Process: Studies In Vitro*, FDA, Rockville, MD, 1997, http://www.fda.gov/cder/guidance/clin3.pdf [accessed Jun 5, 2002].

The kidneys are the most important organs for clearing drugs from the body. Water-soluble drugs are cleared more quickly than lipid-soluble drugs. Volatile and gaseous byproducts of drugs are exhaled by the lungs. Some drugs are re-absorbed into the intestine and colon and later passed out as solid wastes. Another mechanism of clearance is for drugs to be excreted through the skin as perspiration.

The clearance of a drug is given by the following expression:

$$CL = \frac{\text{Rate of drug elimination}}{\text{Drug concentration in blood}}$$

A typical drug clearance curve is shown in Figure 5.8. The curve in Figure 5.8 is a first-order curve, i.e. the elimination rate is proportional to the amount of drug in the bloodstream. As the amount of drug in blood reduces, the elimination rate also reduces. Another term often used is 'half-life'. This is the time taken to clear half (50%) of the remaining drug in the body. Mathematically, it is given by:

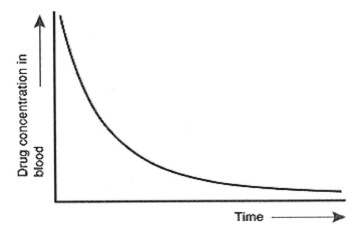

Figure 5.8 Clearance of drug from the bloodstream

$$t_{\frac{1}{2}} = \frac{0.693 \times Vd}{CL}$$

The half-life concept is further illustrated in Table 5.1.

5.3.6 Application of pharmacokinetics results

By combining Figures 5.7 and 5.8, we obtain a situation depicted in Figure 5.9. After a drug is absorbed, it enters the bloodstream and the concentration builds up until a steady state is reached. As time passes, the elimination process takes over and the concentration of the drug decreases.

Table 5.1 Half-life calculations

Number of half lives	Amount of drug in the body	
	% eliminated	% remaining
0	0.0	100.0
1	50.0	50.0
2	75.0	25.0
3	87.5	12.5
4	93.8	6.2
5	96.9	3.1
6	98.4	1.6

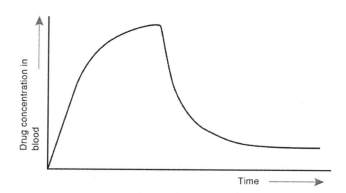

Figure 5.9 Plasma concentration of drug after a single dose

Figure 5.9 would be the situation if a single dose of drug were given, but this is rarely the case. More than one dose is often administered to maintain the therapeutic level of the drug—the level that has been determined from pharmacodynamics studies of dose response versus drug concentration. Before the drug is cleared by the excretion process, another dose is given to keep the drug concentration in a steady state and achieve maximal effects. This is illustrated in Figure 5.10.

Sometimes a larger dose is administered first; this is called a loading dose (see Section 5.3.3). It quickly builds up to the steady state level. After that, smaller doses are given to maintain the steady state.

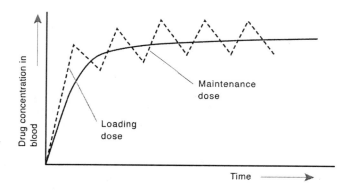

Figure 5.10 Multiple doses to maintain maximal effect

5.4   TOXICOLOGY

In addition to the preclinical research of pharmacodynamics and pharmacokinetics, study of the toxicology of a potential drug is critical to demonstrate that it is safe before it is given to humans in clinical trials. Toxicological studies show the functional and morphological effects of the drug. They are performed by determining the mode, site and degree of action, dose relationship, sex differences, latency and progression and reversibility of these effects.

We summarize in Exhibit 5.5 the International Conference on Harmonization (ICH) guidelines for toxicological and pharmacological studies. Appendix 4 shows the type of information on pharmacodynamics, pharmacokinetics and toxicology that regulatory reviewers examine when a potential drug is filed for Investigational New Drug and New Drug Application approval. The information is extracted from the FDA *Guidance for Reviewers, Pharmacology/Toxicity Review Format* (2001).

Exhibit 5.5   ICH Guidelines on Safety Studies

S1:	*Carcinogenicity studies*
S1A	Guideline on the need for carcinogenicity studies of pharmaceuticals
S1B	Testing for carcinogenicity in pharmaceuticals
S1C	Dose selection for carcinogenicity studies of pharmaceuticals
S2:	*Genotoxicity studies*
S2A	Genotoxicity: specific aspects of regulatory tests
S2B	Genotoxicity: standard battery tests
S3:	*Toxicokinetics and pharmacokinetics*
S3A	Toxicokinetics: guidance on the assessment of systemic exposure toxicity studies
S3B	Pharmacokinetics: Guidance for repeated dose tissue distribution
S4:	*Toxicity testing*
S4	Single dose toxicity tests
S4A	Duration of chronic toxicity testing in animals (rodent and non-rodent)
S5:	*Reproductive toxicology*
S5A	Detection of toxicity to reproduction for medicinal products
S5B(M)	Reproductive toxicology: Male fertility studies
S6:	*Biotechnological products*
S6	Safety studies for biotechnological products
S7:	*Pharmacology studies*
S7A	Safety pharmacology studies for human pharmaceuticals
S7B	Safety pharmacology studies for assessing the potential for delayed ventricular repolarization

5.4.1 Toxicity

It is necessary to determine the toxicity of a drug. The maximum tolerable dose and area under curve are established in rodents and non-rodents. There are two types of toxicity studies: single dose and repeated dose. Single dose acute toxicity testing is conducted for several purposes, including the determination of repeated doses, identification of organs subjected to toxicity, and provision of data for starting doses in human clinical trials.

The experiments are carried out on animals, usually on two mammalian species: a rodent (mouse or rat) and a non-rodent (rabbit). Two different routes of administration are studied; one is the intended route for human clinical trials, and the other is intravenous injection. Various characteristics of the animals are monitored, including weights, clinical signs, organ functions, biochemical parameters, and mortality. At the completion of the study, animals are killed and autopsies are performed to analyze the organs, especially the targeted organ for the drug.

Repeated dose chronic toxicity studies are performed on two species of animals, a rodent and non-rodent. The aim is to evaluate the longer-term effects of the drug in animals. Plasma drug concentrations are measured and pharmacokinetics analyses are performed. Vital functions studied include cardiovascular, respiratory and nervous systems. Animals are retained at the end of the study to check toxicity recovery. Table 5.2 shows the duration of the animal studies, which depends on the duration of the intended human clinical trial. Appendix 4 summarizes the information to be submitted to regulatory authorities.

Table 5.2 Duration of repeated dose toxicity studies to support Phase I and II trials in the European Union and Phase I, II and III trials in the United States and Japan.

Duration of clinical trials	Minimum duration of repeated dose toxicity studies	
	Rodents	**Non-rodents**
Single dose	2–4 weeks	2 weeks
Up to 2 weeks	2–4 weeks (1 month)	2 weeks (1 month)
Up to 1 month	1 month (3 months)	1 month (3 months)
Up to 3 months	3 months (6 months)	3 months (3 months)
Up to 6 months	6 months	6 month (chronic)
>6 months	6 months	6–9 months

NOTE There are slight differences in the requirements for the European Union, the US and Japan. Duration to support Phase III trials in the EU, when they differ from the other data, is given in brackets. Readers are referred to Guidance for Industry: M3 Nonclinical Safety Studies for the Conduct of Human Clinical Trials for Pharmaceuticals, FDA, Rockville, MD, 1997, http://www.fda.gov/cder/guidance/1855fnl.pdf [accessed Jun 9, 2002].

5.4.2   Carcinogenicity

Carcinogenicity studies are carried out to identify the tumor-causing potential of a drug. Drugs are administered to animals continuously for at least six months. Rats are normally used, but another rodent study may be required. The studies are performed using the drug administration route intended for humans. Data for hormone levels, growth factors and tissue enzymatic activities are gathered. At the end of the experiments, the animals are killed and the tissues examined. Appendix 4 summarizes the information to be submitted to regulatory authorities.

5.4.3   Genotoxicity

These studies are to determine if the drug compound can induce mutations to genes. A standard battery of tests is:
- Assessment of genotoxicity in a bacterial reverse mutation test (Ames Test, see Exhibit 5.6)
- Detection of chromosomal damage using *in vitro* method (Mouse Lymphoma tk Test, a test to evaluate the potential of drug in causing mutations to thymidine kinase [tk])
- Detection of chromosomal damage using rodent hematopoietic cells.

Exhibit 5.6 Ames Test

The Ames test is based on the reversion of mutations in the bacterium *Salmonella typhimurium*. Mutant strains of *S. typhimurium*, those with mutations in the *his* operon, are unable to grow without addition of the amino acid histidine. The drug to be tested is mixed with *S. typhimurium* and a small amount of histidine in a nutrient medium. After the histidine is consumed, the growth will stop if the drug is not a mutagen. However, if the drug is a mutagen, it will induce a reversion in the *his* operon and the bacterium will continue to grow.

5.4.4   Reproductive toxicology

The aim of these studies is to assess the effect of the potential drug on mammalian reproduction. All the stages, from pre-mating through conception, pregnancy and birth, to growth of the offspring, are studied. Rats are the predominant species used, and rabbit is the preferred non-rodent model. The route of administration is similar to the intended route for humans. At least three dosage levels and control groups are used (control groups are dosed with drug excipients or vehicles to provide comparable basis for analysis). For the females, effects such as hormonal cycles, pregnancy and embryo development are studied. For the males, effects on the reproductive organs are analyzed. Other parameters studied are detailed in Appendix 4.

5.5   ANIMAL TESTS, *IN VITRO* ASSAYS AND *IN SILICO* METHODS

The use of animals for pharmacological and toxicological studies has yielded invaluable information for drug development. However, many drug candidates failed in Phase I and II clinical trials because the animal models were insufficient to represent human systems and functions for some drugs. Efficacy and acceptable toxicities derived from animal models were not replicated in humans (Exhibit 5.7). In recent years, the direction in development of drugs has shifted towards the use of *ex vivo*, *in vitro* assays and even *in silico* methods. Nevertheless, some tests must still be confirmed in animals.

Exhibit 5.7 Clinical Trial Failures

Only one in 10 Investigational New Drugs (IND) will become approved as drugs. Half the IND failures are due to unacceptable efficacy. Another third fail because of safety issues.

Toxicity failures occur because:
- Toxicity in animals is not fully understood and potential toxicity in humans cannot be estimated
- Toxicity in animals is understood and potential toxicity in humans is not acceptable
- Acceptable therapeutic margins (efficacy versus toxicity) cannot be established
- Toxicities in animals do not predict toxicity in human trials.

SOURCE Johnson, D.E., Predicting human safety: Screening and computational approaches, *Drug Discovery Today*, 5, pp. 445–454 (2000).

Where animals are used, mice and rats are the preferred models. Other species used are hamsters, guinea pigs and rabbits. These animals are bred in a specially controlled environment, under specific pathogen-free conditions, to ensure that they do not carry infections or pathogens before being used in various tests. Different breeds or strains of animals are used, for example, BALB/c mice are used for immunity studies and Fischer – 344 mice for carcinoma evaluation. Nude mice (in addition to the nude gene, which results in the absence of thymus and T-cell function) have two other mutations important in regulating the function of the immune system. More recent additions are transgenic animals with knockout genes. For example, mice with knockout p53 genes have high incidence of tumor growth.

Experimental use of animals is controlled under Good Laboratory Practice (GLP), and study protocols are submitted to the Animal Research Ethics Committee for approval. Studies using animals can only proceed with the approval of the Ethics Committee, which consists of technical personnel, including a veterinarian, as well as lay people who evaluate the study from different perspectives.

In vitro assays are increasingly being used. Reasons are costs, availability of more rapid results, and avoidance of negative publicity. Assays such as cytochrome P-450 enzymes, Ames test and the mouse lymphoma tk test are *in vitro* methods. For absorption studies, Caco-2 (Exhibit 5.8) and Maudin-Darby canine kidney cell assays are now routinely used. Hepatocyte cell lines with metabolism capacity are being developed to test drug metabolism and toxicity. All these examples show that, where possible, pharmaceutical firms are gradually dispensing with animal studies.

Exhibit 5.8 Caco-2 Cell Assays

The Caco-2 cells are derived from human colorectal carcinoma. When these cells are cultured on semi-permeable membranes, they grow into epithelial cells that are very similar to intestinal epithelial cells. The permeability of drugs across these Caco-2 cells provides model tools for the study of drug absorption.

With better understanding of drug functions and information from huge databases, predictive *in silico* ADME algorithms have been designed. These algorithms encompass information derived from *in vivo* and *in vitro* studies; they consider molecular interactions, biological data, pharmacological results and toxicological endpoints. A description of some of these *in silico* methods is given in Exhibit 5.9.

Exhibit 5.9 *In Silico* Predictive Methods

DEREK (Deductive Estimation of Risk from Existing Knowledge; Lhasa Ltd, Leeds, UK) is a rule-based system, which examines toxicity effects of potential drugs.

National Toxicity Program (NTP) is a system that evaluates mutagenicity of potential drugs. *Continued*

Exhibit 5.9 *Continued*

TOKAT (Toxicity Prediction by Komputer Assisted Technology; Oxford Molecular, Hunt Valley, MD, US) uses quantitative structure–activity relationships to predict toxicities in drug molecules.

MCASE (Computer Automated Structure Evaluation; MULTICASE, Cleveland, OH, US) correlates structures and toxicities.

SOURCE Johnson, D.E., Predicting human safety: Screening and computational approaches, *Drug Discovery Today*, 5, pp. 445–454 (2000).

The aim of all the laboratory and animal studies is to understand the effects of the potential drug in living systems. These studies cannot guarantee the safety and efficacy of the drug in humans, but they can enhance the reliability and predictive value. Results from these studies provide a basis for starting dose for clinical trials in humans. The draft *Guidance for Industry and Reviewers: Estimating the Safe Starting Dose in Clinical Trials for Therapeutics in Adult Healthy Volunteers* from the FDA (December 2002) outlines the derivation of the maximum recommended starting dose (MRSD) for a drug to be used in humans for the first time. This dose is based on the following derivation algorithm:

1. Determine the no observed adverse effect level (NOAEL) in animals—the highest dose level that does not produce a significant increase in adverse effects.
2. Convert the NOAEL to human equivalent dose (HED) using the data from Table 5.3 (calculations are based on body surface areas).

5.6 FORMULATIONS AND DELIVERY SYSTEMS

Development of manufacturing processes for the production of drug (active pharmaceutical ingredients), initially to supply enough materials for laboratory testing, then for human clinical trials, and ultimately as production batches of drug products when approved by regulatory authorities. There are two distinct manufacturing processes: synthetic chemistry for pharmaceuticals, and recombinant DNA technology for biopharmaceuticals. Manufacturing processes are discussed in Chapter 10. Apart from pharmacological and toxicological studies, the drug development process encompasses meticulous and methodical work in the following areas:

Table 5.3 Conversion of animal doses to human equivalent doses (HED) based on body surface area

Species	To convert animal dose in mg/kg to dose in mg/m², multiply by kg/m² below:	To convert animal dose in mg/kg to HED[a] in mg/kg, either:	
		Divide animal dose by:	Multiply animal dose by:
Human	37	–	–
Child (20 kg)[b]	25	–	–
Mouse	3	12.3	0.08
Hamster	5	7.4	0.13
Rat	6	6.2	0.16
Ferret	7	5.3	0.19
Guinea pig	8	4.6	0.22
Rabbit	12	3.1	0.32
Dog	20	1.8	0.54
Primates:			
Monkeys[c]	12	3.1	0.32
Marmoset	6	6.2	0.16
Squirrel monkey	7	5.3	0.19
Baboon	20	1.8	0.54
Micro-pig	27	1.4	0.73
Mini-pig	35	1.1	0.95

[a] Assumes 60 kg human. For species not listed or for weights outside the standard ranges, human equivalent dose can be calculated from the formula:
HED = animal dose in mg/kg × (animal weight in kilograms / human weight in kilograms)$^{0.33}$.
[b] This is provided for reference only, as healthy children will rarely be volunteers for Phase I trials.
[c] For example, cynomolgus, rhesus, stumptail.
NOTE Column 2 is for information only. For HED calculations, either column 3 or column 4 is used.

- Formulation of the drug product, which includes active pharmaceutical ingredients and excipients, into final form suitable to be administered to patients.
- Study of drug delivery systems to improve effective delivery of the drug to patients for enhancing certain characteristics and improving patient compliance.

The last two items are discussed below.

5.6.1 Formulations

Most drugs that are prescribed to us are formulated with the active pharmaceutical ingredients and excipients. The formulations of selected drugs are presented in Exhibit 5.10. According to the *US Pharmacopoeia and National Formulary* definition, excipients are 'any component, other than the

active substance(s), intentionally added to the formulation of a dosage form'. There are many reasons for the addition of excipients:
- Control the release of drug substance in the body
- Improve the assimilation process and bioavailability
- Enhance drug dissolution as disintegration promoters
- Extend the stability and shelf life of the drug as antioxidants or preservatives
- Aid in the manufacturing processes in the form of fillers, lubricants, wetting agents and solubilizers
- Mask an unpleasant taste of the active pharmaceutical ingredient
- Use as an aid for identification of the product.

Exhibit 5.10　Selected Drug Formulations

Prilosec

An antiulcerant in 10, 20 and 40 mg doses (see Table 1.2).

Active ingredient: omeprazole

Excipients: cellulose, disodium hydrogen phosphate, hydroxypropyl cellulose, hydroxypropyl methylcellulose, lactose, mannitol, sodium lauryl sulfate, etc.

Prozac

An antidepressant in 10, 20 and 40 mg doses.

Active ingredient: fluoxethine hydrochloride

Excipients: starch, gelatin, silicone, titanium dioxide, iron oxide etc.

Lipitor

Cholesterol reducer in 10, 20, 40 and 80 mg doses (see Table 1.2).

Active ingredient: atorvastatin calcium

Excipients: calcium carbonate, candililla wax, croscarmellose sodium, hydroxypropyl cellulose, lactose monohydrate, magnesium stearate, microcrystalline cellulose, polysorbate 80, simethicone emulsion.

Celebrex

Anti-inflammatory in 100 and 200 mg doses (see Table 1.2).

Active ingredient: celecoxib

Excipients: croscarmellose sodium, edible inks, gelatin, lactose monohydrate, magnesium stearate, povidone, sodium lauryl sulfate and titanium dioxide.

SOURCE　Food and Drug Administration, Center for Drug Evaluation and Research, http://www.fda.gov/cber/ [accessed Jun 27, 2002].

According to the International Pharmaceutical Excipients Council, the most commonly used excipients in the United States are:

- Magnesium stearate
- Lactose
- Microcrystalline cellulose
- Starch (corn)
- Silicon dioxide
- Titanium dioxide
- Stearic acid
- Sodium starch glycolate
- Gelatin
- Talc
- Sucrose
- Calcium stearate
- Pregelatinized starch
- Hydroxypropyl methylcellulose
- Hydroxypropyl cellulose
- Ethylcellulose
- Calcium phosphate.

The FDA maintains a database of approved excipients (*Drug Information: Electronic Orange Book*, http://www.fda.gov/cder/ob/default.htm). Standards and tests for regulatory acceptable excipients are included in the *US Pharmacopoeia and National Formulary*. Two such tests, dissolution and stability, are included in Exhibit 5.11 for reference. For new excipients to be included in a drug formulation, they have to satisfy one of the following criteria:

- Determination by the FDA that the substance is 'generally recognized as safe' (GRAS) according to 21 CFR 182, 184 and 186.
- Approval by the FDA as a food additive under 21 CFR 171
- Excipients referenced in the New Drug Application, showing that they have been tested in laboratory and clinical trials.

5.6.2 Drug delivery systems

Delivery systems have come a long way from pills, syrups and injectables. As we have discussed earlier, the ADME process means that most drugs administered to us have tortuous paths to reach their targets, and in many instances the bioavailability is reduced. A traditional means to overcome the vagaries of ADME is to have larger doses or more frequent administrations.

Exhibit 5.11 Dissolution and Stability Tests

FDA, Guidance for Industry, (1997) *Dissolution Testing of Immediate Release Solid Dosage Forms*

Dissolution tests using the basket method (50/100 rpm) or the paddle method (50/75 rpm) under mild test conditions are used to generate a dissolution profile at 15-minute intervals. The pH range is 1.2–6.8; pH up to 8.0 may be tested with justification. The temperature is 37 ± 0.5 °C. Methods are described in the *US Pharmacopoeia*. Test requirements vary depending on solubility of drug products. *In vitro* test may need validation to confirm *in vivo* results.

Stability Tests on Active Ingredients and Finished Products EU Guidelines (1998) *Medicinal Products for Human Use*, **Vol. 3A, Quality and Biotechnology**

Stability tests on drug products are performed to determine shelf life and storage conditions. Drug products are tested at various temperatures, e.g. <–15 °C, 2–8 °C, 25 °C and 40 °C. High humidity testing at >75% is performed as well, and a combination of 40 °C and 75% relative humidity. Photostability is tested by the exposure of drug products to visible and ultraviolet light sources. Properties and characteristics of the drugs are tested after temperature and humidity exposures to determine the storage conditions and shelf-life.

These types of treatments have complications: (a) potential for adverse events, and (b) ensuring patient compliance to take the medication regularly. New delivery systems are devised to overcome these problems.

The oral route for drug administration is convenient and does not normally require physician's intervention. Most protein-based drugs are, however, not administered via the oral route because they are destroyed by the low pH medium in the stomach. One means to overcome this is the use of enteric coating for some drugs. Drugs are coated with cellulose acetate phthalate, which can withstand the acid environment in the stomach and yet readily dissolves in the slightly alkaline environment of the intestine. In this way, the protein-based drugs can have a safe passage to the intestine for absorption to take place.

Another method is to prolong the release of the drug in the bloodstream. This will reduce the frequency for taking the drug, for example, from several times a day to once per day or even once per week. To achieve this, drug molecules are encapsulated within polymer matrices. These are known as microspheres, polymer micelles, and hydrogels. The polymers are made with biodegradable materials and, through processes of hydrolysis, drug molecules are released at controlled rates as the polymer is degraded. The degradation process can be triggered by pH, temperature, electric field or even ultrasound. Exhibit 5.12 provides further description on these polymeric delivery systems.

Exhibit 5.12 Polymeric Drug Delivery Systems

Two new developments are the dendrimers (highly branched, globular, synthetic macromolecules) and modified buckyballs. Together with hydrogels, they are tailored to provide targeted delivery.

The dendrimers form small micelles, which transport small molecules within their matrices or act as hubs for covalent bonding to drug molecules, extending like dendrites. In this way, they can shepherd high concentrations of drugs to targets.

Buckyballs are cage-like molecules of fullerenes. They are robust and can carry radioactive drugs to targets. Research is directed at using these buckyballs as delivery systems for treatment of cancer.

Hydrogels are 3D cross-linked polymer networks. They can withstand acid conditions and release the entrapped drug molecules. Purdue University researchers have used a poly[methacrylic acid-g-poly(ethylene glycol)] hydrogel to encapsulate insulin, which could be released by pH trigger.

SOURCE Vogelson, C.T., Advances in drug delivery systems, *Modern Drug Discovery*, 4, April, pp. 49–50, 52 (2001); Dorsk Hassani, C.M., Doyle, F.J. and Peppas, N.A., *Molecular Gates Show Promise for Drug Delivery*, Purdue University, 1997, http://www.purdue.edu/UNS/html4ever/970414.Peppas.gate.html [accessed Jun 29, 2002].

Other delivery systems are transdermal patches, metered dose inhalers, nasal sprays, implantable devices and needle-free injections. A description of needleless injection is given in Exhibit 5.13.

Exhibit 5.13 Needleless Injection

The sight of hypodermic syringe is enough to send shivers to most patients, besides the agony for enduring the pain.

Needleless injections are new devices to bypass this problem. Drugs in powder or liquid form can be injected into the subcutaneous layer in the following ways:
Propelled by a jet stream of compressed air
Fired as pallets similar to that of bullets from rifles
Electroporation (a temporary application of direct current, which disturbs the skin surface and allows penetration of the drug molecules).
Needleless injection is ideal for frequent injections, as in the cases of insulin and growth hormone, which are administered routinely.

5.7 FURTHER READING

Atkinson Jr., A.J., Daniels, C.E., Dedrick, R.L. et al., *Principles of Clinical Pharmacology*, Academic Press, San Diego, CA, 2001.

Banakar, U.V. and Makoid, M.C., 'Pharmaceutical issues in drug development', in Welling, P.G., Lasagna, L. and Banakar, U.V. (eds.), *The Drug Development Process, Increasing Efficiency and Cost-Effectiveness*, Marcel Dekker, Inc., New York, 1996.

Bauer, L.A., *Applied Clinical Pharmacokinetics*, McGraw-Hill, New York, 2001.

Butina, D., Segall, M.D. and Frankcombe, K., Predicting ADME properties *in silico*: Methods and models, *Drug Discovery Today*, 7, May, pp. S83–S88 (2002).

Carstensen, J.T., *Advanced Pharmaceutical Solids, Drugs and Pharmaceutical Sciences*, Vol. 110, Marcel Dekker, Inc., New York, 2001.

Gad, S.C., *Drug Safety Evaluation*, Wiley-Interscience, New York, 2002.

Gundertofte, E.K. and Jorgensen, F.S., *Pharmacokinetics Molecular Modeling and Prediction of Bioavailability*, Kluwer Academic/Plenum Publishers, New York, 2000.

Julien, R.M., *A Primer of Drug Action*, 9th edn., Worth Publishers, New York, 2000.

Katzung, B.G. and Trevor, A.J., *Pharmacology, Examination & Board Review*, Prentice-Hill International Inc., US, 1995.

Langer, R., Where a pill won't reach, *Scientific American*, April, pp. 50–57 (2003).

Levine, R.R., *Pharmacology—Drug Actions and Reactions*, 6th edn., Parthenon Publishing Group, New York, 2000.

Page, C.P., Curtis, M.J., Sutter, M.C. et al. (eds.), *Integrated Pharmacology*, 2nd edn., Mosby, Edinburgh, UK, 2002.

Rang, H.P., Dale, M.M. and Ritter, J.M., *Pharmacology*, 3rd edn., Churchill Livingstone, Edinburgh, UK, 1996.

Saunders, L.M. and Hendren, R.W., *Protein Delivery Physical Systems, Pharmaceutical Biotechnology*, Vol. 10, Plenum Press, NY, 1997.

Vogelson, C.T., *Advances in Drug Delivery Systems*, Vol. 4, pp. 49–50, 52 (2001).

Waller, D. and Renwick, A., *Principles of Medical Pharmacology*, Baillere Tindall, London, 1994.

CHAPTER 6

CLINICAL TRIALS

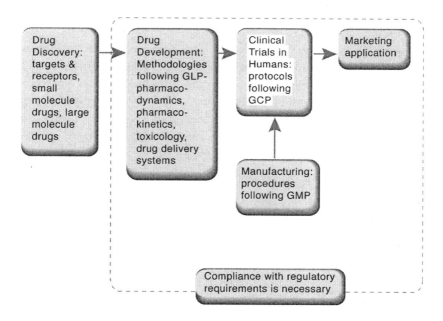

6.1   DEFINITION OF CLINICAL TRIAL

After the lead compound has been optimized and tested in the laboratory, and pharmacological studies have been conducted to show that the lead compound has the potential to become a drug, it is ready for clinical trial in humans. Exhibit 6.1 presents some information about a typical clinical trial.

What is a clinical trial?   According to the International Conference on Harmonization (ICH, see Chapter 7) the definition of a clinical trial or study is:

> Any investigation in human subjects intended to discover or verify the clinical, pharmacological and/or other pharmacodynamic effects of an investigational product, and/or to identify any adverse reactions to an investigational product, and/or to study absorption, distribution, metabolism, and excretion of an investigational product with the object of ascertaining its safety and/or efficacy.

Exhibit 6.1 Typical Clinical Trial

In the past 20 years, the average number of trials per new drug has increased from 30 to more than 70. The number of patients recruited for testing a drug in a typical submission for marketing approval has increased from about 1500 to 5200.

SOURCE Contract Pharma, June 2001.

6.2   ETHICAL CONSIDERATIONS

Before a drug is put forward for a clinical trial, there are ethical and regulatory constraints for the design and conduct of a clinical trial that have to be considered.

The United States National Institutes of Health (NIH) has stipulated seven ethical requirements to ensure that, before the trial begins, there is proper consideration of ethical issues and the trial subjects are protected. The essential tenet is that the potential exploitation of human subjects must be minimized and the risk–benefit ratio must be favorable. These seven ethical requirements are:
- Social value
- Scientific validity
- Fair subject selection

- Informed consent
- Favorable risk–benefit ratio
- Independent review
- Respect for human subjects.

6.2.1   Social value

This requirement is to ensure that the clinical trial is justified based on scientific research, and will result in improvements in health or advancement of scientific knowledge. In this way, resources are not directed at non-meaningful clinical research and human subjects are not being exploited.

6.2.2   Scientific validity

The clinical trial should be conducted methodically with clear objectives and outcomes that are statistically verifiable. The pre-clinical and toxicological data should have been carefully analyzed and should confirm the scientific finding. The trial should not be biased, and should be able to be executed without unreasonable caveats and conditions.

6.2.3   Fair subject selection

Selection of subjects is based on scientific objectives and not on whether the subject is privileged or vulnerable, or because of convenience. Inclusion and exclusion criteria are well thought out and designed solely to satisfy the scientific basis being put forward. There must be documented evidence to support the choice of selection criteria (Exhibit 6.2).

6.2.4   Informed consent

Subjects are to be informed about the aims, methods, risks and benefits of the trial. The availability of alternatives should be explained to the subjects.

Exhibit 6.2 An Example of an Early Clinical Trial

In 1917, comparative studies were carried out in Georgia, US, to evaluate the effects of diets on children with pellagra.

Children were selected from orphanages. This practice would not be allowed today, as institutionalized children who could not defend their rights were taken advantage of.

SOURCE   National Institutes of Health, http://www.nih.gov/ [accessed Nov 9, 2001].

Subjects should not be pressured into enrolling in the trial, but rather should voluntarily join in, and they are able to leave the trial at any time without duress or penalty. For young and incapacitated people who are not able to understand the requirements and implications of the trial, proxy decision from their representatives (parents or guardians) must be obtained.

6.2.5   Favorable risk–benefit ratio

The risk–benefit ratio should be analyzed and, wherever possible, clinical trial subjects should be subjected to minimal risk and maximal benefit. The risk–benefit ratio should be based on proven scientific data gathered at the pre-clinical stage. A clinical trial should not be conducted if there is a doubt about the risk–benefit ratio.

6.2.6   Independent review board/Independent ethics committee (IRB/IEC)

An independent review is to ensure that an independent party assesses the clinical trial so the question of conflict of interest is addressed. The IRB/IEC acts as a third party to oversee the welfare of the trial subjects and ensure that the trial is conducted in accordance to the study being put forward.

The members of IRB/IEC may consist of clinicians, scientists, lawyers, religious leaders and laypeople to represent different viewpoints and protect the rights of the subjects. The investigator is to inform the IRB/IEC if there are changes in the research activity. Such changes, if they present risks to the subjects, have to be approved before the trial continues. The IRB/IEC has the right to stop a trial or require that procedures and methods be changed.

6.2.7   Respect for human subjects

Subjects should be protected and their progress in the trial monitored closely, and appropriate treatments should be provided. New developments in the trial, either risks or benefits, must be relayed to the subjects without prejudice, and the subject's decisions should be honored.

Outcomes from the trial must be communicated to the subjects promptly and in an unbiased way. In addition to the ethical guidelines by the NIH, the World Medical Association has formalized a document called the *Declaration of Helsinki—Ethical Principles for Medical Research Involving Human Subjects* to describe the constraints on research involving human beings. Those countries that have signed this declaration are bound by the ethical principles. An extract of this document is given in Exhibit 6.3.

Exhibit 6.3 World Medical Association Declaration of Helsinki

Ethical Principles for Medical Research Involving Human Subjects

The World Medical Association has developed the Declaration of Helsinki as a statement of ethical principles to provide guidance to physicians and other participants in medical research involving human subjects. Medical research involving human subjects includes research on identifiable human material or identifiable data.

It is the duty of the physician to promote and safeguard the health of the people. The physician's knowledge and conscience are dedicated to the fulfillment of this duty.

The Declaration of Geneva of the World Medical Association binds the physician with the words, 'The health of my patient will be my first consideration,' and the International Code of Medical Ethics declares that, 'A Medical progress is based on research, which ultimately must rest in part on experimentation involving human subjects. In medical research on human subjects, considerations related to the well being of the human subject should take precedence over the interests of science and society.

The primary purpose of medical research involving human subjects is to improve prophylactic, diagnostic and therapeutic procedures and the understanding of the etiology and pathogenesis of disease. Even the best proven prophylactic, diagnostic, and therapeutic methods must continuously be challenged through research for their effectiveness, efficiency, accessibility and quality.

In current medical practice and in medical research, most prophylactic, diagnostic and therapeutic procedures involve risks and burdens.

Medical research is subject to ethical standards that promote respect for all human beings and protect their health and rights. Some research populations are vulnerable and need special protection. The particular needs of the economically and medically disadvantaged must be recognized. Special attention is also required for those who cannot give or refuse consent for themselves, for those who may be subject to giving consent under duress, for those who will not benefit personally from the research and for those for whom the research is combined with care.

Research Investigators should be aware of the ethical, legal and regulatory requirements for research on human subjects in their own countries as well as applicable international requirements. No national ethical, legal or regulatory requirement should be allowed to reduce or eliminate any of the protections for human subjects set forth in this Declaration.

6.3   CLINICAL TRIALS

Clinical trials are divided into four phases. These are Phase I to Phase IV (Figure 6.1). These trials are conducted with specific purposes to evaluate the safety and effectiveness of the drug in defined population groups.

6.3.1   Phase I

The Phase I clinical trial is the first experiment in which a drug is tested on the human body. The primary aim of the trial is to assess the safety of the new drug. Other areas of study include pharmacokinetics (absorption, distribution, metabolism and excretion) and pharmacodynamics.

Normally, healthy volunteers are recruited for the Phase I trial. In many cases, volunteers are compensated financially for participation in the Phase I trial. However, in some situations, patients who are critically ill or with terminal disease are presented with the option to be included in the trial after due consideration of the risk–benefit ratio. Phase I trials are usually conducted with open label, i.e. the subjects are aware of the drugs that they are being given.

The number of subjects is normally between 10 and 100 people. The starting doses are based on the results of preclinical work as described in Chapter 5. Doses are increased as the trial progresses for subjects recruited at later stages, as the effect of the experimental drug becomes apparent. Subjects are monitored closely to check their tolerance of the drug and incidents of side effects. Depending on the study, samples of blood, urine or stool and other physiological information may be obtained for analysis to evaluate absorption, distribution, metabolism and elimination of the drug in the body. Other observations about how the subject feels (e.g. pain, headache, fever, malaise and irritability), and vital signs (blood pressure, heart rate) and behavioral matters are taken into account.

Depending on the complexity of the trial, the cost for Phase I is around US$10 million and the trial may last from several months to a year.

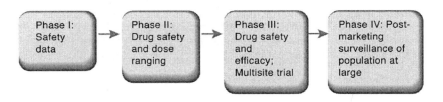

Figure 6.1 The four phases of clinical trials

6.3.2   Phase II

The aim of the Phase II clinical trial is to examine the safety and effectiveness of the drug in the targeted disease group. A series of doses of varying strengths may be used.

It is now common to conduct Phase II trials with a control group in conjunction with the test group given the drug. The control group is given either the current standard treatment or placebo (an inert non-drug substance). Again, the risk–benefit profile has to be assessed as to whether the trial should use placebo or standard treatment to ensure the subjects' well being is not compromised during the trial. Patients are randomized to either the control group or the drug group without bias. The randomization procedure is important, because the information will provide comparative data about the safety and effectiveness of the drug versus placebo or standard treatment. Phase II clinical trials can be divided into IIa and IIb, with IIb being an extension to the safety and efficacy studies assessed in IIa.

Another practice is to blind the trial, which means that the subjects are not privy to whether they receive the placebo or drug. In some trials, even the investigator is unaware of whether the subject is in the control or active group. This is called a double-blind trial. The rationale is to eliminate the possibility of bias affecting the trial results.

The result of the Phase II trial is information needed to determine the effective dose and the dosing regimen of frequency and duration. Specific clinical endpoints or markers are used to assess interaction of drug and disease. There are two types of markers: definitive and surrogate. For example, in the case of cancer or hypertension, the definitive markers are mortality and stroke, respectively, and the surrogate markers may be tumor size, or cancer-associated proteins p53, TGF-α in the case of cancer, and blood pressure or cholesterol level in hypertension. Statistical analysis is carried out to evaluate the influence of the drug on different patient groups, to determine the optimum conditions.

For Phase II, the number of patients is normally in the vicinity of 50–500. The trial may take 1–2 years or more to complete, depending on the study numbers and availability of patients. The cost for such a trial can be more than US$20 million.

The success rate of Phase I and II studies is estimated as around 30%. An example of a Phase II trial is presented in Exhibit 6.4.

Exhibit 6.4 Phase II Studies: Tolerability and Primary Efficacy of CX516 in Alzheimer's Disease

This is a Phase II trial sponsored by the National Institute of Neurological Disorders and Stroke to determine the effectiveness and safety of a drug called CX516 (Ampalex) in patients with Alzheimer's disease.

Brain cells release glutamate, an amino acid, which attaches itself to a receptor called AMPA (alpha-amino-2,3-dihydro-5-methyl-3-oxo-5-isoxazolepropanoic acid). The attachment to the receptor activates other cells. The clinical trial is to find out how CX516 affects the AMPA receptors.

SOURCE ClinicalTrials.gov, http://www.clinical trials.gov [accessed Oct 1, 2001].

6.3.3   Phase III

After the successful completion of the Phase II trial, the objective of Phase III is to confirm the efficacy of the drug in a large patient group. Phase III is an extension of Phase II, and the trial is normally conducted in several hospitals in different demographic locations, to determine the influence of ethnic responses, together with incorporation of new criteria for fine-tuning the trial. This trial is also known as a multi-site trial.

Because the results are crucial to the determination of the drug's effectiveness, the Phase III trial is referred to as the pivotal trial, as it can make or break the success of a drug. The methodology of the trial has to be carefully prepared so that meaningful results can be gathered at the conclusion of the trial. Extensive statistical analyses are performed to evaluate the data. If for any reason the drug does not show significant advantage over current treatment, the result may be refined and certain subgroups are analyzed to determine if the effects are greater in one group than the other. The study results provide comprehensive data for understanding the critical parameters of safety and effectiveness of the drug.

These results enable the pharmaceutical company to set the dosage, treatment frequency, duration and target patient groups for the drug. The information and analyses gathered, together with Chemistry, Manufacturing and Control (CMC, see Chapter 8), are submitted to regulatory authorities to seek approval to market the drug. An example of a Phase III trial is presented in Exhibit 6.5.

Patient numbers for Phase III can vary from several hundreds to thousands. The larger number is normally for trials involving infectious diseases such as influenza or vaccines, as these can recruit up to tens of thousands of people to provide a larger sample size for detecting 'rare' serious effects. Statistical proof to show the efficacy of the drug at the targeted patient group has to be established. At least two Phase III trials need to be conducted. Because of the magnitude of the trial, the duration may be 3–5 years and the cost is around US$50–100 million.

> **Exhibit 6.5 Phase III Study: Combination Therapy with IL-2 (interleukin-2) plus Antiretroviral Drugs to Treat HIV Infection**
>
> This trial is sponsored by the National Institute of Allergy and Infectious Disease.
>
> In this study, the patients are divided into two groups. One group receives the antiretroviral drug alone, and the other receives IL-2 and the antiretroviral drug together. IL-2 is a protein that can activate the immune system.
>
> This is a randomized trial, and is open-label (not blinded). Patients are to be examined physically during the trial and their blood samples collected for analysis.
>
> SOURCE ClinicalTrials.gov, http://www.clinical trials.gov [accessed Oct 2, 2001].

6.3.4   Phase IV

Phase IV clinical trials are post-marketing approval trials to monitor the efficacy and side effects of the drug in an uncontrolled real-life situation. This is also known as a post-market surveillance trial. Information about the effectiveness of the drug compared with established treatment, side effects, patient's quality of life, and cost-effectiveness is collated.

Any adverse events are reported and acted on to ensure patients' welfare is not compromised by the drug. Serious events are reported to regulatory authorities within a specified time and, if deemed necessary, the drug is recalled or doctors and patients are notified.

6.4   REGULATORY REQUIREMENTS FOR CLINICAL TRIALS

Clinical trials are performed under Good Clinical Practice (GCP). Up to now, there has been no reference to the regulatory requirement. The reality is that every trial has to be approved and carried out under regulatory compliance to comply with GCP requirements. Otherwise, the trials may be considered as non-compliant and become invalid.

A normal course of event in initiating a clinical trial is for the Sponsor (see below) to prepare an Investigator's Brochure and select an Investigator to conduct the trial. The Sponsor and Investigator then prepare the trial protocol, which is submitted to the Institutional Review Board or Independent Ethics Committee for approval. An approval from the regulatory authority, such as the US Food and Drug Administration (FDA) or the Medicines Control Agencies (MCA) of the United Kingdom, is then sought (see Chapter 8).

Different countries have different requirements for clinical trials. However, the two main documents that most clinical trials are based on are the documents from the FDA and the ICH. The relevant documents are:

- FDA 21 CFR Parts 50, 56, 312
- ICH Harmonized Tripartite Guideline for Good Clinical Practice.

In the US, an IND (Investigational New Drug) application has to be filed with the FDA. For other countries, a notification has to be submitted to the respective regulatory authorities. For example, Clinical Trial Exemption (CTX) applications are required for the UK, Clinical Trial Notification (CTN) and CTX for Australia, and a Clinical Trial Certificate (CTC) for Singapore and the European Agency for the Evaluation of Medicinal Products (EMEA). A more extensive discussion concerning regulatory authorities and the processes and procedures of applications is presented in Chapters 7 and 8. The relevant authority will review the application. A positive response from the authority is required before the trial can commence.

The scope of this book does not allow a discussion about all the requirements for GCP here. Readers are referred to Exhibit 6.6 for the headings in the relevant regulatory documents to gain further understanding of the requirements. Some important issues are, however, discussed below to clarify the important aspects and requirements for clinical trials in accordance to GCP. Some of these aspects are:

- Investigator
- Investigator's brochure
- Informed consent
- Protocol
- Inclusion and exclusion criteria
- Case report form
- Randomization, placebo-controlled and double-blinded
- Monitoring
- Adverse events

- Statistics
- Sponsor
- Clinical research organization
- Surrogate markers.

Exhibit 6.6 Examples of GCP Requirements

Main Heading from 21CFR Part 50 Protection of Human Subjects

Subpart A – General Provisions

Subpart B – Informed Consent of Human Subjects

Subpart C – Protection Pertaining to Clinical Investigations Involving Prisoners as Subjects

Main Heading from 21CFR Part 312 – Investigational New Drug Application

Subpart A – General Provisions

Subpart B – IND

Subpart C – Administrative Actions

Subpart D – Responsibilities of Sponsors and Investigators

Subpart E – Drugs Intended to Treat Life-threatening and Severely-debilitating Illnesses

Subpart F – Miscellaneous

Subpart G – Drugs for Investigational Use in Laboratory Research Animals or In Vitro Tests.

Main Heading from 21CFR Part 56 – Institutional Review Board

Subpart A – General Provisions

Subpart B - Organization and Personnel

Subpart C – IRB Functions and Operations

Subpart D – Records and Reports

Subpart E – Administrative Action for Noncompliance

ICH Harmonized Tripartite Guideline for Good Clinical Practice

Section II

Introduction

Glossary

The Principle of ICH GCP

Institutional Review Board/Independent Ethics Committee (IRB/IEC)

Investigator

Sponsor

Clinical Trial Protocol and Protocol Amendments

Investigator's Brochure

Essential Documents for the Conduct of a Clinical Trial

6.4.1   Investigator

The Investigator is the person who conducts the trial. If there is a team in the investigation, then there is a Principal Investigator. This person is normally an expert in the field of the disease to be investigated. The Investigator's responsibility is to ensure that GCP is being implemented in the course of the trial and the subjects' rights and welfare are respected. Another important point is that the Investigator has to maintain impartiality. He or she is not an employee of the company (the sponsor where the drug is developed), to show that there is transparency and no conflict of interest, nor there is financial gain if the drug is successful.

6.4.2   Investigator's brochure

The Investigator's Brochure is a collection of information prepared and updated by the sponsor for the Investigator. The information consists of all the data relevant to the drug under investigation (Exhibit 6.7). The data

---

Exhibit 6.7 Investigator's Brochure

Description of the drug

        Physical, chemical and biological properties

        Dosage form, storage conditions, stability

Pharmacology

        Pharmacodynamics

        Pharmacokinetics

        Toxicology

An Investigator's Brochure under 21CFR312.23(a)(5) is being developed by the FDA under the auspices of the ICH.

SOURCE   Food and Drug Administration, Center for Drug Evaluation and Research, http//www.fda.gov/cder/ [accessed Oct 12, 2001].

6.4.3   Informed consent

This is described earlier, and is a fundamental aspect that has to be included in a clinical trial.

6.4.4   Protocol

This document sets out how a trial is to be conducted. It contains the rationale for the clinical trial, methodology on how the trial is designed, the number of subjects to be recruited, the markers or endpoints to show effectiveness of the drug, statistical methods to be used to analyze the data, how the subjects are protected in the trial, informed consent and confidentiality, as well as welfare and frequency of monitoring. Exhibit 6.8 summarizes the required information for a protocol.

6.4.5 Inclusion and exclusion criteria

These criteria set out the conditions under which a person may or may not be included in the trial. The criteria may include the disease type, medical history, age group, sex, and so on. It is necessary to set out the parameters for the criteria to enable meaningful analysis to be made for assessment of the safety and effectiveness of the experimental drug. Subjects are screened before commencement to ensure that they meet the recruitment criteria before being admitted to the trial.

Exhibit 6.8 Clinical Trial Protocol

Information to be included (ICH GCP)

Protocol title

Name and address of Sponsor and Monitor

Name of authorized person

Name of Sponsor's medical expert

Name of Investigator responsible for the trial

Name of physician responsible for trial-related medical decisions

Name of Clinical Laboratory, and other Institutions involved in the trial

Name and description of the clinical trial protocol

Summary of results from non-clinical studies

Potential risks and benefits to human subjects

Description and justification for route of administration, dosage and treatment plan

Compliance to GCP

Description of the population to be studied

Reference literature and related data

Standard Operating Procedures.

SOURCE International Conference for Harmonization, *Good Clinical Practice*, http://www.ich.org/ [accessed Oct 29, 2001].

6.4.6   Case report form

All the information relating to a subject is recorded in the Case Report Form. The commencement of the trial will include gathering baseline data from the subjects. Then at each defined stage of a trial, the designed markers or endpoints are analyzed and recorded. These may include dosing information, observations, vital signs, blood analysis, targeted enzyme levels, hormonal changes and so on. There are also records for patient's comments, adverse events and investigator's spontaneous comments. The Case Report Forms are part of the regulatory document, and the data are statistically analyzed and submitted to regulatory authorities for marketing approval of the drug. An example of a hypothetical case report form is presented in Exhibit 6.9.

Exhibit 6.9 Example of a Case Report Form

Personal Data
Patient's Last name: _____   First name: _____   Middle initial: _____
Address: _____
Telephone number: _____   Address: _____

Study Data
Study number: _____   IRB number: _____   Patient number: _____
Date of visit: _____
Age: _____ years   Sex: _____ M/F   Race: _____   Ethnicity: _____

Clinical Data
Height: _____   Weight: _____
Symptoms, signs and adverse reactions: _____
Associated disease history: _____
Medication taken: _____

Laboratory Analysis
Hemoglobin: _____   Platelet count: _____
Bilirubin: _____   ALT: _____
Cholesterol/LDL: _____   Cholesterol/HDL: _____

Other Details
Patient's comments: _____
Physician's name: _____
Address and Telephone number: _____
Person completing this form: _____
Signature: _____   Date: _____

6.4.7   Randomization, placebo-controlled and double-blinded

Some trials are conducted with open labels, that is, the subjects are aware of the type of drugs that they have been provided. However, in most trials, the subjects are divided into treatment and control groups using statistical randomization process (Exhibit 6.10). The aim is to reduce bias in the studies. Subjects are divided into control and active groups.

In a double-blinded study, both the Investigator and the subjects are unaware of whether they receive the drug or the placebo. The randomization code is held in confidence and is opened at the end of the trial for data analysis or in cases where adverse events occurred.

Exhibit 6.10 Randomization Techniques

Randomized parallel group fixed dose: Subjects are divided into several groups, such as Placebo, 10 mg, 20 mg and 40 mg. Subjects continue with this regimen for the duration of the trial.

Randomized parallel group forced titration: Subjects are divided into placebo and active groups. Active groups all start with the same dose, for example, 10 mg. One group continues with 10 mg, another group later increases to 20 mg and stays at this dose. A third active group then increases from 10 mg to 20 mg and finally to 40 mg progressively.

Randomized parallel group optional titration: Subjects are divided into placebo and active groups. Active groups all start with the same dose, say, 10 mg. Depending on response and safety assessment, dose can be increased to 20 mg and then 40 mg for selected subjects.

Randomized crossover design: Subjects are divided into placebo and active groups. After some time these two groups crossover, the initial placebo group now becoming the active group and vice versa. There may be a washout period before the crossover to enable the effect of the placebo and active to washout. This method requires a smaller number of subjects and is useful in cases for studying rare or more stable illnesses.

Randomized Latin square design: This is a crossover design with dose ranging. For example the regimens for six separate groups are: (a) Placebo, 10 mg, 20 mg, (b) Placebo, 20 mg, 10 mg, (c) 10 mg, 20 mg, Placebo, (d) 10 mg, Placebo, 20 mg, (e) 20 mg, Placebo, 10 mg, and (f) 20 mg, 10 mg, Placebo. This is a very powerful method to show the efficacy of the drug under trial.

SOURCE Monkhouse, D.C., and Rhodes, C.T. (eds.), *Drug Products for Clinical Trials*, Marcel Dekker, Inc., New York, 1998.

6.4.8 Monitoring

An important aspect of the trial is the meticulous monitoring required. This is a process to interact with the subjects: monitoring their well being, the effects of drug and placebo, adverse events, and so on. Information is recorded in the Case Report Forms. All the processes are recorded in accordance with Standard Operating Procedures, which describe how the trial is to be conducted, and GCP.

6.4.9 Adverse events

These are the unintended reactions of the subjects as a consequence of taking the drug or placebo. Subjects are checked and, if the adverse events are serious, subjects may be temporarily removed from the trial. If there is a persistence of adverse event, the subject may be withdrawn from the trial. The randomization code may be broken (opened) to determine whether the subject has been given the drug or placebo.

6.4.10 Statistics

Statistics plays a major role in the design of the clinical trial. The groups or subgroups to be studied, the frequencies, dosages, and the markers to monitor drug efficacy are all important factors to consider. The statistical analysis provides the tool to demonstrate, at a certain confidence level, whether the drug is effective. This is normally reported in the form of a statistical power test, analyzing the Type I and Type II errors.

6.4.11 Sponsor

This is the organization or individual that initiates the clinical trial and finance the study. The organization may be a government department, pharmaceutical company, university or individual. Normally, however, the sponsor is a pharmaceutical company.

6.4.12 Clinical research organization

This is the organization that is contracted by the Sponsor to conduct and monitor the trial. It also provides a certain measure of independence to the trial and enhances the validity of the trial results to be unencumbered by conflict of interest.

6.4.13 Surrogate markers

Sometimes it is not possible to measure the direct effect of the drug. Endpoints or surrogate markers are used to monitor the pharmacodynamics and pharmacokinetics of the drug. These markers may be changes in blood pressure, cholesterol level, concentration of certain enzymes, proteins, blood glucose levels and similar factors.

6.5 ROLE OF REGULATORY AUTHORITIES

Government bodies have on occasion accelerated clinical trials against advice from researchers, in response to public demands (Exhibit 6.11). The climate today is that due diligence regarding safety has to be performed before the drug is administered to human subjects and that clinical trial submissions have to be approved by the regulatory authorities before the trial commences.

Exhibit 6.11 Polio Vaccine Trial

In the 1950s, Dr. Jonas Salk and Dr. Albert Sabin from the University of Pittsburgh in the US worked on polio vaccines. Salk used inactivated polio virus, whereas Sabin developed a live form of polio virus.

Scientists differed as to which method provided the better vaccine. Both Salk and Sabin agreed that more tests were needed before a mass vaccination program could begin.

The National Foundation, which funded the research, and the American public wanted a mass vaccination urgently. The average incidence of polio in the US in 1949–1953 was 25.7 cases per 100 000 children. The National Foundation ordered 27 million doses of the Salk vaccine for a trial, and close to one million children were vaccinated (749 236 children from Grades 1, 2 and 3 were offered vaccine, and 401 974 completed the trial).

The trial was one of the greatest triumphs in medical history. Church bells rang across the country when the trial results were announced. Within five years, polio was wiped out from the US.

SOURCE   Meier, P., *The Salk Vaccine Trials*, http://www.math.uah.edu/ siegrist/ma487/salk.html [accessed Jan 2, 2002].

Regulatory authorities play an important and active role to ensure regulatory compliance in the conduct of a clinical trial. Agencies such as the FDA inspect clinical studies. An inspection of a trial may reveal that the protocol is not being followed strictly, the investigator may not be involved with the project as much as is expected, there may be a lack of patient care, changes to the protocol may not have been relayed to the IRB, and so on. In such cases, corrective actions have to be implemented immediately and the FDA satisfied before the trial can continue. Deficiencies found are reported on Form 583.

6.6   GENE THERAPY CLINICAL TRIAL

As genomic research progresses, the possibility of replacing a person's faulty genes with normal genes becomes a reality (Chapter 4). Currently, there are many ethical and scientific issues facing gene therapy.

For a gene therapy clinical trial, the FDA requires that the IND be filed as for normal drug trials. However, there are more stringent requirements on the source and tests being carried out on the gene to be inserted to the subject. There is also the need for closer monitoring, from both the investigator and the FDA. In addition, the FDA has been conducting safety symposia to educate the investigator on the safety issues of gene therapy. Exhibit 6.12 describes a Phase I gene therapy trial on Alzheimer's disease.

Exhibit 6.12   Gene Therapy

Ceregene has begun enrolling patients in a Phase I study of its Alzheimer's disease gene therapy. The trial is sponsored by the University of California, San Diego School of Medicine. Ceregene is the exclusive licensee of the technology, which involves surgical implantation of cells that produce nerve growth factor.

SOURCE Contract Pharma, June 2001.

6.7   FURTHER READING

Cato, A., Sutton, L. and Cato III, A. (eds.), *Clinical Drug Trials and Tribulations*, 2nd edn., Marcel Dekker, Inc., New York, 2002.

Center for Drug Evaluation and Research, *Guideline for the Format and Content of the Clinical and Statistical Sections of an Application*, FDA, Rockville, MD, 1998.

Cohen, A. and Posner, J. (eds.), *A Guide to Clinical Drug Research*, 2nd edn., Kluwer Academic Publishers, The Netherlands, 2000.

Dawson, B. and Trapp, R.G., *Basic and Clinical Biostatistics*, McGraw-Hill, Singapore, 2001.

Friedman, L.M. and Furberg, C., *Fundamentals of Clinical Trials*, 3rd edn., Mosby, St. Louis, 1996.

Gad, S.C., *Drug Safety Evaluation*, John Wiley & Sons, Inc., New York, 2002.

Good, P.I., *A Manager's Guide to the Design and Conduct of Clinical Trials*, John Wiley & Sons, Inc., New York, 2002.

Guarino, R.A. (ed.), *New Drug Approval Process—Clinical and Regulatory Management*, Marcel Dekker, Inc., New York, 1987.

International Conference on Harmonization, *Guideline for Industry—Structure and Content of Clinical Study Reports*, ICH E3, 1996, http://www.fda.gov/cder/guidance/iche3.pdf [accessed Nov 3, 2001].

Mathieu, M. (ed.), *Biologics Development: A regulatory Overview*, Parexel International Corporation, Waltham, MA, 1993.

Monkhouse, D.C. and Rhodes, C.T. (eds.), *Drug Products for Clinical Trials, An International Guide to Formulation, Production, Quality Control*, Marcel Dekker, Inc., New York, 1998.

Piantodosi, S., *Clinical Trials—A Methodologic Perspective*, John Wiley & Sons, Canada, 1997.

CHAPTER 7

REGULATORY AUTHORITIES

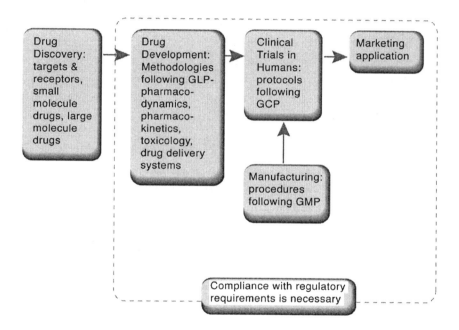

7.1   ROLE OF REGULATORY AUTHORITIES

All of us want the drugs that are prescribed for us to be safe and effective to treat our ailments. It is the role of public regulatory authorities to ensure that pharmaceutical companies comply with regulations. There is legislation that requires drugs to be developed, tested, trialed and manufactured in accordance to guidelines so that they are safe and patients' well being is protected. There have been several occasions when drugs were not safe and people's health has been compromised; there were times when unscrupulous people or firms wrongly or carelessly manufactured drugs; children or vulnerable people have been recruited to clinical trials without consent, and insufficient tests were carried out on some drugs during development, leading to untold damage (see Exhibit 7.1 for an account of the thalidomide tragedy).

Exhibit 7.1 Thalidomide

Thalidomide was synthesized in Germany and became available in late 1957. It was prescribed for the treatment of insomnia and nausea in pregnant women.

However, it had not been discovered that the thalidomide drug molecule could cross the placental barrier and affect fetal development. As a result, thousands of babies were born with crippled extremities, disfigurement and disabilities. Numerous fetuses were stillborn or died soon after birth.

The drug was banned in early 1962, but by then the lives of many people had been severely affected.

Refer to Exhibit 10.7 for the chemical structure of thalidomide.

Regulatory authorities perform the watchdog role to ensure that animal studies comply with Good Laboratory Practice (GLP), clinical trials are performed in accordance with Good Clinical Practice (GCP) and drugs are manufactured under current Good Manufacturing Practice (cGMP) conditions. The regulatory authorities also carry out surveys to ensure that labels and advertising materials are accurate and in accordance with approved claims. Advertising materials should have clear explanations about the drug, dosage and frequency of medication.

In this chapter, we explain the regulatory authorities in the major countries. The regulatory process is complicated and lengthy; this is especially the case where major industrialized nations have independently over the years set up their own systems of regulations and controls, which invariably have different requirements to those in other countries. Processes are, however, in place to harmonize the regulatory procedures in the major industrialized countries. In this way, regulatory requirements and review processes are consistent and can be mutually recognized by member countries. Eventually, harmonization will reduce duplicate requirements and the cost and time for regulatory reviews. This will translate to patients receiving access to new drugs more speedily and at less cost than now.

We will follow up in Chapter 8 to examine more closely the regulatory processes for testing, trialing and approving a drug for marketing.

7.2   US FOOD AND DRUG ADMINISTRATION

The United States Food and Drug Administration (FDA) is required by the US Federal Food, Drug, and Cosmetic Act to regulate drug products in the US. Its role is to ensure that drugs are developed, manufactured and marketed in accordance with regulatory requirements so that they are safe and effective. The FDA has four centers and a regulatory office:

- Center for Drugs Evaluation and Research (CDER)
- Center for Biologics Evaluation and Research (CBER)
- Center for Devices and Radiological Health
- Center for Veterinary Medicine
- Office of Regulatory Affairs

Exhibit 7.2 presents a brief history of the FDA. For the purpose of regulation on drugs, the relevant centers are CDER and CBER.

7.2.1   Center for Drug Evaluation and Research

The CDER oversees the research, development, manufacture and marketing of synthetic small molecule drugs (drugs that are described in Chapter 3). As of June 30, 2003, the CDER is also responsible for the regulation of biologic therapeutic products. Most of these drugs are large protein-based molecules generated by hybridoma or recombinant DNA technology, such as monoclonal antibodies, cytokines (interferon, interleukin), tissue growth factors and other proteins described in Chapter 4. These products are:

- Monoclonal antibodies for *in vivo* use
- Cytokines, growth factors, enzymes, immunomodulators and thrombolytics

Exhibit 7.2 A Brief History of the FDA

The FDA started from a single chemist in the US Department of Agriculture in 1862, with the appointment of Charles M. Wetherill by President Lincoln. By 2001, it had a staff of about 9100 and a budget of $1.294 billion. The FDA now has employees from diverse disciplines, including chemists, pharmacologists, physicians, microbiologists, veterinarians, pharmacists, and lawyers.

About a third of the agency's employees are stationed outside of the Washington, D.C., area in over 150 field offices and laboratories, including five regional offices and 20 district offices.

The FDA regulates:

Drugs (e.g. prescriptions, OTCs, generics)

Biologics (e.g. vaccines, blood products)

Medical devices (e.g. pacemakers, contact lenses)

Food (e.g. nutrition, dietary supplements)

Animal feed and drugs (e.g. livestock, pets)

Cosmetics (e.g. safety, labeling)

Radiation emitting products (e.g. cell phones, lasers)

- Proteins intended for therapeutic use that are extracted from animals or microorganisms, including recombinant versions of these products
- Other non-vaccine therapeutic immunotherapies.

The CDER's involvement starts with the Phase I clinical study via the approval of an Investigational New Drug (IND) application. In its review process for the IND, CDER checks that preclinical tests have been performed in compliance with GLP. When the clinical trials commence, CDER monitors the conduct of the clinical trials through Phases I, II and III, based on adherence to GCP. At the conclusion of Phase III trials, marketing applications from sponsor pharmaceutical organizations are evaluated by CDER, relying on scientific data and clinical results. The marketing applications are:

- New Drug Applications (NDAs) for synthetic drugs
- Biologics License Applications (BLAs) for therapeutic biologic drugs.

Risks (drugs have potential risks as they interfere with our body functions) and benefits evaluations are undertaken before drugs are approved for marketing. Expert reviews from external personnel are sought from time to time, to ensure that decisions are based on the latest scientific opinions. It also ensures that advertising and marketing of drugs are in accordance with claims approved. Marketed drugs are monitored for unexpected health risks. If unexpected health risks or adverse reactions are confirmed, the CDER informs the public or, in severe cases, directs the suppliers to remove drugs from the market. The manufacture of drugs is monitored to ensure compliance with cGMP.

The three categories of drugs regulated by the CDER are:

- Prescription drugs
- Generic drugs
- Over-the-counter (OTC) drugs.

7.2.2 Center for Biologics Evaluation and Research

The CBER regulates non-therapeutic biologics—drugs that are described in Chapter 4, which are not regulated by the CDER. These include:

- Viral-vectored gene insertions (e.g. gene therapy)
- Drugs composed of human or animal cells or from physical parts of those cells
- Allergen patch tests
- Allergenics
- Antitoxins, antivenins and venoms
- *In vitro* diagnostics
- Vaccines, including therapeutic vaccines
- Toxoids and toxins intended for immunization.

In addition, the CBER controls the approval of human tissue for transplantation, blood and blood products, and devices related to blood products. These devices include automated cell separators, empty plastic containers, and blood storage refrigerators and freezers.

In contrast to the synthetic drugs, biologics are complex, large compounds with molecular weights >500 kDa and they are not easily characterized. They are dissimilar to synthetic drugs, which are chemically well-defined entities. Biologics are also labile (that is, heat and shear sensitive), and are very dependent on the manufacturing process parameters.

The regulatory process is the filing of IND for clinical trials. At the conclusion of clinical trials, the sponsor files Biological License Approval (BLA) application for marketing approval. The CBER evaluates a biologic in terms of risk versus benefits before approving it for marketing.

7.2.3   Pertinent FDA processes and controls

Drugs (synthetic drugs) are regulated in the US as required by the Food, Drug and Cosmetic Act (FDCA) of 1938. Biologics are, however, regulated by the Public Health Service Act (PHSA) of 1944 and the FDCA. This is because the PHSA is concerned with medical products that are less well defined, necessitating more control in the handling and manufacturing processes.

The applicable regulations for drugs are codified in Title 21 of the US *Code of Federal Regulations* (CFR). These regulations promulgate the FDA's requirement in many aspects of drug clinical research, manufacturing and marketing. Table 7.1 lists some of these applicable regulations. Readers should note that these regulations are updated by the FDA as a result of new requirements or information.

In addition, the FDA publishes Guidelines and Points to Consider (PTCs) documents to guide pharmaceutical organizations in many relevant areas, from testing methodologies, manufacturing requirements and drug stability information, to filling in of forms and the requisite data.

In 2001, the CDER approved 66 new drugs, 24 of which were new molecular entities (NMEs) or new chemical entities (NCEs). The median approval time was 14 months. In the same period, the CBER reviewed and approved 16 BLAs. The median approval time was 20.3 months.

Under the Prescription Drug User Fee Act (PDUFA), the FDA collects fees from applicants to expedite the review and approval processes under strict guidelines. The PDUFA rates for the fiscal year 2003 (1 October 2002 to 30 September 2003) are shown in Table 7.2.

The FDA also carries out inspections on establishments to ensure compliance with regulations. The establishments include laboratories, clinical trial centers and manufacturing facilities. Further information on establishment inspection is discussed in Chapter 10.

In some circumstances, the FDA processes drug reviews under the accelerated scheme. This mechanism is to review and approve drugs speedily for cases where effective therapies are lacking or in situations of rare diseases. One of the fastest approval times to date is the case of imatinib mesylate (Gleevec, Novartis) (Exhibit 7.3) for the treatment of chronic myeloid leukemia (CML); it was approved in less than three months after the filing of an NDA with the FDA. Another example is the new AIDS drug indinavir (Crixivan, Merck), which was approved in just 42 days.

Table 7.1 Selected regulations from 21 CFR

Document number	Description
21 CFR Part 11	Electronic Records, Electronic Signatures
21 CFR Part 50	Protection of Human Subjects
21 CFR Part 56	Institutional Review Board
21 CFR Part 58	Good Laboratory Practices for Non-clinical Laboratory Studies
21 CFR Part 202	Prescription Drug Advertising
21 CFR Part 203	Prescription Advertising
21 CFR Part 210	Current Good Manufacturing Practice in Manufacturing, Processing, Packaging or Holding of Drugs; General
21 CFR Part 211	Current Good Manufacturing Practice for Finished Pharmaceuticals
21 CFR Part 312	Investigational New Drug Applications
21 CFR Part 314	Applications for FDA Approval to Market a New Drug
21 CFR Part 600	Biological Products: General
21 CFR Part 610	General Biological Products Standards

Table 7.2 PDUFA fees

Application	Fee
Applications requiring clinical data	US$533 400
Applications not requiring clinical data	US$266 700
Supplements requiring clinical data	US$266 700
Establishments	US$209 900
Products	US$32 400

Exhibit 7.3 Imatinib Mesylate (Gleevec)

Chronic myeloid leukemia (CML) occurs when there is a translocation of chromosomes 9 and 22. These two different chromosomes break off and reattach on the opposite chromosome. A consequence is that the activity of the Bcr-Abl gene, which encodes the enzyme tyrosine kinase, is turned on all the time. With this heightened activity, high levels of white blood cells are produced in the bone marrow.

Imatinib mesylate is a tyrosine kinase inhibitor (see Chapter 2 on receptors). It is used to block the growth of white blood cells.

Imatinib mesylate is manufactured by Novartis. Clinical trials showed that patients had their white blood cells reduced substantially after being treated with Gleevec.

Continued

Exhibit 7.3 *Continued*

The long-term effects of Imatinib mesylate are still unknown. However, its significant results in the trials to date convinced the FDA to approve it under the accelerated approval regulations for the treatment of CML.

SOURCE *FDA Approves Gleevec for Leukemia Treatment*, http://www.fda.gov/ bbs/ topics/NEWS/2001/NEW00759.html [accessed May 21, 2001].

7.3 EUROPEAN AGENCY FOR THE EVALUATION OF MEDICINAL PRODUCTS

There are two avenues for drug approval in Europe:

- *Centralized procedure:* Under the European Union (EU) Council Regulation (EEC No. 2309/93), a Centralized Community Procedure for the authorization of medicinal products was created. The European Agency for the Evaluation of Medicinal Products (EMEA) was formed in 1995 to coordinate scientific evaluation of the safety, efficacy and quality of medicinal products under this procedure. All biologics are under the purview of EMEA evaluation, and it is optional for other conventional drug products (synthetic drugs).

- *Mutual recognition procedure:* This applies to conventional drugs. Applications are made to individual Member States selected by the applicant. A system is put in place whereby mutual recognition of the evaluations is observed by other Member States. When there is a dispute between Member States on the issue of mutual recognition, the EMEA is called upon to arbitrate, and its decision is binding on the Member States.

The EMEA's key aims, according to the EU Enterprise Directorate-General publication, are to:

- Protect and promote public health by providing safe and effective medicines for human and veterinary use
- Give patients quick access to innovative new therapy
- Facilitate the free movements of pharmaceutical products throughout the EU
- Improve information for patients and professionals on the correct use of medicinal products

- Harmonize scientific requirements to optimize pharmaceutical research worldwide.

There are two committees within the EMEA; they are:

- Committee for Proprietary Medicinal Products (CPMP)
- Committee for Veterinary Medicinal Products (CVMP).

For our purposes, the committee for drug approval is the CPMP. Applications are submitted to the EMEA according to the centralized procedure. The review process is described in Chapter 8. From 1995 to June 2002, the EMEA received 353 applications. The CPMP has provided 237 opinions (decisions) on 179 medical compounds, of which five were negative opinions.

Another relevant Council Regulation is EEC/2309/93, and together with Directive 75/319/EEC, it requires Member States to establish national pharmacovigilance system to collect and evaluate information on adverse reactions to medicinal products and to take appropriate actions.

Clinical trial applications are not centralized. Submissions are made through individual Member States. Refer to Chapter 8 for details of clinical trial application in Europe.

7.4 JAPAN'S MINISTRY OF HEALTH, LABOR AND WELFARE

The Japanese pharmaceutical market is the second largest in the world. It is larger than the combined markets of the United Kingdom, France and Germany.

Marketing and manufacturing of drugs in Japan is under the control of the Ministry of Health, Labor and Welfare (MHLW). The MHLW has set up an advisory body, the Central Pharmaceutical Affairs Council (CPAC), to advise the ministry from a scientific viewpoint. There are three requisites in the approvals of drugs in Japan:

- *Shonin:* this is a product approval for the manufacturing or import of drugs based on the documentation provided to demonstrate the safety and effectiveness of drugs evaluated in clinical trials
- *Kyoka:* this is a license to manufacture a drug in Japan or for the importation of a drug into Japan
- *Pricing scheme:* the Japanese pharmaceutical market relies heavily on reimbursement. Companies have to negotiate a pricing scheme with the MHLW according to rules formulated by the Social Insurance

Medical Affairs Council (Chuikyo).

There are no restrictions on foreign companies applying for and holding the *shonin* in their own names. However, in terms of ease of marketing, the *kyoka* is usually held by the local importer or distributor in Japan.

Foreign clinical results are acceptable except in areas where there are immunological and ethnic differences between Japanese and foreigners. The ethnic factors are divided into two components: intrinsic factors such as racial factors and physiological differences; and extrinsic factors, which include cultural and environmental issues. In these cases, the MHLW may require that some bridging comparative clinical trials be performed with dose ranging protocols. This will enable absorption, distribution, metabolism and excretion studies to be carried out on Japanese and provide a better dosage and indication for the Japanese people. The MHLW also requires that application be accompanied with one year of real-time stability data and that sterility test results be included.

Standard processing period according to the MHLW is as follow:

- New drugs: 18 months
- Generics: 2 years
- OTC drugs: 10 months
- *In vitro* diagnostic reagents: 6 months.

The MHLW has enacted the *Standards on the Implementation of Clinical Trials on Drugs* in 1998 to detail the requirements for scientific and ethical data.

7.5   CHINA'S STATE DRUG ADMINISTRATION

China's pharmaceutical market is quite modest at present. The 1999 record shows that total market was around US$8 billion, with 'Western' drugs accounting for two-thirds of the amount (US$5 billion). The Chinese government maintains price control on imported drugs. With China's entry into the World Trade Organization (WTO), tariffs will be reduced from 20% to 6.5%. Deregulation of the domestic market will be completed by 2003. The projection is that the market size will reach US$60 billion by 2010, and China will be the world's largest market by 2020.

The regulation of drugs in China is under the jurisdiction of the State Drug Administration (SDA). The SDA was formed in March 1998 and is under the control of the State Council. The SDA manages the regulation for

'Western' drugs and Traditional Chinese Medicine (TCM), as well as medical devices. These regulations include the approval of clinical trials (Exhibit 7.4) and registration, distribution, and marketing surveillance of new drugs, generic drugs, OTC drugs, TCM products and medical devices. It also controls GMP manufacturing compliance, monitors adverse events, and prosecutes illicit and forgery and unlicensed drug manufacturers.

Exhibit 7.4 Clinical Trials in China

Unlike in the US and Europe, only certain research centers and hospitals are especially designated by the Chinese SDA for the conduct of clinical trials.

In May 2001, the SDA approved the conduct of a multicenter Phase II trial on liver cancer. The compound is MTC-Doxorubicin from FeRx Inc., US. It was the first time that a trial had been approved in China for a compound that was not previously approved for commercial use in the US, Europe or Japan.

SOURCE   *FDA Approves First TCM Drug for Phase II Clinical Trials,* http:www.asiabiotech.com.sg/kh-biotech/readmore/vol5/v5n16/fda.html [accessed Dec 3, 2001].

Drugs are classified into several categories. These are synthetic drugs, TCM, and biological products. The SDA stipulates compliance to cGMP for medical products, GCP for clinical trials and GLP for non-clinical drug safety research.

Foreign drugs require import registration. Foreign drug manufacturers and distributors file for examination and registration of their products with relevant data and documents. Clinical trials may need to be conducted based on evaluation by the Department of Drug Registration (DDR).

The SDA has set up fines for the manufacture and distribution of fake and inferior drugs. There are also strict controls on advertising drugs; these prohibit the use of certain words, phrases and unscientific claims.

7.6   OTHER REGULATORY AUTHORITIES

Table 7.3 shows the regulatory authorities in selected countries.

Table 7.3 Selected international regulatory authorities

Country	Regulatory authority
Argentina	National Administration of Drugs, Foods and Medical Technology
Australia	Therapeutic Goods Administration
Brazil	Ministry of Health
Canada	Health Protection Branch
Chile	Institute of Public Health
Denmark	Laegemiddelsturelsen
Egypt	Ministry of Health and Population
Finland	National Agency for Medicines
France	Agence du Medicament
Germany	Federal Institute of Drugs and Medical Devices
Greece	Ministry of Health and Welfare
ndia	Ministry of Health and Family Welfare
Indonesia	Ministry of Health
Israel	Ministry of Health
Italy	Ministry of Health
Jamaica	Ministry of Health
Kenya	Ministry of Health
Korea	Food and Drug Administration
Malaysia	Ministry of Health
Mexico	Ministry of Health
Netherlands	Medicines Evaluation Board
New Zealand	Medicines and Medical Devices Safety Authority
Norway	Norwegian Board of Health
Philippines	Ministry of Health
Russia	Ministry of Health
Singapore	Centre for Pharmaceutical Administration
South Africa	Department of Health
Spain	Spanish Drug Agency
Sweden	National Board of Health and Welfare
Switzerland	International Office for Control of Medicaments
Taiwan	Department of Health
Thailand	Food and Drug Administration
UK	Medicines Control Agency
US	Food and Drug Administration
Zimbabwe	Ministry of Health

7.7   AUTHORITIES OTHER THAN DRUG REGULATORY AGENCIES

Although pharmaceutical organizations have to comply with requirements of regulatory agencies, there are other authorities that control the manufacturing and marketing of drugs. For example, in the US these include:

- State health authorities

- Occupational Safety and Health Administration (OSHA)
- Environmental Protection Agency (EPA)
- Local regulatory bodies.

Compliance with all these authorities would assist in smoother paths towards approval of drugs for manufacturing and marketing.

7.8 INTERNATIONAL CONFERENCE ON HARMONIZATION

Specific plans for the formation of the International Conference on Harmonization (ICH) were conceived at the WHO International Conference of Drug Regulatory Authorities (ICDRA) in Paris in 1989. In April 1990, the ICH was formed in Brussels, with the aim of formulating a joint regulatory–industry initiative on international harmonization of drug regulations. The ICH is composed of representatives from the regulatory agencies and industry associations of the US, Europe and Japan. The ICH Steering Committee meets at least twice a year, with the location rotating among the three regions. It is charged with the responsibilities to prepare harmonized Common Technical Documents (CTDs) that can be accepted by each region.

There are four major categories of CTDs. They are topics on Quality, Safety, Efficacy, and Multidisciplinary. Details are provided in Exhibit 7.5.

The intention is that these CTDs are to be implemented by the three partners of ICH by 1 July 2003. The CTDs are format-based documents for submission to the regulatory authorities; the process of review, for example via IND, NDA, or the Centralized Procedure is not affected. The harmonized CTDs help to reduce cost and accelerate approval time.

7.9 WORLD HEALTH ORGANIZATION

The World Health Organization (WHO) is a specialized agency of the United Nations. There are 191 Member States. WHO is headquartered in Europe with four regional offices in Africa, the Americas, the Eastern Mediterranean, South East Asia and the Western Pacific. WHO is not a regulatory agency; its functions are:

- To give worldwide guidance in the field of health
- To set global standards for health
- To cooperate with governments in strengthening national health programs

- To develop and transfer appropriate health technology, information and standards.

WHO works with regulatory authorities in member states in setting up policies and training programs to ensure drugs are safe, pure and effective, and are being distributed and administered as specified.

Exhibit 7.5 CTDs

Current Status of Harmonization: (over 50 topics harmonized)

      Efficacy: 12 topic headings; 16 guidelines

      Safety: 7 topic headings; 10 guidelines

      Quality: 7 topic headings; 18 guidelines

      Medical Dictionary: MedDRA

      Electronic Standards: ESTRI

      Timing of Preclinical Studies

      Common Technical Document: CTD

E = Efficacy Topics: those relating to clinical studies in human subjects. Examples: E4 Dose Response Studies, Carcinogenicity Testing, E6 Good Clinical Practices. (Note: Clinical Safety Data Management is also classified as an 'Efficacy' topic, E2).

S = Safety Topics: those relating to *in vitro* and *in vivo* preclinical studies. Examples: S1 Carcinogenicity Testing, S2 Genotoxicity Testing.

Q = Quality Topics: those relating to chemical and pharmaceutical Quality Assurance. Examples: Q1 Stability Testing, Q3 Impurity Testing.

M = Multidisciplinary Topics: cross-cutting topics that do not fit uniquely into one of the above categories.

7.10 PHARMACEUTICAL INSPECTION COOPERATION SCHEME

The Pharmaceutical Inspection Cooperation Scheme (PIC/S) was formed in 1995 to enhance the work set up under the Pharmaceutical Inspection Convention (PIC) in 1970. The purpose of the PIC/S is:

- To pursue and strengthen the cooperation established between the participating authorities in the field of inspection and related areas, with a view to maintaining the mutual confidence and promoting quality assurance of inspections

- To continue common efforts for the development, harmonization and maintenance of GMP.

The member countries are Australia, Austria, Belgium, Canada, Czech Republic, Denmark, Finland, France, Germany, Greece, Hungary, Iceland, Ireland, Italy, Liechtenstein, Malaysia, Netherlands, Norway, Portugal, Romania, Singapore, Slovak Republic, Spain, Sweden, Switzerland and the United Kingdom. Inspection of pharmaceutical facilities by one member is mutually recognized by another member to streamline regulatory inspection processes.

7.11 FURTHER READING

Center for Biologics Evaluation and Research, *CBER's Report to the Biologics Community—2000*, FDA, Rockville, MD, 2000, http://ww.fda.gov/cber/inside/biolrpt.htm [accessed Mar 7, 2002].

Center for Drug Evaluation and Research, *Center for Drug Evaluation and Research Fact Book*, FDA, Rockville, MD, 1997, http://www.fda.gov/ cder/reports/cderfact.pdf [accessed Feb 25, 2002].

European Agency for the Evaluation of Medicinal Products website, http://www.emea.eu.int/.

European Commission Enterprise Directorate-General, *Pharmaceuticals in the European Union*, Office for Official Publications of the European Communities, Luxembourg, 2000.

Food and Drug Administration website, http://www.fda.gov/.

Food and Drug Administration, *Activities of FDA's Medical Product Centers in 2001*, FDA, Rockville, MD, 2001, http://www.fda.gov/bbs/topics/ANSWERS/2002/ANS01132.html [accessed Apr 1, 2002].

Food and Drug Administration, Center for Biologics Evaluation and Research website, http://www.fda.gov/cber/.

Food and Drug Administration, Center for Drugs Evaluation and Research website, http://www.fda.gov/cder/.

International Conference on Harmonization website, http://www.ifpma.org/ich1.html.

Japan Pharmaceuticals, http://www.tradeport.org/ts/countries/japan/isa/isar0061.html [accessed Jun 13, 2001].

Mathieu, M. (ed.), *Biologics Development: A Regulatory Overview*, Parexel International

Corporation, Waltham, MA, 1993.

National Trade Data Bank, Japan – US Department of Commerce, 2000.

Trade Compliance Center, *Japan Report on Medical Equipment and Pharmaceuticals Market-oriented,   Sector   Selective   (MOSS)   Discussions,*   http://199.88. 185.106/tcc/data/commerce_html/TCC_Documents/Japan_Moss/Japan_Moss.html [accessed Jun 13, 2001].

CHAPTER 8

REGULATORY APPLICATIONS

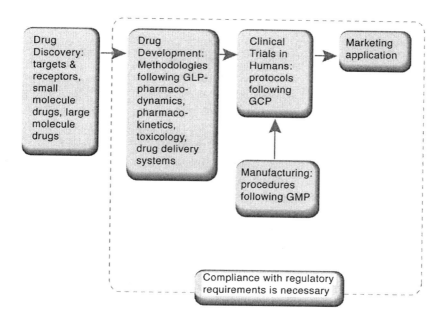

8.1   INTRODUCTION

There are very few regulatory requirements that stipulate how an organization or institution should conduct drug discovery. In general, organizations and institutions are relatively unencumbered on the methods and techniques they adopt to discover new drugs, except in the case of gene therapy and stem cell research, where the regulations are specific and ethical limits are set. However, as drugs move along the pipeline from discovery to preclinical and clinical trials, there are strict procedures to follow.

In Chapter 5, we discussed the use of animals in preclinical studies. The applicable regulatory requirement is Good Laboratory Practice (GLP). In Chapter 6, we discussed clinical trials in humans. Here Good Clinical Practice (GCP) is required. Further along the pipeline, assuming that the drug shows efficacy with acceptable adverse events in the clinical trials, the drug will be registered and manufactured in compliance with Good Manufacturing Practice (GMP) for commercial sale. The processes for all these steps are governed by regulatory authorities.

The United States Food and Drug Administration (FDA) has one of the most comprehensive and transparent regulatory systems in the world. In this chapter, we base our discussion on the FDA system. The emphasis in this chapter is to introduce the processes for regulatory approvals. Before any new drug is trialed on human subjects, an Investigational New Drug (IND) application has to be filed. At the conclusion of clinical trials, the marketing approval for a drug is filed using a New Drug Application (NDA) for synthetic drugs or a Biologics License Application (BLA) for protein-based drugs.   Other regulatory processes for Europe, Japan and China are introduced in later sections of this chapter.

8.2   FOOD AND DRUG ADMINISTRATION

8.2.1   Drug development process

Figure 8.1 shows the drug development processes and the applicable regulatory steps. Before a drug is administered to humans, the FDA requires that preclinical research on animals be carried out. The information is necessary to assess the safety level of the drug. Based on this information, clinical trials on humans can be designed. The trial protocol will consider the safe dose, methods for dose ranging, route of drug administration, and toxicity effects.

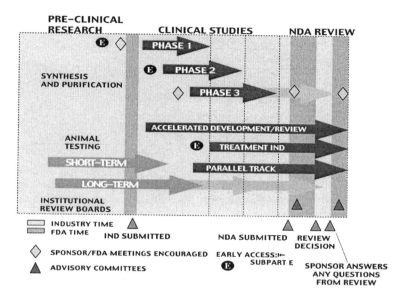

Figure 8.1 Drug development process. SOURCE Center for Drug Evaluation and Research, 'The new drug development process' in *The CDER Handbook*, FDA, Rockville, MD, http://www.fda.gov/cder/handbook/develop.htm [accessed Jul 10, 2002].

8.2.2 Investigational New Drug

Investigational New Drug (IND) is an application to the FDA to seek permission for a human clinical trial to be conducted. An IND application is detailed under 21 CFR Part 312. The process for an IND is summarized in Figure 8.2.

A firm or institution, called a sponsor, is responsible for submitting the IND application. The relevant authorities are the Center for Drug Evaluation and Research (CDER) for small molecule synthetic drugs and therapeutic biologics, and the Center for Biologics Evaluation and Research (CBER) for non-therapeutic biologics (see Sections 7.2.1 and 7.2.2). The pre-IND meeting is to discuss a number of issues:

- The design of animal research, which is required to lend support to the clinical studies
- The intended protocol for conducting the clinical trial
- Discussion on chemistry, manufacturing and control of the investigational drug.

Such a meeting will help the sponsor to organize animal research, gather data and design the clinical protocol based on suggestions by the FDA.

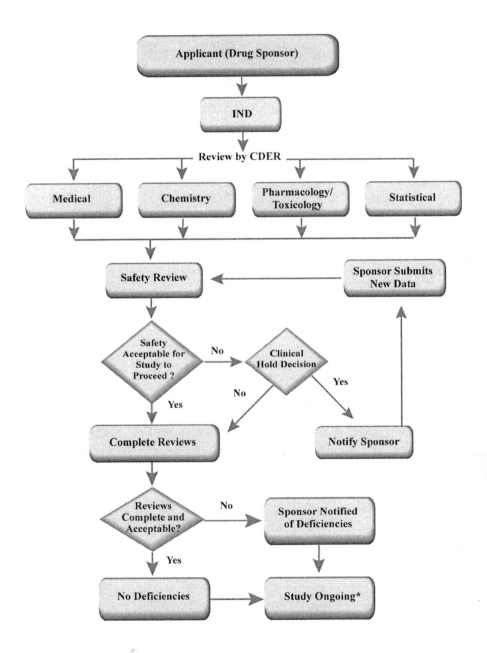

Figure 8.2 The IND process. SOURCE Center for Drug Evaluation and Research, 'IND review process' in *The CDER Handbook*, FDA, Rockville, MD, http://www.fda.gov/cder/handbook/ind.htm [accessed Jul 10, 2002].

An IND is submitted on Form 1571. The materials to submit to the FDA are stated in Form 1571, Section 12 of Page 2 of this form. These are:

1. Form 1571 *[21CFR 312.23(a)(1)]*
2. Table of Contents *[21 CFR 312.23(a)(2)]*
3. Introductory Statement *[21 CFR 312.23(a)(3)]*
4. General Investigational Plan *[21 CFR 312.23(a)(3)]*
5. Investigator's brochure *[21 CFR 312.23(a)(5)]*
6. Protocols *[21 CFR 312.23(a)(6)]*
    a. Study protocols *[21 CFR 312.23(a)(6)]*
    b. Investigator data *[21 CFR 312.23(a)(6)(iii)]*
    c. Facilities data *[21 CFR 312.23(a) (6)(iii)]*
    d. Institutional Review Board data *[21 CFR 312.23(a)(6)(iii)(b)]*
7. Chemistry, manufacturing, and control data *[21 CFR 312.23(a)(7)]* Environmental assessment or claim for exclusion *[21 CFR 312.23(a)(7)(iv)(e)]*
8. Pharmacology and toxicology data *[21 CFR 312.23(a)(8)]*
9. Previous human experience *[21 CFR 312.23(a)(9)]*
10. Additional information *[21 CFR 312.23(a)(10)]*.

Items 1 to 4 and 9 and 10 are self-explanatory and will not be discussed further. Items 5, 6, 7 and 8 on Investigational Plan, Investigator's Brochure and Protocols are covered in Chapter 6, and Pharmacology and Toxicity data are discussed in Chapter 5. We will concentrate our discussion on Item 9.

Chemistry, manufacturing and control   As stated in 21 CFR Part 312, chemistry, manufacturing and control (CMC) information is to 'describe the composition, manufacture, and controls of the drug substance and the drug product...sufficient information is required to be submitted to assure the proper identification, quality, purity and strength of the investigational drug...'.

The FDA has various guidelines pertaining to the requirements of the data to be presented in the CMC for different drugs. In general, the CMC describes the drug, its chemistry and characterization. Other requirements are the manufacturing processes, quality control testing and storage, stability and labeling. We will highlight an example of a vaccine CMC according to the contents presented in *Guidance for Industry, Content and Format of Chemistry, Manufacturing and Controls Information and Establishment Description Information for a Vaccine or Related Product* (CBER, January 1999):

A.   Description and Characterization

       1.   Description

       2.   Characterization   (Physicochemical   characterization, biological activity)

B.   Manufacturer

       1.   Identification

       2.   Floor Diagrams

       3.   Manufacture of Other Products

C.   Method of manufacture

       1.   Raw Materials

       2.   Flow Charts

       3.   Detailed Description (Sources, Cell Growth, Harvesting, Purification etc.)

       4.   Batch Records

D.   Process Controls

       1.   In-process Controls

       2.   Process validation

       3.   Control of Bioburden

E.   Manufacturing Consistency

       1.   Reference Standards

       2.   Release Testing

F.   Drug Substance Specification

       1.   Specifications

       2.   Impurities profile

G.   Reprocessing

H.   Container and Closure System

I.   Drug Substance Stability

       1.   Contamination Precautions

The sponsor has to explain how the drug is to be manufactured, tested and stored. The important criterion is to ensure that it is safe for the subjects of the clinical trials. The CMC is a 'living' document; it is updated as the clinical trials proceed from Phase I to Phases II and III and eventually to a licensed product. In essence, the CMC describes the adherence to Good Manufacturing Practice (GMP) for the manufacture of the trial drug. The subject of GMP is described in Chapters 9 and 10.

IND review   Following submission of Form 1571, the FDA has 30 days to review the application. The topics reviewed include medical, chemistry, pharmacology and toxicology, and statistics. Medical review focuses on design of the clinical trial protocol, risk–benefit issues for the trial subjects and supporting safety data from preclinical research. Chemistry review is based on the CMC to determine that appropriate controls are in place to manufacture, test, package and label the drug for the trial. Pharmacological and toxicological review considers the mechanism of drug action, absorption, distribution, metabolism and excretion (ADME), organs targeted or affected by the drug, and toxicological studies, including acute toxicity doses. Statistical review examines the design of the protocol with respect to subject numbers, doses, markers or indicators to demonstrate that sufficient data will be gathered for meaningful statistical analysis of the outcomes.

At the end of 30 days, the FDA informs the sponsor of its review finding. There may be additional information that the FDA requires the sponsor to submit, in which case the trial is put on clinical hold until all queries are satisfactorily answered. If the FDA considers the information provided does not support the conduct of a trial or subjects may be at risk in a trial, the clinical hold is not lifted and the IND is not approved.

Phase I, II and III trials   An IND is submitted for each phase of clinical trial, Phases I to III. At any stage of the trial, the FDA has the authority to put clinical hold on the trial until deficiencies or safety issues are resolved. The sponsor can request meetings with the FDA at various stages as below:

- *End of Phase I meeting:* After completing Phase 1, sponsor meets with FDA to discuss results of the trial and agree on plan for Phase 2 studies.
- *End of Phase II/pre-Phase III meeting:* The meeting will evaluate the data obtained from Phase II studies. If the results are encouraging, Phase III is planned to gather further confirmation of the safety and efficacy of the drug. A more extensive protocol may need to be devised.
- *Pre-NDA/BLA meeting:* This meeting is to prepare for the filing of the New Drug Application (NDA, for synthetic drug) or Biologics License Application (BLA, for protein-based drug). Results from Phase III are discussed. These data should support the safety and efficacy of the drug. A meeting at this stage can help to facilitate the FDA review process when the NDA or BLA is submitted.

Other review mechanisms   Although most drugs go through all the stages of Phases I, II and III, there are special mechanisms in place to expedite development and approval of certain drugs. These mechanisms are divided into the following:

- *Accelerated development/review:* A drug for the treatment of serious or life-threatening diseases for which there are no alternative therapies may receive expedited review and approval. A condition for the approval is that the sponsor undertakes to continue with further clinical trials after approval to confirm the efficacy of the drug.

- *Treatment investigational new drugs:* The FDA allows certain drugs to be administered to patients who have life-threatening illnesses that will lead to death without suitable treatment. An example is cancer patients receiving treatments with investigational new drugs (Exhibit 8.1).

- *Parallel track:* Some patients do not fulfill the criteria to be enrolled in clinical trials, but their conditions qualify them to be treated in parallel with an ongoing clinical trial. AIDS patients are an example for this group.

Exhibit 8.1 Alimta

Recently, the FDA agreed to the use of a drug for treating a rare form of cancer under 'compassionate' purposes before an NDA is submitted. The drug pemetrexed (Alimta, Eli Lilly) has shown positive Phase III results in prolonging the lifespan of patients with pleural mesothelioma (a cancer linked to asbestos). Patients in trials, when treated with pemetrexed together with chemotherapy and vitamins, showed an average 13 months lifespan extension after being diagnosed with pleural mesothelioma. This compares with seven months for the current standard treatment of chemotherapy and vitamins courses.

SOURCE Washington drug letter, *FDA News.com*, 34, No. 22, June, p. 4.

8.2.3   New Drug Application/Biologics License Application

At the conclusion of the Phase III clinical trial, if the results demonstrate that the drug is safe and efficacious over existing treatment drugs, an application is made to the FDA to seek approval for marketing the drug. A New Drug Application (NDA) or a Biologics License Application (BLA) is filed. The process for filing and reviewing of the NDA/BLA is presented in Figure 8.3. The application is submitted using Form 356h (Figure 8.4).

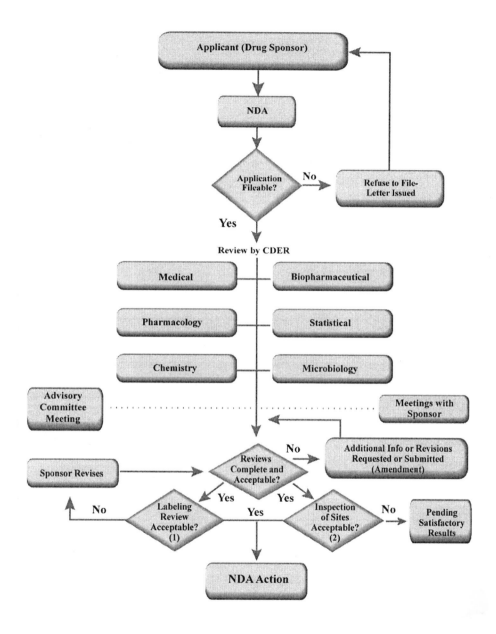

Figure 8.3 The NDA Process. SOURCE Center for Drug Evaluation and Research, 'NDA review process', in *The CDER Handbook*, FDA, Rockville, MD, http://www.fda.gov/cder/handbook/nda.htm [accessed Jul 10, 2002].

DEPARTMENT OF HEALTH AND HUMAN SERVICES FOOD AND DRUG ADMINISTRATION APPLICATION TO MARKET A NEW DRUG, BIOLOGIC, OR AN ANTIBIOTIC DRUG FOR HUMAN USE (Title 21, Code of Federal Regulations, 314 & 601)	Form Approved: OMB No. 0910-0338 Expiration Date: April 30, 2000 See OMB Statement on page 2. **FOR FDA USE ONLY** APPLICATION NUMBER

APPLICANT INFORMATION

NAME OF APPLICANT	DATE OF SUBMISSION
TELEPHONE NO. *(Include Area Code)*	FACSIMILE (FAX) Number *(Include Area Code)*
APPLICANT ADDRESS *(Number, Street, City, State, Country, ZIP Code or Mail Code, and U.S. License number if previously issued):*	AUTHORIZED U.S. AGENT NAME & ADDRESS *(Number, Street, City, State, ZIP Code, telephone & FAX number)* IF APPLICABLE

PRODUCT DESCRIPTION

NEW DRUG OR ANTIBIOTIC APPLICATION NUMBER, OR BIOLOGICS LICENSE APPLICATION NUMBER (If previously issued)

ESTABLISHED NAME *(e.g., Proper name, USP/USAN name)*	PROPRIETARY NAME *(trade name)* IF ANY
CHEMICAL/BIOCHEMICAL/BLOOD PRODUCT NAME *(If any)*	CODE NAME *(if any)*
DOSAGE FORM:	STRENGTHS:	ROUTE OF ADMINISTRATION:

(PROPOSED) INDICATION(S) FOR USE:

APPLICATION INFORMATION

APPLICATION TYPE
(check one) ☐ NEW DRUG APPLICATION (21 CFR 314.50)   ☐ ABBREVIATED APPLICATION (ANDA, AADA, 21 CFR 314.94)
☐ BIOLOGICS LICENSE APPLICATION (21 CFR part 601)

IF AN NDA, IDENTIFY THE APPROPRIATE TYPE   ☐ 505 (b) (1)   ☐ 505 (b) (2)   ☐ 507

IF AN ANDA, OR AADA, IDENTIFY THE REFERENCE LISTED DRUG PRODUCT THAT IS THE BASIS FOR THE SUBMISSION
Name of Drug   Holder of Approved Application

TYPE OF SUBMISSION
(check one)   ☐ ORIGINAL APPLICATION   ☐ AMENDMENT TO A PENDING APPLICATION   ☐ RESUBMISSION
☐ PRESUBMISSION   ☐ ANNUAL REPORT   ☐ ESTABLISHMENT DESCRIPTION SUPPLEMENT   ☐ SUPAC SUPPLEMENT
☐ EFFICACY SUPPLEMENT   ☐ LABELING SUPPLEMENT   ☐ CHEMISTRY MANUFACTURING AND CONTROLS SUPPLEMENT   ☐ OTHER

REASON FOR SUBMISSION

PROPOSED MARKETING STATUS (check one)   ☐ PRESCRIPTION PRODUCT (Rx)   ☐ OVER THE COUNTER PRODUCT (OTC)

NUMBER OF VOLUMES SUBMITTED _____	THIS APPLICATION IS ☐ PAPER ☐ PAPER AND ELECTRONIC ☐ ELECTRONIC

ESTABLISHMENT INFORMATION

Provide locations of all manufacturing, packaging and control sites for drug substance and drug product (continuation sheets may be used if necessary). Include name, address, contact, telephone number, registration number (CFN), DMF number, and manufacturing steps and/or type of testing (e.g. Final dosage form, Stability testing) conducted at the site. Please indicate whether the site is ready for inspection or, if not, when it will be ready.

Cross References (list related License Applications, INDs, NDAs, PMAs, 510(k)s, IDEs, BMFs, and DMFs referenced in the current application)

FORM FDA 356h (7/97)   Created by Electronic Document Services/USDHHS: (301) 443-2454   EF

PAGE 1

Figure 8.4 Form 356h (Page 1)

Form 356h is a harmonized form, and a sponsor can use it for NDA, BLA and Abbreviated New Drug Application (ANDA, see Section 8.2.5). Page 1 of the form requires Applicant Information, Product Description, Application Information and Establishment Information. Page 2 requires the provision of a number of items to substantiate the application. The items to be submitted under Form 536h are:

1. Index
2. Labeling
3. Summary
4. Chemistry section
   - Chemistry, manufacturing, and controls information
   - Samples
   - Methods validation package
5. Non-clinical pharmacology and toxicology section
6. Human pharmacokinetics and bioavailability section
7. Clinical microbiology
8. Clinical data section
9. Safety update report
10. Statistical section
11. Case report tabulations
12. Case report forms
13. Patent information on any patent which claims the drug
14. A patent certification on any patent which claims the drug
15. Establishment description
16. Debarment certification
17. Field copy certification
18. User fee cover sheet
19. Other.

The submission of Form 356h is the culmination of all the work and effort that has been put into discovering, developing and trialing the drug. The information submitted is substantial, with many volumes prepared for separate sections; literally truckloads of documents are delivered to the FDA. However, the submission can now be streamlined through electronic means. Instructions for electronic submission are detailed in the FDA document *Regulations and Instructions for Submitting Drug Applications Electronically*. It should be noted that every new drug in the US has been approved via the NDA process since 1938, although there have been changes to the requirements for submission over the years. Before the introduction of BLA in 1998, biologics were approved under two separate submissions of Product License Application (PLA) and Establishment License Application (ELA).

Details for the required information to be submitted with Form 356h are stated in 21 CFR Part 314 for synthetic drugs and 21 CFR Part 601 for biopharmaceutical drugs. We will select a few key items for discussion.

Index   The index of Form 356h sets out how the extensive numbers of documents are to be referenced. A well-organized index system is important for the reviewers to search for the required information. This will assist to expedite the review process, without the necessity for the FDA to stop the review time clock to seek clarification.

Labeling   Labeling is reviewed following requirements of 21 CFR Part 201. The requirements are as listed in Table 8.1.

Summary   The summary presents the case for the drug's approval. It includes discussion about the drug's mechanism of action, its effect on animals, results of clinical trials, manufacturing and tests methods, its stability and proposed dosage and treatment protocol. The summary may run into hundreds of pages. It is one of the few documents being read by all the different reviewers; as such, a good summary will assist with the review process.

Chemistry section   This is the CMC with updated information pertaining to the chemistry, manufacturing and controls of the drug. The FDA recognizes that manufacturing processes and test methods go through various stages of optimization and refinement as the drugs are produced for Phases I and II clinical trials. By the Phase III stage, however, all the manufacturing processes are expected to be defined and test methods validated. A detailed explanation of the drug manufacturing processes is presented in Chapter 10. Some pertinent data are given below:
- *Drug molecule:* chemical composition, physical and chemical characteristics and specifications.
- *Raw materials:* list of all materials used, specifications and tests for these raw materials.
- *Equipment:* list of equipment used, validation of the equipment, validated methods for cleaning and procedures for contamination control.
- *Analytical methods:* validation to assure that the analytical methods are appropriate for the tests.

Table 8.1 Review of labeling

Item	Explanatory notes
Description	Proprietary and established name of drug; dosage form; ingredients; chemical name; and structural formula.
Clinical pharmacology	Summary of the actions of the drug in humans; *in vitro* and *in vivo* actions in animals if pertinent to human therapeutics; pharmacokinetics.
Indications and usage	Description of use of drug in the treatment, prevention or diagnosis of a recognized disease or condition.
Contraindications	Description of situations in which the drug should not be used because the risk of use clearly outweighs any possible benefit.
Warnings	Description of serious adverse reactions and potential safety hazards, subsequent limitation in use, and steps that should be taken if they occur.
Precautions	Information regarding any special care to be exercised for the safe and effective use of the drug. Includes general precautions and information for patients on drug interactions, carcinogenesis/mutagenesis, pregnancy rating, labor and delivery, nursing mothers, and pediatric use.
Adverse reactions	Description of undesirable effect(s) reasonably associated with the proper use of the drug.
Drug abuse/ dependence	Description of types of abuse that can occur with the drug and the adverse reactions pertinent to them.
Over dosage	Description of the signs, symptoms and laboratory findings of acute over dosage and the general principles of treatment.
Dosage/ administration	Recommendation for usage dose, usual dosage range, and, if appropriate, upper limit beyond which safety and effectiveness have not been established.
How to be supplied	Information on the available dosage forms to which the labeling applies.

SOURCE Adapted from Center for Drug Evaluation and Research, *New Drug Application (NDA) Process*, FDA, Rockville, MD, http://www.fda.gov/cder/regulatory/applications/nda.htm [accessed Jul 10, 2002].

- *Manufacturing processes:* flow charts for production steps, controls of contamination, removal of impurities, purification steps, in-process tests and batch records.
- *Facility:* controls on equipment, calibration policies, security of access, maintenance of clean environment, flow of materials, equipment and products.
- *Drug stability:* data to substantiate the stability of the drug for storage and transportation.
- *Product release criteria:* specifications, test methods, storage and shipping conditions.

For biopharmaceuticals, further information is required. Listed below are some examples.

- *Cell line:* source, species, history, characteristics, cloning methods, vectors used, genotype and phenotype of host cell system.
- *Cell bank:* controls for working and master cell banks.
- *Assays:* validated methods of analysis, e.g. ELISA for MAb.
- *Production:* culture medium used, cell culture and fermentation techniques, in-process controls, purification steps and cleaning of chromatographic columns and matrices.

The CMC details all the manufacturing steps and controls being introduced, to ensure that the drug product is pure, consistent, safe and effective. The sponsor has to demonstrate that the manufacturing facility is set up and complies with cGMP regulations for the production of the drug when it is approved. The FDA has the right to obtain samples from the sponsor for evaluation and test.

Non-clinical pharmacology and toxicology section   This section is to present data in addition to that included in the IND. Long-term toxicology data are required. The sponsor is also expected to provide study results of the drug on reproduction and effects on fetuses.

Clinical results   Items 6 to 12 of Form 356h are all related to the clinical results. These are perhaps the most important sections of the submission to demonstrate the safety and efficacy of the drug for treating the target disease. Detailed analyses of clinical data are presented to support the application. Some of these analyses include:

- Kinetics studies to show the ADME mechanisms on target organs and tissues
- For anti-infective agents, *in vivo* and *in vitro* tests and the effects of the drug on the microorganisms have to be reported
- Description of the statistical model adopted for analyses
- Statistical analyses of results from the clinical trials, showing statistical power of the test
- Comparison of the therapeutic index and safety data
- Report on adverse events, incapacity and death, if any, and investigation of the cause.

Drug Master File   As stated by the FDA, the Drug Master File (DMF) is submitted to the FDA to provide confidential information relating to the facilities and manufacturing processes and techniques for producing the drug material. It is, however, not required by law or FDA regulations that a DMF be submitted accompanying the IND or NDA/BLA applications. In reality, however, most organizations prepare and submit the DMF with their applications.

The FDA *Guideline for Drug Master Files* (21 CFR Part 314.420) consists of the following sections:

- Contents
- Definitions
- Types of Drug Master Files
    - Type I: Not applicable. Provision removed by FDA
    - Type II: Drug substance, drug substance intermediate, and materials used in their preparation, or drug product
    - Type III: Packaging materials
    - Type IV: Excipient, colorant, flavor, essence, or materials used in their preparation
    - Type V: Facilities for production, contract manufacturing facilities and testing facilities.
- Authorization to Refer to a Drug Master File
- Processing and Reviewing Policies
- Holder Obligations
- Closure of a Drug Master File.

The Type V DMF enables confidential information to be submitted to the FDA, for example, a contract manufacturing facility may provide proprietary information to the FDA without divulging it to the sponsor client. The FDA reviews the DMF, but the DMF is never approved or disapproved. The holder of the DMF is notified of deficiencies for rectification. It is the holder's responsibility to update the DMF on an annual basis.

NDA/BLA review Review is undertaken by FDA staff from different offices within CDER and CBER. These staff members are trained physicians, statisticians, chemists, biologists, pharmacologists and other scientists. The FDA may consult with external review committees and experts, but is not bound by their recommendations.

Since the introduction of the Prescription Drug User Fee Act (PDUFA, Chapter 7) in 1992, the FDA has set a target time for the review of NDA/BLA. In general, the review time for the NDA/BLA is 12 months, including FDA time and sponsor time to respond to deficiencies. The target for priority NDA/BLA is six months. An example is the approval of imatinib mesylate (Gleevec, Novartis), which took less than three months (see Chapter 7). Figure 8.5 shows the review time of the NDA/BLA application. Drugs are eligible for priority review if they show significant improvement compared with marketed products in the treatment, diagnosis, or prevention of a disease.

For a new facility being set up to manufacture a drug under NDA/BLA, the FDA is likely to perform a pre-approval inspection (PAI) to ensure the facility has adequate procedures and controls to manufacture the drug under GMP according to *Compliance Program Guide 7346.832*. For an existing facility already manufacturing the drug, with the NDA/BLA for extension of treatment indications or other non-manufacturing related matters, the FDA may waive the PAI.

When the NDA/BLA is approved, the sponsor has the license to market the drug. It is the sponsor's responsibility to inform the FDA of adverse

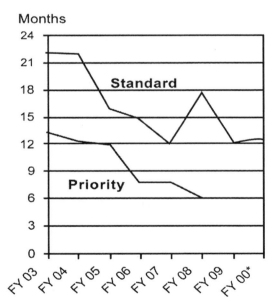

Median Approval Times

Months

24
21
18   **Standard**
15
12
9
6   **Priority**
3
0

FY 03   FY 04   FY 05   FY 06   FY 07   FY 08   FY 09   FY 00*

FY of Submission
* Projected

Figure 8.5 NDA/BLA drug approval time. SOURCE Food and Drug Administration, *FY 2001   Performance   Report   to   Congress*,   FDA,   Rockville,   MD, http://www.fda.gov/oc/pdufa/report2001/pdufareport.html [accessed Jul 10, 2002].

events or any unexpected findings. The FDA has the responsibility to safeguard the public's health. It monitors adverse events, advertising and manufacturing in accordance with GMP.

Review outcome   The outcomes from the review can be classified into three categories:

- *Not approvable letter:* application cannot be approved and deficiencies are detailed.
- *Approvable letter:* deficiencies are minor and can be corrected or supplementary information has to be provided. Eventually the drug is approved.
- *Approval letter:* the drug is approved.

8.2.4   Orphan drugs

Drugs are designated as orphan drugs for those diseases with patient population of less than 200 000 in the US. The FDA has a special provision for the development, marketing approval and marketing of orphan drugs (refer to 21 CFR Part 316). The Orphan Drug Act provides incentives to organizations to research and test drugs that have limited commercial returns because of the small size of the patient group. In return for the commercial risks undertaken, there is assistance in the forms of NDA fee waivers, tax credits for clinical research, and grants for the research. The FDA also provides market exclusivity (monopoly) to the organization to market the drug for seven years.

8.2.5   Generics

A generic drug is defined as a drug that is equivalent to a prescription drug approved by the FDA, but for which the patent validity has expired. An ANDA approval is required (Figure 8.6).

There is no requirement to provide preclinical or clinical data to demonstrate safety and efficacy of generic drug. However, the review is based on bioequivalence and manufacturing control information. The sponsor provides data to establish that the generic drug is equivalent to the off-patent prescription drug in terms of chemistry, dosage, bioavailability, absorption, distribution, metabolism and excretion (ADME) characteristics and toxicology. Information on manufacturing and control is submitted to demonstrate that production of generics complies with GMP.

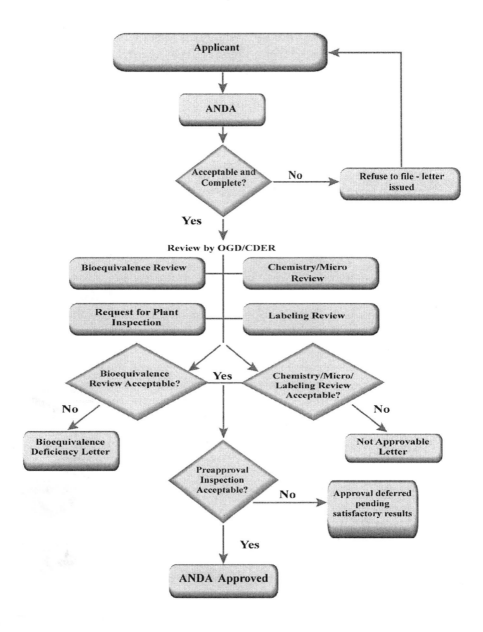

Figure 8.6 Approval process for generics. SOURCE   Center for Drug Evaluation and Research, 'Generic drug (ANDA) approval process', in *The CDER Handbook*, FDA, Rockville, MD, http://www.fda.gov/cder/handbook/anda.htm [accessed Jul 10, 2002].

8.2.6   Over-the-counter drugs

The approval process for over–the-counter (OTC) drugs is presented in Figure 8.7. Some of the important points are the review of labeling to ensure it is clear and understandable by consumers, and public comment on the listing of the OTC drug. Monographs are prepared for OTC drugs; they list the raw materials used in the drug, dosage, indications of use and labeling information.

8.3   EUROPEAN UNION

Similar to the US requirements, there are two regulatory steps to go through before a drug is approved to be marketed in the European Union. These two steps are clinical trial application and marketing authorization application. There are more than 12 Member States in the European Union; clinical trial applications are approved at the Member State level, whereas marketing authorization applications are approved at both the Member State or centralized levels.

8.3.1   Clinical trial application

EU Directive 2001/20/EC (April 2001) sets out the new rules and regulations for the approval and conduct of clinical trials in Europe. Member States had until 1 May 2003 to enact the Directive into national legislation and put it into effect by 1 May 2004.

A sponsor submits a clinical trial application to the Competent Authority in each Member State where the trials are to be conducted. The Competent Authority has 60 days to review and approve or reject the application. Application is in prescribed forms and covers the proposed clinical trial protocol, manufacturing and quality controls on the drug, and supporting data, such as (a) chemical, pharmaceutical and biological data, (b) non-clinical pharmacological and toxicological data and (c) clinical data and previous human experience. The supporting data are submitted in the Common Technical Document (CTD) format (Section 7.8).

Most of the information sought is similar to FDA's IND requirements. One major difference is that a Qualified Person has to certify that the investigational medicinal product (IMP) is manufactured according to GMP. The Competent Authority has the right to inspect the manufacturing facility for GMP compliance, the preclinical facility for GLP compliance, and the clinical trial sites for GCP compliance.

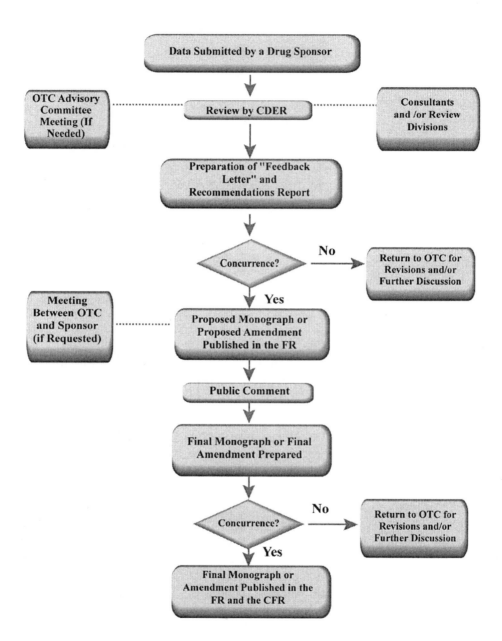

Figure 8.7 Approval process for OTC drugs. SOURCE Center for Drug Evaluation and Research, 'OTC drug monograph review process' in *The CDER Handbook*, FDA, Rockville, MD, http://www.fda.gov/cder/handbook/otc.htm [accessed Jul 10, 2002].

In the UK, clinical trial applications are submitted to the Medicines Control Agency (MCA). There are several schemes for clinical trial application; the major two are the Clinical Trial Certificate (CTC) and Clinical Trial Exemption (CTX) schemes.

The CTC system was the scheme used for the control of clinical trials before the introduction of CTX in 1981. Most clinical trials are now conducted under the CTX scheme. The CTX scheme was devised to speed up review and approval of clinical trials to allow important drugs to enter trials with minimum delay. Identical data are submitted for the filing of CTC and CTX; the difference is that, for CTX, only a summary of raw data is required. Information for submission is in three parts:

- *Part I:* Application Form: Introduction, Background and Rationale for Trial
- *Part II:* Composition, Method of Preparation, Controls of Starting Materials, Control Tests on Intermediate Products, Control Tests on the Finished Product, Stability and Other Information (Placebos, Comparator Products, Adventitious Agents, etc.)
- *Part III:* Experimental and Biological Studies: Non-clinical Pharmaceutical and Toxicological Studies.

A CTC application is submitted on Form MLA 202; the approval is for two years. A CTX application is submitted on Form MLA 164; the approval is for three years. The conditions associated with the CTX scheme are:

- A registered medical practitioner must certify the accuracy of the summary information
- The sponsor must inform MCA of any refusal by an ethics committee to permit the trial
- The sponsor must inform MCA of any adverse events and safety issues.

8.3.2 Marketing authorization

Following successful clinical trials, the sponsor has to apply for authorization to market the drug in Europe. Depending on the type of drug product and the intended market, there are four different types of marketing authorization applications (Figure 8.8).

Centralized Procedure This procedure, according to Council Regulation (EEC) No. 2309/93 and Directive 93/41/EEC, is for drugs developed using biotechnology processes to be classified as Part A products, and other

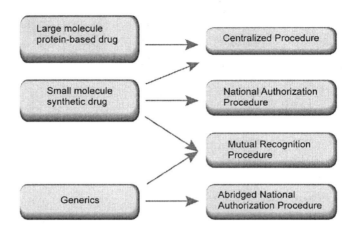

Figure 8.8 Marketing authorization procedures

drugs to be classified as Part B products (see Exhibit 8.2 for a description of Parts A and B products). The marketing authorization is for the entire European community. It is summarized in Table 8.2.

Exhibit 8.2 Drug Products according to Council Regulation (EEC) No. 2309/93

Part A Products

Drugs developed by one of the following processes:
      Recombinant DNA technology
      Expression of proteins in prokaryotes and eukaryotes cells
      Hybridoma and monoclonal antibody methods

Part B Products

Drugs of the following categories are classified as Part B products:
      Developed by other biotechnological processes
      Administered by means of new delivery systems
      New therapeutic indications
      Based on radioisotopes
      Derived from human blood or plasma
      New manufacturing processes
      New active substance

An application is submitted to the European Agency for the Evaluation of Medicinal Products (EMEA). The EMEA evaluates the application and forwards its opinion (positive or negative for granting of a marketing authorization) to the European Commission. The opinion is supported by the European Public Assessment Report, which summarizes the scientific analyses and discussions during the evaluation process. The European Commission consults the relevant Standing Committees before granting the marketing authorization. The process may take up to 300 days.

Mutual Recognition Procedure The Mutual Recognition Procedure is stated in Council Directive 93/39/EEC. In essence, once a drug is approved for marketing authorization by one Member State, it is eligible to apply for marketing authorization in other Member States through the mutual recognition procedure in place since 1998. The procedure is depicted in Figure 8.9.

Table 8.2 Centralized Procedure

Day	Action
1	Start of the procedure
70	Receipt of Assessment reports from (Co-)Rapporteur(s) by CPMP members and EMEA.
100	(Co-)Rapporteur(s), other CPMP members and EMEA receive comments from members of CPMP.
115	Receipt of draft questions from (Co-)Rapporteur(s) by CPMP members and EMEA.
120	CPMP validates questions and review scientific data to be sent to Applicant by EMEA.
121	Submission of the response; restart of the clock.
150	Common response Assessment Report from (Co-)Rapporteur(s) received by CPMP members and EMEA.
170	Deadline for comments from CPMP members back to (Co-)Rapporteur(s)
180	CPMP decision on need of oral explanation by Applicant
181	Restart the clock and oral explanation
185	Final draft of English SPC, Leaflet and Labeling by Applicant to the (Co-)Rapporteur(s), EMEA and other CPMP members.
Before 210	CPMP opinion and CPMP draft Assessment Report.
Day 5 at the latest after opinion	Applicant provides the EMEA and CPMP members with all translations of SPC, labeling and package leaflets.

Table 8.2 *Continued*

Day	Action
Day 15 after opinion	Preparation by the Application of final revised translations of SPC, labeling and package leaflets taking into account comments by EMEA and CPMP.
Day 20 at the latest after opinion	Applicant provides EMEA with final translations of SPC, labeling and package leaflets in all official languages of the EU.
Before 240	Finalization of CPMP Assessment Report to be transmitted to the Applicant.
Before 300	Finalization of European Public Assessment Report in consultation with (Co-)Rapporteur(s), CPMP and company (for confidentiality aspects).

Identical applications are submitted to those Member States where marketing authorizations are sought. The first Member State that reviews the application is called the 'Reference Member State'. It notifies other states, called 'Concerned Member States'. Concerned Member States may suspend their own evaluations to await assessment by the Reference Member State. The decision of the Reference Member State is forwarded to the Concerned Member States. If the Concerned Member States reject mutual recognition, the matter is referred to the CPMP of the EMEA for arbitration. The EMEA forwards its opinion to the European Commission, which makes the final decision. Altogether, the decision process may take up to 300 days if there is no objection, and 600 days when objections are raised.

National Authorization Procedure   To obtain marketing authorization in a country, the application must be submitted to the Competent Authority of that Member State in its own language. For National Authorizations in more than one country, submissions have to be sent to each country in its own language. In many ways, the National Authorization system is superseded by the Centralized and Mutual Recognition Procedures.

Abridged National Authorization Procedure   This procedure is for generics, and there is no necessity to provide preclinical or clinical results. However, evidence of bioavailability and bioequivalence, and GMP manufacturing compliance have to be submitted. If the applicant has an abridged approval from a Member State, the Mutual Recognition Procedure can be used.

Submission details for Centralized Procedure   This procedure was effective from 1995. Six months before submission, the pharmaceutical

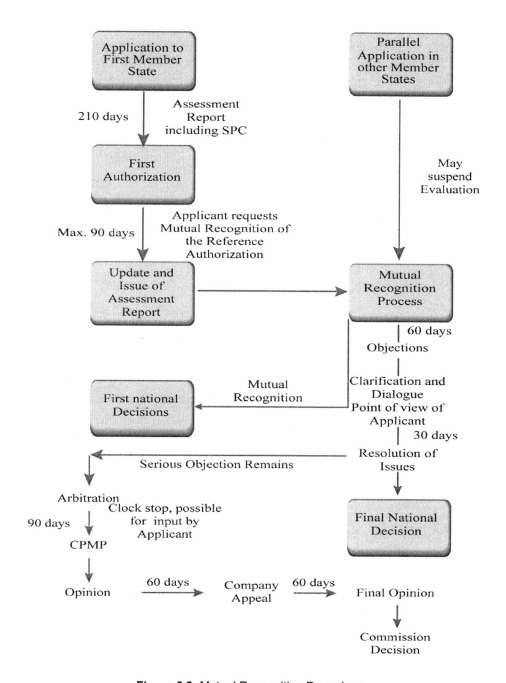

Figure 8.9 Mutual Recognition Procedure

company wishing to apply for marketing authorization via the Centralized Procedure notifies EMEA of its intention and expected submission date. This notification is required to be accompanied by a number of items, for example:

- Draft Summary of Product Characteristics (SPC)
- Justification for evaluation under the Centralized Procedure (refer to Part A and B Products designation)
- Proposed DMF
- Manufacturing location.

A Rapporteur and Co-rapporteur, whose role is to coordinate the evaluation of the application, are appointed by the EMEA three months before the submission.

Submission for marketing authorization is in a prescribed format. It is accompanied by the payment of fees (see Exhibit 8.3). Details for the submission dossier are described later.

Exhibit 8.3 Application Fees, 2003

Full Application: Euro 200 000 basic fees

Abridged Application: Euro 100 000 basic fee

Renewal: Euro 10 000

Inspection: Euro 15 000 within Europe, travel expenses additional outside Europe

Annual fee: Euro 60 000

Scientific Advice Fee: up to Euro 60 000

There are two stages for the Centralized Procedure. The first phase is the evaluation phase. The Rapporteur and Co-rapporteur coordinate the evaluation within the EMEA and communicate with the applicant. The EMEA has the right to request drug samples for testing. The EMEA may also perform pre-authorization inspection of the drug manufacturing facility to ensure compliance to GMP. At the end of stage 1, the EMEA sends its opinion to the European Commission for decision-making, which is the second stage. Documents in eleven languages are sent by the EMEA to the European Commission. The European Commission checks to ensure the marketing authorization complies with European Community law, and formalizes the EMEA decision into a decision for the entire European Community.

Preparation of marketing authorization application dossier   The application dossier is divided into four parts:
Part I: Summary of the dossier
Part II: Chemical/pharmaceutical/biological documentation
Part III: Toxico-Pharmaceutical documentation
Part IV: Clinical documentation.

Part I: There are three sub-sections:
Part IA: Administrative data, packaging, samples
Part IB: SPC, package leaflets
Part IC: Expert reports.
EU Directive 75/319/EEC requires that documents submitted for marketing authorization be drawn up and signed by experts with technical and professional qualifications.
Part IA is self-explanatory and will not be discussed further.
The major headings for Part IB are:

- Trade name of the medicinal product
- Qualitative and quantitative composition
- Pharmaceutical form
- Clinical particulars
- Pharmacological properties
- Pharmaceutical particulars
- Marketing authorization holder
- Marketing authorization number
- Date of first authorization/renewal of authorization
- Date of revision of text.

Part IC is divided into three sub-parts: Part IC1, IC2 and IC3, containing expert reports in prescribed format:

Part IC1 contains an expert report on the chemical, pharmaceutical and biological documentation. Topics presented include composition, method of preparation, control of starting materials, control tests on intermediate products, control tests on finished product, stability, and information on the pharmaceutical expert. An example is given in Exhibit 8.4.

Part IC2 contains an expert report on the toxico-pharmacological (preclinical) documentation. Topics presented include pharmacodynamics, pharmacokinetics, toxicity, and information on the preclinical expert. An example is given in Exhibit 8.5.

Part IC3 contains an expert report on the clinical documentation. Topics presented include clinical pharmacology, clinical trials, post-marketing experience, and information on the clinical expert (see Exhibit 8.6).

Part II: Part II is the report concerning chemical, pharmaceutical and biological documentation. The report details the composition, method of

---

Exhibit 8.4 Expert Report on the Chemical, Pharmaceutical and Biological Documentation

Part II Concerning Chemical, Pharmaceutical and Biological Documentation for Chemical Active Substances

Part II A: Composition
1.   Composition of the Medicinal Product
2.   Container (Brief Description)
3.   Clinical Trial Formula(e)
4.   Development Pharmaceutics

Part II B: Method of Preparation
1.   Manufacturing Formula
2.   Manufacturing Process
3.   Validation of the Process

Part II C: Control of Starting Materials
1.   Active Substance(s)
       a.   Specifications and Routine Tests
       b.   Scientific Data
2.   Excipient(s)
       a.   Specifications and Routine Tests
       b.   Scientific Data
3.   Packaging Material
       a.   Specifications and Routine Tests
       b.   Scientific Data

Part II D: Control Tests on Intermediate Products (if necessary)

Part II E: Control Tests on the Finished Product
1.   Specifications and Routine Tests
       a.   Product Specifications and Tests for Release
       b.   Control Methods
2.   Scientific Data
       a.   Analytical validation of Methods
       b.   Batch Analysis

Part II F: Stability
1.   Stability Tests on Active Substance(s)
2.   Stability tests on the Finished Product

Part II G: Bioavailability/Bioequivalence

Part II H: Data Related to the Environmental Risk Assessment for Products containing, or consisting of Genetically Modified Organisms

Part II Q: Other Information

Exhibit 8.5 Expert Report on the Toxico-pharmacological (Preclinical) Documentation

Part III Toxico-Pharmacological Documentation

Part III A: Toxicity
1. Single Dose Toxicity Studies
2. Repeated Dose Toxicity Studies

Part III B: Reproductive Function

Part III C: Embryo-Fetal and Perinatal Toxicity

Part III D: Mutagenic Potential
1.   In vitro
2.   In vivo

Part III E: Carcinogenic Potential

Part III F: Pharmacodynamics
1.   Pharmacodynamics Effects Relating to the Proposed Indications
2.   General Pharmacodynamics
3.   Drug Interactions

Part III G: Pharmacokinetics
1.   Pharmacokinetics after a Single Dose
2.   Pharmacokinetics after Repeated Dose
3.   Distribution in Normal and Pregnant animals
4.   Biotransformation

Part III H: Local Tolerance

Part III Q: Other Information

Part III R: Environmental Risk Assessment/Ecotoxicity

development of formulation, manufacturing processes under GMP, analytical test procedures, bioavailability and bioequivalence. It should be noted that all analytical test procedures need to be validated, and the validation studies must be provided.

There are four different drug products under Part II: chemical active substance(s), radiopharmaceutical products, biological medicinal products, and vegetable medicinal products. For example, the GMP production report for biological medicinal products includes description of the genes used, strain of cell line, cell bank system, fermentation and harvesting, purification, characterization, analytical method development, process validation, impurities, and batch analysis (GMP production of biopharmaceuticals is described in Chapter 10). A DMF (Exhibit 8.7) is submitted.

Exhibit 8.6 Expert Report on the Clinical Documentation

Part IV Clinical Documentation
Part IV A: Clinical Pharmacology
  1.   Pharmacodynamics
     a.   A Summary
     b.   The Detailed Research Design (Protocol)
     c.   The Results Including:
        i.   Characteristics of the population studied
        ii.   The results in terms of efficacy
        iii.   The clinical and biological results relevant to safety
        iv.   The analysis of results
     d.   Conclusions
     e.   Bibliography
  2.   Pharmacokinetics

     a.   A Summary

     b.   The Detailed Research Design
     c.   The Results
     d.   The Conclusions
     e.   Bibliography
Part IVB: Clinical Experience
  1.   Clinical Trials
     a.   A Summary
     b.   A Detailed Description of the Research Design
     c.   The Final Results Including:
        i.   Characteristics of the population studied
        ii.   The results in terms of efficacy
        iii.   Clinical and biological results concerning safety
        iv.   Statistical evaluation of the results
        v.   Tabulated patient data, including clinical and laboratory
               monitoring results
     d.   Possible Discussion
     e.   Conclusion
  2.   Post-Marketing Experience (if available)
     a.   Adverse Reaction and Monitoring Event and Reports
     b.   Number of Patients Exposed
  3.   Published and Unpublished Experience
Part IV Q: Other Information

Exhibit 8.7 European DMF

The DMF is used for the following active substances:
  •   New active substances
  •   Existing active substances not described in the *European
      Pharmacopoeia*, but described in the pharmacopoeia of a Member State

Exhibit 8.7 *Continued*

Existing active substances, not described in the *European Pharmacopoeia* or the pharmacopoeia of a Member State.

The DMF consists of a confidential part and a non-confidential part. The confidential part is to protect valuable intellectual property or 'know-how' of the active substance manufacturer.

Content of the DMF	Restricted part (expert report) confidential	Applicants part (expert report) non-confidential
Names and Sites of Active Substance Manufacturer	+	+
Specification and Routine Test		+
Nomenclature		+
Description		+
Previous Use in Medicinal Products	+	
Manufacturing Method		
- Brief Outline (flow-chart)		+
- Detailed Description	+	
Quality Control during Manufacture	+	
Process Validation and Evaluation of Data	+	
Development Chemistry		
- Evidence of Structure		+
- Potential Isomerism		+
- Physicochemical Characterization		+
Analytical Validation		+
Impurities		+
Batch analysis		+
Stability		+

Part III: This part is to ensure that safety tests have been carried out according to GLP. The data to be submitted are toxicity (single dose and repeated dose), reproduction function, embryo–fetal and perinatal toxicity, mutagenic potential, carcinogenic potential, pharmacodynamics, pharmacokinetics and local tolerance.

Part IV: This is the clinical documentation. All phases of clinical trials must be carried out in accordance with GCP. The clinical data are pharmacodynamics, pharmacokinetics, clinical trials (including all individual data) and post-marketing experience.

8.4   JAPAN

Drug approval processes go through IND and NDA procedures in Japan. The MHLW of Japan has set up the Organization for Pharmaceutical Safety & Research (OPSR), which provides technical consultation services for clinical trials. There are four types of consultations: before IND, at end of Phase II studies, before NDA, and consultation on individual protocols.

Japan has adopted the ICH GCP guidelines for clinical trials since 1997. It upholds the Helsinki Declaration to ensure the rights, welfare and privacy of subjects are protected in clinical trials. Japan accepts foreign clinical trials, but bridging trials may need to be performed to take into consideration effects of ethnic factors.

An NDA submitted to the MHLW is reviewed by the OPSR. OPSR personnel have the authority to inspect the drug manufacturing facility and clinical trial sites to assess compliance. Results of the review are forwarded to the Pharmaceutical and Medical Devices Evaluation Center (PMDEC), which prepares the approval procedures. The Central Pharmaceutical Affairs Council (CPAC) gives the final approval. Figure 8.10 shows the drug approval process in Japan.

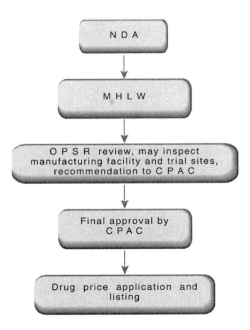

Figure 8.10 Drug approval process in Japan

8.5   CHINA

The regulations regarding the registration of Western drugs, both synthetic and protein-based, are complex, with several different levels of reviews. We discuss below (Figure 8.11) the application for registration to import a 'Western' drug into China.

An application on the prescribed form is submitted to the Department of Drug Registration (DDR) of the State Drug Administration (SDA). The DDR evaluates completion of document and then forwards it to the Drug Evaluation Division (DED) for technical review. External experts may be consulted, and the DED compiles a technical report for the DDR.

The National Institute for the Control of Pharmaceutical & Biological Products (NICPBP) performs tests on the drug samples submitted. Based on the test results and report from the DED, the DDR approves the conduct of clinical trials at designated hospitals in China.

At the conclusion of clinical trials, the results are evaluated by the DED, which submits a report to the DDR. Based on the report, the DDR makes a final recommendation to the Director of the SDA for approval to import the drug into China. The overall process may take one to two years.

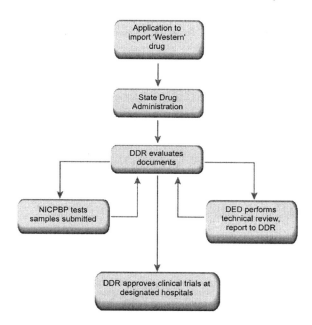

Figure 8.11 Imported 'Western' drug approval process in China

8.6 FURTHER READING

Cameron, A.M., The European Clinical Trials Directive, *Global Outsourcing Review*, 4, pp. 50–52 (2002).

European Commission, 'Notice to Applicants, Medicinal Products for Human Use, Presentation and Content of Dossier', Volume 2B of *The Rules Governing Medicinal Products in the European Union*, EC, 1998.

European Commission, 'Notice to Applicants, Medicinal Products for Human Use, Procedures for Marketing Authorization', Volume 2A of *The Rules Governing Medicinal Products in the European Union*, EC, 1998.

Food and Drug Administration, *Accelerated Approvals*, FDA, 21 CFR Parts 314.500 and 601.4.

Food and Drug Administration, *Application for FDA Approval to Market a New Drug*, FDA, 21 CFR Part 314.

Food and Drug Administration, Center for Biologics Evaluation and Research website, http://www.fda.gov/cber/index.html.

Food and Drug Administration, Center for Drug Evaluation and Research website, http://www.fda.gov/cder/.

Food and Drug Administration, *Cover Form for the Technical Review of Drug Master Files*, FDA, Rockville, MD, 1998.

Food and Drug Administration, *Guidance for Industry, Changes to an Approved Application: Biological Products*, FDA, Rockville, MD, 1997.

Food and Drug Administration, *Guidance for Industry, Content and Format of Chemistry, Manufacturing and Controls Information and Establishment Description Information for a Vaccine or Related Product*, FDA, Rockville, MD, 1999.

Food and Drug Administration, *Guidance for Industry, Cooperative Manufacturing Arrangements for Licensed Biologics*, FDA, Rockville, MD, 1999.

Food and Drug Administration, *Guidance for Industry, Forms for Registration of Producers of Drugs and Listing of Drugs in Commercial Distribution*, FDA, Rockville, MD, 2001.

Food and Drug Administration, *Guidance for Industry, IND Meetings for Human Drugs and Biologics*, FDA, Rockville, MD, 2001.

Food and Drug Administration, *Guidance for Industry, Providing Regulatory Submissions in Electronic Format—General*, FDA, Rockville, MD, 1999.

Food and Drug Administration, *Guidance for Industry, Submitting Type V Drug Master Files to the Center for Biologics Evaluation and Research*, FDA, Rockville, MD, 2001.

Food and Drug Administration, *Guidance to Industry, IND Meetings for Human Drugs and Biologics—Chemistry, Manufacturing, and Controls Information*, FDA, Rockville, MD.

Food and Drug Administration, *Guideline for Drug Master Files*, FDA, Rockville, MD, 1989.

Food and Drug Administration, *Implementation of Biologics License; Elimination of Establishment License and Product License Public Workshop*, FDA, Rockville, MD, 1998.

Food and Drug Administration, *Investigational New Drug Application*, FDA, 21 CFR Part 312.

International Conference on Harmonization, 'Organization of the Common Technical Document for the Registration of Pharmaceuticals for Human Use', *Harmonized Tripartite Guideline*, ICH, 2002.

International Conference on Harmonization, 'The Common Technical Document for the Registration of Pharmaceuticals for Human Use: Quality, Quality Overall Summary of Module 2, Module 3: Quality', *Harmonized Tripartite Guideline*, ICH, 2002.

International Conference on Harmonization, 'The Common Technical Document for the Registration of Pharmaceuticals for Human Use: Safety, Nonclinical Overview and Nonclinical Summaries of Module 2, Organization of Module 4', *Harmonized Tripartite Guideline*, ICH, 2002.

Japan Pharmaceutical Manufacturers Association, *New Drug Development and Approval Process*, http://www.jpma.or.jp/12english/guide_industry/new_drug/new_drug.html [accessed Aug 8, 2002].

Lehman, Lee & Xu, *Food & Drug FAQ*, http://www.lehmanlaw.com/FAQ/ faq/FD.htm [accessed Dec 22, 2002].

Maeder, T., The orphan drug backlash, *Scientific American*, May, pp. 80–87 (2003).

Medicines Control Agency, *Guidance Notes on Applications for Clinical Trial Exemptions and Clinical Trial Certificates*, http://www.mca.gov.uk/ [accessed Dec 21, 2002].

Medicines Control Agency, *Marketing Authorisations: Abridged Licensing*, http://www.mca.gov.uk/ourwork/licensingmeds/types/abridged.htm [accessed Dec 21, 2002].

Medicines Control Agency, *Types of Licence/Certificate: Clinical Trials*, http://mca.gov.uk/ourwork/licensingmeds/types/clintrials.htm [Accessed Dec 21, 2002].

Medicines Control Agency, *Types of Licence/Certificate: Marketing Authorisations*, http://mca.gov.uk/ourwork/licensingmeds/types/marketauth.htm [Accessed Dec 21, 2002].

CHAPTER 9

GOOD MANUFACTURING PRACTICE: REGULATORY REQUIREMENTS

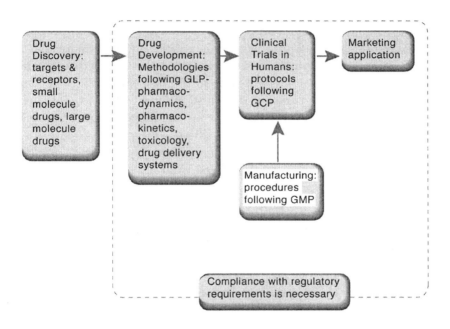

9.1   INTRODUCTION

In the earlier chapters, we discussed how a drug is discovered, followed by research on pharmacodynamics and pharmacokinetics, then by clinical trials on humans, leading finally to filing of the application and approval being given for the drug to be marketed. This is a long journey of some 10–12 years, with many risks of failures along the way. Now, after having been granted the marketing approval, a pharmaceutical firm is ready to manufacture the drug for sale, but it must do so in accordance with Good Manufacturing Practice (GMP).

GMP is a quality concept, and consists of a set of policies and procedures for manufacturers of drug products. These policies and procedures describe the facilities, equipment, methods and controls for producing drugs with the intended quality. The guiding principle for GMP is that quality cannot be tested into a product, but must be designed and built into each batch of the drug product throughout all aspects of its manufacturing processes. Manufacturers are required to abide by the GMP regulatory guidelines to ensure drugs are pure, consistent, safe and effective. Regulatory guidelines are dynamic; they are revised and updated from time to time to implement new research, data or information. Therefore, manufacturers have to keep abreast with regulatory developments by following current Good Manufacturing Practice (cGMP).

On a global level, GMP regulations are very similar for various countries. There are, however, differences in emphasis and implementation in specific areas. We will explain the GMP regulations from the United States, Europe and the International Conference on Harmonization (ICH) in this chapter. In Chapter 10, we will discuss the manufacturing processes for synthetic and protein-based drugs.

9.2   UNITED STATES

GMP regulations came into effect in the US in 1963. They have since undergone several major revisions. The implementation of GMP is the result of a number of tragedies to ensure that drugs are safe for the patients and effective for treatments. Some of these tragedies are described in Exhibit 9.1.

The Food and Drug Administration (FDA) is charged with the responsibility for ensuring drug manufacturers comply with GMP regulations in the US. GMP is defined by the FDA as:

Exhibit 9.1 Some Drug Tragedies

In 1902, several children died after being administered contaminated diphtheria antitoxin.

In 1937, 107 people died when the drug sulfanilamide was wrongly formulated.

In 1955, 10 children died after being given improperly inactivated polio vaccine.

In 1960s, untold physical damage was caused by thalidomide (see Chapter 6).

"a federal regulation setting minimum quality requirements that drug, biologics and device manufacturers must meet. It describes in general terms known and accepted quality assurance principles for producing these products. Its components are scientific understanding, documentation, analysis and measurements and personnel matters. Its intended result is total quality assurance and product control".

The US FDA GMP is codified in the following regulations:
- 21 CFR Part 210: Current Good Manufacturing Practice in Manufacturing, Processing, Packing, or Holding of Drugs; General
- 21 CFR Part 211: Current Good Manufacturing Practice for Finished Pharmaceuticals
- 21 CFR Part 600: Biological Products: General
- 21 CFR Part 610: General Biological Products Standards.

Further details for each of these sets of regulations are presented in Exhibit 9.2. We elaborate on selected items of these regulations (as part of ICH Q7A) in later sections. It should be noted that the applicable regulations for synthetic drugs are 21 CFR Parts 210 and 211, and for protein-based drugs the regulations are 21 CFR Parts 210, 211, 600 and 610. The reason is that protein-based biopharmaceuticals are less well defined chemically and they are sensitive to storage and manufacturing environment as well as the manufacturing processes. Biopharmaceuticals are normally prepared under aseptic conditions, as they are sensitive to degradation under normal sterilization processes. Special techniques and analytical methods are required for the production and testing of biopharmaceuticals.

According to 21 CFR 210.1 (a), the regulations 'contain the minimum current good manufacturing practice for methods to be used in, and the facilities or controls to be used for, the manufacture, processing, packing, or holding of a drug to assure that such drug meets the requirements…'.

In addition to the regulations under 21 CFR, the FDA publishes Guidance to Industry and documents called Points to Consider (PTCs) as guidelines and recommendations to industry to adopt as part of the compliance program.

Exhibit 9.2   FDA Current Good Manufacturing Practice

21 CFR Part 210: Current Good Manufacturing Practice in Manufacturing, Processing, Packing, or Holding of Drugs; General

210.1	Status of current good manufacturing practice regulations
210.2	Applicability of current good manufacturing practice regulations
210.3	Definitions

21 CFR Part 211: Current Good Manufacturing Practice for Finished Pharmaceuticals

Subpart A: General Provisions

211.1	Scope
211.3	Definitions

Subpart B: Organization and Personnel

211.22	Responsibilities of quality control unit
211.25	Personnel qualifications
211.28	Personnel responsibilities
211.34	Consultants

Subpart C: Building and Facilities

211.42	Design and construction features
211.44	Lighting
211.45	Ventilation, air filtration, air heating and cooling
211.48	Plumbing
211.50	Sewerage and refuse
211.52	Washing and toilet facilities
211.56	Sanitation
211.58	Maintenance

Subpart D: Equipment

211.63	Equipment design, size, and location
211.65	Equipment construction
211.67	Equipment cleaning and maintenance
211.68	Automatic, mechanical, and electronic equipment

Exhibit 9.2 *Continued*

211.72   Filters

Subpart E: Control of Components and Drug Product Containers and Closures

211.80   General requirements

211.82   Receipt and storage of untested components, drug product containers, and closures

211.84   Testing and approval or rejection of components, drug product containers, and closures

211.86   Use of approved components, drug product containers, and closures

211.89.1   Rejected components, drug product containers, and closures

211.94   Drug product containers and closures

Subpart F: Production and Process Controls

211.100   Written procedures; deviations

211.101   Charge-in of components

211.103   Calculation of yield

211.105   Equipment identification

211.110   Sampling and testing of in-process materials and drug products

211.111   Time limitation on production

211.113   Control of microbiological contamination

211.115   Reprocessing

Subpart G: Packaging and Labeling Control

211.122   Materials examination and usage criteria

211.125   Labeling issuance

211.130   Packaging and labeling operations

211.132   Tamper-resistant packaging requirement for over-the counter human drug products

211.134   Drug product inspection

211.137   Expiration dating

Subpart H: Holding and Distribution

211.142   Warehousing procedures

211.150   Distribution procedures

Subpart I: Laboratory Controls

211.160   General requirements

211.165   Testing and release for distribution

211.166   Stability testing

Continued

Exhibit 9.2 *Continued*

211.167   Special testing requirements

211.170   Reserve samples

211.173   Laboratory animals

211.176   Penicillin contamination

Subpart J: Records and Reports

211.182   Equipment cleaning and use log

211.184   Component, drug product container, closure, and labeling records

211.186   Master production and control records

211.188   Batch production and control records

211.192   Production, control, and laboratory record review and investigation of discrepancies

211.194   Laboratory records

211.196   Distribution records

211.198   Compliant files

Subpart K: Returned and Salvaged Drug Products

211.204   Returned drug products

211.208   Drug product salvaging

Subpart L: Validation

211.220   Process validation

211.222   Methods validation

Subpart M: Contamination

211.220   Control of chemical and physical contaminants

21 CFR Part 600: Biological Products: General

600.36   Definitions

600.10   Personnel

600.11   Physical establishment, equipment, animals and care

600.12   Records

600.13   Retention samples

600.15   Temperature during Shipment

600.20   Inspector

600.21   Time of Inspection

600.22   Duties of Inspector

600.80   Postmarketing Reporting of Adverse Experiences

Exhibit 9.2 *Continued*

600.16	Distribution Reports
600.81	Reporting of Errors
600.9	Waivers

21 CFR Part 610: General Biological Products Standards

610.1	Test prior to release required for each lot
610.2	Requests for samples and protocols; official release
610.9	Equivalent methods and processes
610.10	Potency
610.11	General safety
610.11a	Inactivated influenza vaccine, general safety test
610.12	Sterility
610.13	Purity
610.14	Identity
610.15	Constituent materials
610.16	Total solids in serums
610.17	Permissible combinations
610.18	Cultures
610.19	Status of specific products; Group A streptococcus
610.20	Standard preparations
610.21	Limits of potency
610.30	Test for mycoplasma
610.40	Test for hepatitis B surface antigen
610.41	History of hepatitis B surface antigen
610.45	Human Immunodeficiency Virus (HIV) requirements
610.46	'Lookback' requirements
610.47	'Lookback' notification requirements for transfusion services
610.50	Date of manufacture
610.53	Dating periods for licensed biological products
610.60	Container label
610.61	Package label
610.62	Proper name; package label; legible type
610.63	Divided manufacturing responsibility to be shown
610.64	Name and address of distributor
610.65	Product for export

9.3   EUROPE

The principles and guidelines for GMP for human medicinal products were laid down in EU Directive 91/356/EEC on 13 June 1991. The basic requirements are:

- Quality management
- Personnel
- Premises and equipment
- Documentation
- Production
- Quality control
- Contract manufacture and analysis
- Complaint and product recall
- Self-inspection

- Including Annexes –

    1.   Manufacture of sterile medicinal products
    2.   Manufacture of biological medicinal products for human use
    3.   Manufacture of radiopharmaceuticals
    4.   Manufacture of veterinary medicinal products other than immunologicals.

9.4   INTERNATIONAL CONFERENCE ON HARMONIZATION

We discussed in Section 7.8 the tripartite harmonization of common technical documents (CTDs) by the US, Europe and Japan. The GMP Guidance is one of these CTDs; it is described in the ICH Q7A document called *GMP Guidance for Active Pharmaceutical Ingredients*. Because of the wide implications of this guide, the Steering Committee of ICH invited experts from Australia, India and China and industrial representatives from the generics industry, self-medication industry and PIC/S (Pharmaceutical Inspection Cooperation Scheme, Section 7.10) to participate in the preparation of this document. Hence, the Q7A document has been endorsed as a truly international document for GMP.

The US, EU and Japan have implemented this GMP Guide, and the details are presented in Exhibit 9.3.   The Q7A GMP Guidance sets out the requirements for GMP manufacturing.   Details are summarized in Exhibit 9.4. Most of the requirements of ICH Q7A are derived from the 21 CFR and EU GMP Directive. The important additional sections in ICH Q7A are

Internal Audits (Self Inspection), Contract Manufacturers and Agents, Brokers, Traders, Distributors, Repackers and Relabelers. The section on APIs for Use in Clinical Trials clarifies the regulatory authorities' expectations for drugs designated for clinical trials, as opposed to approved drugs manufactured on a routine production basis.

Exhibit 9.3 Implementation of ICH Q7A GMP Guide

European Union
Adopted by CPMP, November 2000, issued as CPMP/ICH/1935/00
http://dg3.eudra.org/

Ministry of Health, Labor and Welfare, Japan
Adopted November 2, 2001, PMSB Notification No. 1200
http://www.nihs.go.jp/dig/ich/ichindex.htm

Food and Drug Administration
Published in the Federal Register, Vol. 66, No 186, September 25, 2001, Pages 49028 to 49029
CDER: http://www.fda.gov/cder/guidance/index.htm
CBER: http://www.fda.gov/ cber/guidelines.htm

Exhibit 9.4 ICH Q7A—GMP Guide for Active Pharmaceutical Ingredients

Introduction
Objective
Regulatory Applicability
Scope

Quality Management
Principles
Responsibilities of the Quality Unit(s)
Responsibilities for Production Activities
Internal Audits (Self Inspection)
Product Quality Review

Personnel
Personnel Qualifications
Personnel Hygiene
Consultants

Buildings and Facilities
Design and Construction
Utilities
Water
Containment

Continued

Exhibit 9.4 *Continued*

Lighting
Sewerage and Refuse
Sanitation and Maintenance

Process Equipment
Design and Construction
Equipment Maintenance and Cleaning
Calibration
Computerized System

Documentation and Records
Documentation System and Specifications
Equipment Cleaning and Use Record
Records of Raw Materials, Intermediates, API Labeling and Packaging Materials
Master Production Instructions
Batch Production Records
Laboratory Control Records
Batch Production Record Review

Materials Management
General Controls
Receipt and Quarantine
Sampling and Testing of Incoming Production Materials
Storage
Re-evaluation

Production and In-Process Controls
Production Operations
Time Limits
In-process Sampling and Controls
Blending Batches of Intermediates or APIs
Contamination Control

Packaging and Identification Labeling of APIs and Intermediates
General
Packaging Materials
Label Issuance and Control
Packaging and Labeling Operations

Storage and Distribution
Warehousing Procedures
Distribution Procedures

Laboratory Controls
General Controls
Testing of Intermediates and APIs
Validation of Analytical Procedures
Certificate of Analysis
Stability Monitoring of APIs
Expiry and Retest Dating
Reserve/Retention Samples

Exhibit 9.4 *Continued*

Validation
Validation Policy
Validation Documentation
Qualification
Approaches to Process Validation
Process Validation Program
Periodic Review of Validated Systems
Cleaning Validation
Validation of Analytical methods

Change Control

Rejection and Re-use of Materials
Rejection
Reprocessing
Reworking
Recovery of Materials and Solvents

Returns Complaints and Recalls

Contract Manufacturers (Including Laboratories)

Agents, Brokers, Traders, Distributors, Repackers, and Relabelers
Applicability
Traceability and Distributed APIs and Intermediates
Quality Management

Repackaging, Relabeling, and Holding of APIs and Intermediates
Stability
Transfer of Information
Handling of Complaints and Recalls
Handling of Returns

Specific Guidance for APIs Manufactured by Cell Culture / Fermentation
General
Cell Bank Maintenance and Record Keeping
Cell Culture/Fermentation
Harvesting, Isolation and Purification
Viral Removal/Inactivation Steps

APIs for Use in Clinical Trials
General
Quality
Equipment and Facility
Control of Raw materials
Production
Validation
Changes

Laboratory Controls

Documentation

Glossary

9.5 CORE ELEMENTS OF GMP

The core elements of the ICH Q7A GMP Guidance are discussed below.

9.5.1　Introduction: Scope

The Guidance applies to the manufacture of active pharmaceutical ingredients (APIs) for use in human drug products. It is detailed in Table 9.1.

9.5.2　Quality management

The first and foremost element for GMP is the quality system. This can be divided into Quality Assurance (QA) and Quality Control (QC). QA is a total system approach. It sets out the compliance policies and procedures for all facets of drug manufacturing. QC is the practical extension of QA. The role of QC is concerned with inspection and testing of environment, raw materials, in-process intermediates, and finished products.

All personnel involved in GMP production of drugs have to take ownership of quality. It is a requirement that processes and equipment for

Table 9.1 Application of ICH Q7A to API manufacturing

Type of manufacturing	Application of the Guidance to steps (shown in gray) used in this type of manufacturing			
Chemical manufacturing	Introduction of the API starting material into process	Production of intermediates	Isolation and purification	Physical processing and packaging
API derived from animal sources	Cutting, mixing, and/or initial processing	Introduction of the API starting material into process	Isolation and purification	Physical processing and packaging
API extracted from plant sources	Cutting and initial extractions	Introduction of the API starting material into process	Isolation and purification	Physical processing and packaging
Biotechnology: fermentation/ cell culture	Maintenance of working cell bank	Cell culture and/or fermentation	Isolation and purification	Physical processing and packaging
'Classical' fermentation to produce an API	Maintenance of the cell bank	Introduction of the cells into fermentation	Isolation and purification	Physical processing and packaging

SOURCE Adapted from International Conference for Harmonization, *GMP Guidance for Active Pharmaceutical Ingredients*, ICH Q7A.

drug manufacturing must be approved and operated by qualified personnel. Quality-related activities have to be recorded to enable traceability of data and information. Deviations and excursions of processes and results from specified conditions or criteria have to be reported, investigated and resolved. Drug products have to be tested and meet specifications before being released by an authorized person, normally from the QA department. Responsibilities for the QA and QC departments and production activities need to be defined. Approved procedures are to be followed and processing conditions and data recorded.

Two important aspects are internal audits and product quality review. Internal audits are to regularly monitor the compliance activities in drug manufacture and to ensure rectification to these activities if deviations occur. Trending and statistical analysis of data provide early warning of impending problems. Product quality review is to check the relevance and adequacy of the manufacturing activities. It provides input to update and improve the quality system.

9.5.3   Personnel

Personnel engaged in GMP manufacturing of drug products are required to be formally trained in quality practices. They are only assigned to tasks for which they have been trained. This is to guarantee that drugs are manufactured by qualified personnel and quality is built into each step of the manufacturing process.

Personnel are the main source of contaminants to drug products, and hence personnel cleanliness is an important factor (see Exhibit 9.5). Any personnel suffering from infectious diseases or having open wounds are assigned to non-GMP production activities to reduce possibility of contamination.

Exhibit 9.5 Human-Caused Particles

About 10^7 dead cells are shed each day

About 2000 microorganisms per square centimeter

Number of 0.3 μm particles shed during specific activities:

Motionless	100 000
Getting-up	1 000 000
Walking	5 000 000

SOURCE Adapted from Hofmann, F.K., *GMP Compliance*, Centre for Continuous Education, Vista, CA, 2001.

9.5.4   Buildings and Facilities

Buildings must be designed with regard to the needs for manufacturing with minimum risk of contamination. There must be demarcation of areas for different activities. Such segregation reduces the possibility of contamination and materials mix-ups.

For the manufacture of drug products, certain processes have to be performed in clean areas. Specifications for environmental airborne particulates and viable microorganisms in cleanrooms are provided in EU Directive 91/356/EEC, Annex 1 and ISO 14644-1:1999 (which replaced FS 209E in January 2002). Details for these specifications are summarized in Table 9.2.

The cleanliness is graded in accordance to the nature of operations: for example, Grade A for aseptic preparation and filling, Grade B for aseptic preparation and filling, Grade C for preparation of solutions to be filtered and Grade D for handling of components after washing. The 'at rest' condition is defined as the condition where installation is complete with

Table 9.2 Airborne environmental cleanliness requirements

	Maximum permissible number of particles per microorganisms			
	Aseptic core	Aseptic process area	Clean preparation area	Support area
EU 91/356/EEC Annex 1	*Grade A*	*Grade B*	*Grade C*	*Grade D*
At rest				
0.5 μm particles/m^3	3 500	3 500	350 000	3 500 000
5 μm particles/m^3	None	None	2 000	20 000
In operation				
0.5 μm particles/m^3	3 500	350 000	3 500 000	unclassified
5 μm particles/m^3	None	2 000	20 000	unclassified
Viable organisms cfu/m^3	<1	<10	<100	<200
ISO 14644-1: 1999	*ISO 5*	*ISO 7*	*ISO 8*	
In operation				
0.5 μm particles/m^3	3 520	352 000	3 520 000	unclassified

production equipment installed and operating, but with no operating personnel present. The 'In operation' condition is when equipment is functioning and a specified number of personnel are present. The viable microorganisms are the permissible number of colony forming units (cfu) on a culture plate for a cubic meter of air sample. There are other limits for microorganisms present on surfaces and personnel that need to be monitored. Specifications for these microorganism limits for clearances in operation are recommended in EU Directive 91/356/EEC Annex 1 (Table 9.3).

To control the cleanliness levels, the heating, ventilation and air-conditioning system (HVAC) circulates air that is filtered through high efficiency particulate air (HEPA) filters, which remove up to 99.97% of particles 0.3 μm and larger. The number of air exchanges is also controlled, at a minimum of 20 air changes per hour, depending on room classifications.

Cleanrooms are pressurized to prevent contaminant from entering. The FDA specifies a minimum of 0.05 inch water (12.5 Pa) difference in pressure between cleanrooms of different classifications, with the more critical, cleaner rooms having higher pressures. A schematic diagram showing the pressure gradient through air locks is shown in Figure 9.1.

Both the temperature and relative humidity are normally controlled by the HVAC to, for example, 21 ± 2 °C and 30%–50%, respectively, for operator comfort and to reduce growth of microorganisms. The facility is also designed to prevent product from escaping into the environment. Wastes (both solids and liquids) are decontaminated and exhaust air is filtered before discharge. In some facilities, the direction of flow of personnel, materials and equipment is controlled to prevent cross-contamination.

For a facility manufacturing biopharmaceuticals, appropriate designs according to biosafety level (BSL1 to BSL4; refer to Exhibit 9.6 for biosafety definitions) have to be implemented.

Table 9.3 Recommended limits for microbial contamination

Grade	Air sample (cfu/m^3)	Settle plate, diameter 90 mm (cfu/4 hours)	Contact plate, diameter. 55 mm (cfu/plate)	Personnel glove print, 5 fingers (cfu/glove)
A	<1	<1	<1	<1
B	<10	<5	<5	<5
C	<100	<50	<25	N/A
D	<200	<100	<50	N/A

N/A = Not applicable.

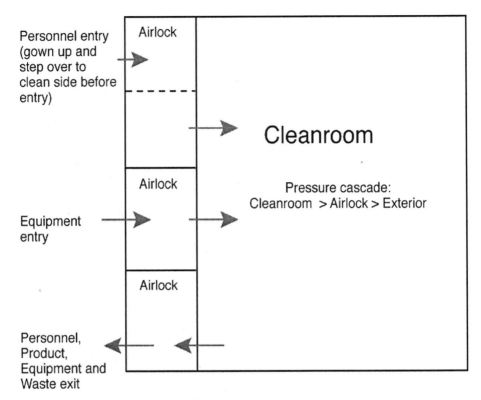

Figure 9.1 Cleanroom pressure scheme

Utilities such as gases and air piped to reaction vessels are filtered (≤0.2 µm filters) to control the risk of microbial contamination. Water is considered a raw material in the manufacture of drug products. It requires a more detailed discussion, and is presented in Section 9.6.1.

9.5.5   Process equipment

Appropriate equipment is used for manufacturing drugs. The equipment must be maintained and calibrated at defined periods to ensure it functions as intended. After each production batch, equipment is cleaned to prevent cross-contamination from residues. A discussion of cleaning is given in Section 9.6.2.

For computerized systems, the regulatory requirements are very specific, and these are detailed in Section 9.6.3.

Exhibit 9.6 Biosafety Levels

BSL 1: Biosafety Level 1 is suitable for work involving well-characterized microorganisms not known to consistently cause disease in healthy adults, and of minimal potential hazard to laboratory personnel and the environment. Safety equipment: none required. Microorganisms include *Bacillus subtilis, Naegleria gruberi*, and infectious canine hepatitis virus.

BSL 2: Biosafety Level 2 is suitable for work involving microorganisms of moderate potential hazard to personnel and the environment. Safety equipment: Class I or II biosafety cabinets or other physical containment devices; laboratory coats, gloves, face protection as needed. Microorganisms include hepatitis B virus, HIV, salmonellae and mycoplasma.

BSL 3: Biosafety Level 3 is for work with indigenous or exotic microorganisms, which may cause serious or potentially lethal disease if inhaled. Safety equipment: Class I or II biosafety cabinets or other physical containment devices; protective laboratory clothing, gloves, respiratory protection as needed. Microorganisms include *Mycobacterium tuberculosis, B. anthracis* and *Coxiella burnetii.*

BSL 4: Biosafety Level 4 is for work with dangerous and exotic microorganisms that pose a high individual risk of aerosol-transmitted laboratory infections and life-threatening disease. Safety equipment: Class III biosafety cabinet or Class I or II biosafety cabinets with full-body, air-supplied, positive pressure personnel suit. Microorganisms include Marburg virus, Ebola virus, Congo-Crimean hemorrhagic fever virus and Nipah virus.

SOURCE National Institutes of Health, *Biosafety in Biological and Microbiological Laboratories*, http://bmbl.od.nih.gov/sect2.htm [accessed Aug 22, 2002].

9.5.6 Documentation and records

Documentation comprises procedures, instructions, test methods, batch records, etc. that are documented and controlled. Documentation is prepared, reviewed and approved by qualified personnel. Approved copies of documents are distributed to relevant departments and superseded copies are retrieved and archived. The retention period for each type of document is specified. Documents are issued with document and version numbers for ease of identification and reference. Master copies of documents are filed at secured locations with authorized access. Master copies stored in electronic media require validation in accordance with FDA regulation in 21 CFR Part 11 (see Section 9.6.3) to assess the security of access and data integrity.

Records include materials transfer records, batch records, materials/intermediates/finished product test records, shipping records, water test records and environmental test records. They provide an audit trail for reviewing all the information related to the production of any batch of drug product. The data are required to be reviewed for product release.

9.5.7   Materials management

Materials are managed to assure:
- Materials received match those that were ordered
- Identification labels are attached
- Where required, certificates of approval are provided
- Materials are quarantined and stored in specified conditions prior to QC inspection and test
- Segregation of approved materials from rejects
- Transfer of materials to relevant departments for use
- Receipt and quarantine of finished products
- Storage of approved products pending shipment
- Shipment of products to designated receivers.

It is necessary to ensure suppliers of materials have in place appropriate quality systems and that they are reliable. External audits may be required to inspect and confirm the supplier's facility and quality system.

9.5.8   Production and in-process controls

Materials, processes and control parameters for drug production are stated in written documents. Production personnel follow procedures and record materials used, amounts weighed and date of operation. Equipment, reaction vessels and the production area are cleaned and their status recorded in logbooks. Throughout the production stages, equipment conditions (for example pH, pressure, stirring speed and temperature) are also recorded. Adjustments to in-process control parameters, if permitted, are entered onto batch records.

Samples of intermediates and finished products taken for analysis are recorded, stating the time, date and conditions for these samples. Deviations in operating conditions and out of specifications (OOS) in samples are reported and investigated. Figure 9.2 shows a mechanism for production and in-process controls.

Equipment, raw materials, intermediates, finished products and packaging materials may require sterilization. A discussion of the sterilization process is presented in Section 9.6.4.

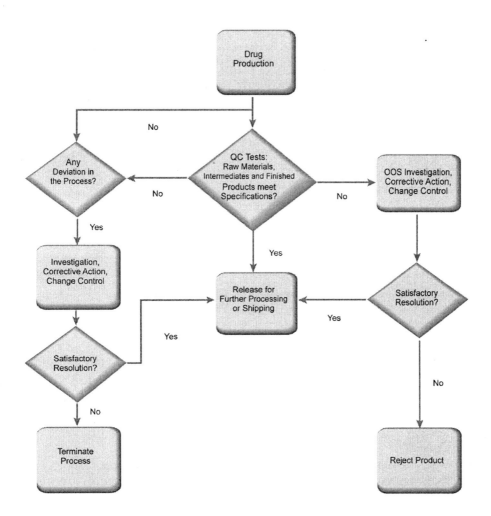

Figure 9.2 Production and in-process control mechanism

9.5.9 Packaging, identification and labeling of APIs, intermediates and finished products

Proper identification of raw materials, intermediates and finished products is necessary to prevent misuse and mix-ups. Labels are controlled and accounted for to prevent mislabeling. If required, packages may be sealed to provide an alert of mishandling or unauthorized tempering.

9.5.10 Laboratory controls

The aim of laboratory controls is to ensure that only approved materials are used and only drug products that meet specifications are released.

Laboratory controls commence with sampling and testing of incoming materials according to written procedures. Some aspects of the tests include identity, quantity, purity, activity, heterogeneity, stability, sterility and safety. Intermediates and finished products are tested in accordance with pre-set specifications. Out of specification (OOS) results are investigated. OOS may be due to analyst or operator error, inappropriate method, production problems or an inherent problem with the samples.

Test methods used in the laboratory are generally derived from pharmacopeias such as the *US Pharmacopoeia*, *British Pharmacopoeia* or *European Pharmacopoeia*. For test methods that are not from recognized pharmacopoeias, validation of the analytical methods is required. The validation includes testing for accuracy, specificity, ruggedness, robustness, precision, detection limit, quantitation limit and range. A discussion of analytical methods validation is presented in Section 9.6.5.

Samples are retained for possible future evaluation, normally they are retained for one year after the expiry date of the batch or three years after distribution of the production batch, whichever is longer. Drug stability governs the effectivity date and storage conditions of the drug. Programs to evaluate stability of drug are an integral part of tests. Details for stability programs are discussed in Section 9.6.6.

9.5.11 Validation

The FDA definition for Process Validation (FDA *Guidelines on General Principles of Process Validation*, May 1987) is:

> Process validation is establishing documented evidence which provides a high degree of assurance that a specific process will consistently produce a product meeting its predetermined specifications and quality attributes.

A pharmaceutical company has to adopt a proactive policy of validation for its facilities, production processes, production equipment and support systems, analytical methods and computerized systems. A properly validated approach will help to assure drug product quality, optimize the processes and reduce manufacturing cost.

The approach to validation commences with the Validation Master Plan (VMP), which details:

- Validation policy
- Organization of validation activities
- Personnel responsibilities
- Facilities, systems, equipment and processes to be validated
- Documentation structure and formats
- Change control processes
- Planning and scheduling.

There are various phases of validation, as defined below:

- *Design Qualification (DQ):* providing documented verification that the design of the facilities, equipment, or systems meets the requirements of the user specifications and GMP.
- *Installation Qualification (IQ):* providing documented verification that the equipment or systems, as installed or modified, comply with the approved design and that all the manufacturer's recommendations have been duly considered.
- *Operational Qualification (OQ):* providing documented verification that the equipment or systems perform as intended throughout the anticipated operating ranges.
- *Performance Qualification (PQ):* providing documented verification that the equipment and ancillary systems, when connected together, can perform effectively and reproducibly based on the approved process method and specifications.

DQ is performed by the supplier of the equipment or system at the supplier's factory as part of factory acceptance test. IQ (based on site acceptance test), OQ and PQ are performed on-site at the GMP facility. For a GMP manufacturing facility, the validation activities include the facility design, HVAC system, environment control, laboratory and production equipment, water system, gases and utilities, cleaning and analytical methods. Validation protocols (IQ, OQ and PQ) are prepared for each item, listing all critical steps and acceptance criteria. Deviations are reviewed and resolved before the validation activity proceeds to the next phase.

9.5.12 Change controls

Regulatory authorities recognize that, in spite of all the control systems put in place, deviations and changes are sometimes inevitable. A robust GMP system includes procedures to handle, review and approve changes in raw materials, specifications, analytical methods, facilities, equipment, processes, computer software, and labeling and packaging. All the changes have to be documented with references for traceability.

Proposed changes have to be reviewed and approved before being implemented. There may be justification to re-test or re-validate the affected system, equipment or process to ensure that quality of the drug product is not compromised. It is necessary to perform ongoing monitoring of changes for a period and assess the long-term impact of the changes to ensure control system is put in place.

9.6   SELECTED GMP SYSTEMS

In this section, we describe selected systems to illustrate the implementation of GMP concepts for these systems.

9.6.1   Water system

Two grades of water are used in drug manufacture: Purified Water (PW) and Water-for-Injection (WFI). In general, oral dosage drugs are prepared using PW, and parenteral injection drugs using WFI. Figure 9.3 illustrates a typical water system for generating pharmaceutical PW and WFI.

Incoming potable water (drinkable water) normally contains undissolved particulate matter and dissolved organic and inorganic compounds, as well as microorganisms. Several stages of treatment and purification are needed to produce PW and WFI.

Multimedia filters, which consist of a top layer of coarse and low density anthracite, layers of silicas, and then dense finest media vitreous silicate, remove about 98% of particulates >20 μm. These filters are regularly backwashed to avoid build-up of particulates. Finer filters (5–10 μm) are used to remove suspended matter and colloidal materials. To prevent scaling due to water hardness, sodium ions generated from brine are exchanged with calcium and magnesium ions in the water. Activated carbon or metabisulfite is used to remove chlorine.

In some cases, reverse osmosis is applied, and this removes almost all the particulates and organic materials, as well as microorganisms and endotoxins. Electrodeionization, which combines ion exchange membranes and resins, removes the last traces of dissolved ions from water under influence of a direct electric current. The last stage of the purification is ozone sterilization of water to inactivate residual microorganisms, as ozone is an efficient disinfectant (UV at 254 nm wavelength is then used to break up the spent ozone). The PW generated is then circulated to each point where it is used (point of use; POU).

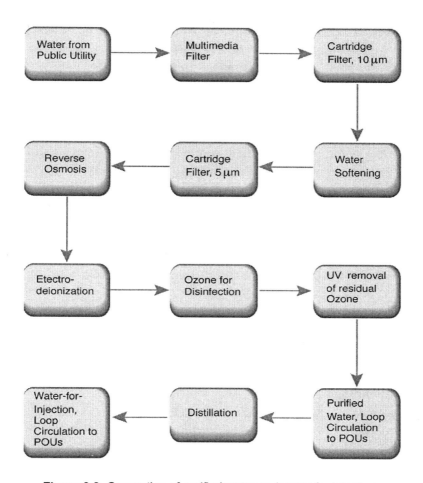

Figure 9.3 Generation of purified water and water for injection

To obtain WFI, the PW is distilled via several stills. Similarly, WFI is circulated to the POUs.

Several important points should be noted:

- PW and WFI are never stagnant; they are recirculated at 1–3 m/s to prevent growth of microorganisms.
- Pipeworks are designed to be self-draining with a slope of at least 1% over its length to prevent accumulation of water.
- Spray balls are used to continuously wash the PW and WFI storage tanks.

- Plastics such as polypropylene and acrylonitrile butadiene styrene are used for the construction of pre-treatment tanks and pipeworks.
- After purification, 316L grade stainless steel is used. This is resistant to corrosion and is electropolished and passivated to reduce roughness, which may act as sites for bacterial growth and future corrosion.
- There should be no deadlegs, i.e. areas where water may stagnate. The length of pipes without continuous flow of water should be less than six times the internal diameter of the pipe.
- WFI is circulated hot at about 80°C as hot water is self-sanitizing.

The quality of PW and WFI is constantly monitored. The FDA has provided guidance for the validation of water systems. The validation program consists of three phases. Phases 1 and 2 are for two to four weeks each of continuous sampling and testing of water to establish the effectiveness of the pretreatment and purification and distillation processes. Phase 3 is routine monitoring of the water quality over the remainder of a one-year period to gauge the influences of seasonal conditions on the water quality.

The specifications for PW and WFI according to the *US Pharmacopoeia* are given in Table 9.4.

9.6.2   Cleaning

Cleaning of product contact surfaces such as reaction and storage vessels is an important aspect of pharmaceutical manufacturing. Residual materials are contaminants and may provide fertile grounds for microorganisms to grow. This is especially the case for biopharmaceutical production, because the soiled materials are normally protein-based, and, unlike synthetic drugs, biopharmaceutical drugs are not generally subjected to terminal sterilization.

Table 9.4   The *US Pharmacopoeia* specifications for purified water and water for injection

	Purified water	Water for injection
pH	5.0–7.0	5.0–7.0
Conductivity (μS/cm)	≤1.1 at 20°C	≤1.1 at 20°C
Total organic carbon (parts per billion)	<500	<500
Microbial	<100 cfu/mL	<10 cfu/100 mL
Endotoxin (EU/mL)	—	0.25

cfu = colony forming unit

There are several approaches to cleaning. The favored approach is clean-in-place (CIP), in which cleaning solutions are piped to the vessel under computer control. In cases where CIP is not suitable, clean-out-of-place (COP) is used. This approach is mostly for smaller items. COP may be carried out manually or with automated tanks. A third approach is manual cleaning, although this is prone to human error and is not generally adopted.

Different types of cleaning solutions are used. They include acids, bases and detergents (Table 9.5).

The effectiveness of cleaning needs to be validated. The types of cleaning agents, concentrations, cleaning cycle and temperature have to be determined. This is achieved by performing IQ, OQ and PQ for each piece of equipment that has product contact surfaces. After cleaning, final rinse water samples using PW or WFI are collected. Direct surface sampling using swabs can be used as well. The samples are analyzed for pH, conductivity, microorganism levels, endotoxin, total organic carbon (TOC), residual materials and other appropriate tests to determine levels of contaminants carried over from previous batches and residuals left by cleaning agents.

Other systems and areas that require cleaning are chromatographic columns and surfaces in the facilities, especially cleanrooms. A rigorous cleaning program has to be implemented to minimize potential product contamination. This includes a limit being set for the maximum carryover of contaminants and validated by the validation process (Exhibit 9.7).

9.6.3 Computer validation

The pervasiveness of computerized systems within the pharmaceutical manufacturing facilities requires that these systems be validated to prevent potential problems from computer software 'bugs' and incompatible

Table 9.5 Types of cleaning agents

Cleaning agent	Concentration
Acetic acid	100–200 ppm
Peracetic acid	100–200 ppm
Phosphoric acid	1000–2500 ppm
Sodium hydroxide	1500–7500 ppm
Sodium hypochlorite	25–50 ppm
Solubilizing detergents	According to manufacturer's directions

SOURCE Vos, J.R. and O'Brien, R.W., 'Cleaning and validation of cleaning in biopharmaceutical processing: A survey' in Avis, K.E., Wagner, C. M. and Wu, V.L. (eds.), *Biotechnology: Quality Assurance and Validation, Drug manufacturing Technology Series*, Volume 4, Interpharm Press, Inc., Buffalo Grove, IL, 1999.

Exhibit 9.7 Maximum Allowable Carryover

Equipment is cleaned after a production batch. The maximum allowable carryover (MAC) of materials from one production batch to the next batch is given by the formula:

$$MAC = TD \times BS \times SF / LDD$$

where TD = a single therapeutic dose, BS = batch size of next product to be manufactured in the same equipment, SF = safety factor, and LDD = largest daily dose of the next product to be manufactured in the same equipment

If the therapeutic dose is 100 mg, batch size is 10 kg, largest daily dose is 800 mg and the safety factor is 1/1000, the MAC is:

$$MAC = (100 \text{ mg} \times 10\,000\,000 \text{ mg} \times 1/1000) / 800 \text{ mg}$$

$$= 1250 \text{ mg}.$$

SOURCE   Parenteral Drug Association, Technical report No. 29, Points to consider for cleaning validation, *PDA Journal of Pharmaceutical Science and Technology*, 52, Nov–Dec Supplement (1998).

interfaces between software and hardware. FDA regulations under 21 CFR Part 11 (effective August 20, 1997) spell out the regulatory requirements for electronic signatures and electronic records to ensure that they are trustworthy and reliable (Exhibit 9.8). In February 2003, the FDA undertook to re-examine certain provisions of Part 11 as a result of response from the pharmaceutical industry. Currently, the FDA enforces a narrow interpretation of Part 11, which applies when electronic records are used in place of paper records. However, Part 11 does not apply when computers are used for producing printouts and the regulated activities are based on a paper system. For systems that predate August 1997, the FDA applies discretion in its enforcement, although these systems must comply with predicate rules effective at the time.

Another industry guide for development and testing of computerized systems is the Good Automated Manufacturing Practice by the International Society for Pharmaceutical Engineering. This document sets out the various lifecycle stages for software systems design, testing and validation (Figure 9.4).

User requirement specifications (URS) for the computerized system are provided by the pharmaceutical firm to the computer systems vendor. The vendor generates functional and design specifications as a basis for

Exhibit 9.8   21 CFR Part 11 Electronic Records; Electronic Signatures—Maintenance of Electronic Records

This regulation is far reaching and contains explicit requirements for computerized systems validation. It 'applies to electronic records and electronic signatures that persons create, modify, maintain, archive or transmit ...'. As such, it requires persons to 'employ procedures and controls designed to ensure the authenticity, integrity, and, when appropriate, the confidentiality of electronic records, and to ensure that the signer cannot readily repudiate the signed record as not genuine'.

Examples of some selected requirements are:

Section 11.10(a): Validation of systems to ensure accuracy, reliability, consistent intended performance, and the ability to discern invalid or altered records.

Section 11.10(b): The ability to generate accurate and complete copies of records in both human readable and electronic form suitable for inspection, reviews, and copying by the agency (FDA).

Section 11.10(d): Limiting system access to authorized individuals.

Section 11.10(e): Use secured, computer generated, time-stamped, audit trails.

Section 11.50: Signed electronic records shall contain information associated with the signing that clearly indicates the printed name of the signer, the date and time of signing and what the signature means.

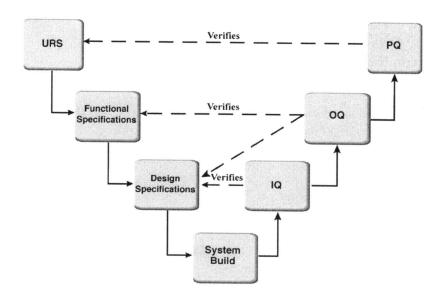

Figure 9.4 Framework for specification and qualification of computerized systems

designing and coding software for the computerized system. The system is then built, together with all the interfaces to the hardware, and tested by the vendor. After installation of the computerized system, IQ, OQ and PQ are performed at the pharmaceutical facility to verify that the system is able to meet the URS, design and functional specifications.

Computer validation is to establish documented evidence to show that the computerized system will consistently function and meet its predetermined specification and quality attributes with a high degree of assurance. Some of the parameters tested in the validation process include:

IQ: Proper installation of system
      Correct software version
      All parts are present and connected correctly
      Software virus check
      Integrity of hard disk
      Availability of source code, manuals

OQ: Start –up routine
      Calibration routine
      Data transfer/backup
      Data integrity
      Power failure
      Auto lock off
      Human–machine interface
      Security access/audit trail
      System Stress test in event of power failure
      Alarm tests
      Operator data entry tests

PQ: System compatibility tests under operational conditions at defined limits.

In accordance with GAMP, there are different validation strategies depending on the categories of software (Exhibit 9.9).

9.6.4   Analytical methods validation

Generally, GMP manufacturers use compendial methods from the *US Pharmacopoeia*, *British Pharmacopoeia* or *European Pharmacopoeia* as much as possible, as these methods have been validated and accepted by regulatory authorities. However, manufacturers are expected to demonstrate that the compendial methods are suitable for the conditions under which the tests are performed.

Exhibit 9.9 Categories of Software

Category 1: Operating systems

These are established commercially available operating systems. They are not subject to specific validation; their features are functionally tested and challenged indirectly during testing of the application. Name and version number are documented and verified during IQ.

Category 2: Firmware

Instrumentation and controllers often incorporate firmware. The name, version and any configuration and calibration for the firmware should be documented and verified during IQ, and functionality tested during OQ.

Category 3: Standard software packages

These are commercial, 'off-the-shelf' software packages. The package is not configured, and process parameters may be input into the application. The name and version should be documented and verified during IQ. Compliance to URS should be tested during OQ. Supplier documentation should be assessed and used.

Category 4: Configurable software packages

These software packages can be configured according to user requirements. A supplier audit is usually required to confirm software has been developed according to documented quality system. Validation should ensure software meets URS requirements. Full life cycle validation is needed.

Category 5: Custom (bespoke) software

These software packages are developed to meet specific requirements of the user. A supplier audit is usually required to confirm the software has been developed according to a documented quality system. Validation should ensure the software meets URS requirements. Full life cycle validation is needed.

SOURCE International Society for Pharmaceutical Engineering, *Guide for Validation of Automated Systems: GAMP 4—Good Automated Manufacturing Practice*, ISPE, 2001.

There are occasions where new analytical methods have to be developed specifically for testing raw materials, intermediates and finished products that are not covered by compendial methods. In these situations, the analytical methods are required to undergo a validation process to ensure they are suitable. One or more of the following parameters as defined in Exhibit 9.10 must be validated for newly developed analytical methods:

- Specificity
- Accuracy
- Precision

Exhibit 9.10 Analytical Methods Validation

Specificity: ability to assess unequivocally the analyte in the presence of components that may be expected to be present.

Accuracy: expresses the closeness of agreement between the value that is acceptable, either as a conventional time value or an acceptable reference value and the value found.

Precision: expresses the closeness of agreement between a series of measurements obtained from multiple sampling of the same homogenous sample under the prescribed conditions.

Repeatability: expresses the precision under the same operating conditions over a short interval of time.

Limit of detection: the lowest amount of analyte that can be detected in a sample.

Limit of quantitation: the lowest amount of analyte that can be quantitatively determined in a sample with suitable precision and accuracy.

Linearity: ability to obtain test results that are proportional to the concentration of analyte in the sample.

Ruggedness: interval between upper and lower concentration of analyte in the sample for which it has been demonstrated that the analytical procedure has a suitable level of precision, accuracy and linearity.

Robustness: a measurement of its capacity to remain unaffected by small, but deliberate, variations in method parameters; provides an indication of its reliability during normal use.

SOURCE   International Conference for Harmonization, 'Text on validation of analytical procedure', ICH Q2A, and 'Analytical methods', ICH Q2B, in *Harmonized Tripartite Guideline*, ICH, 1994.

- Repeatability
- Limit of Detection
- Limit of Quantitation
- Linearity
- Ruggedness
- Robustness.

A rationale should be generated to explain and support the reasoning for validating the selected parameters. The use of reference standards during validation helps to reinforce the reliability of the analytical method developed. The conditions of how a test is performed may have a strong influence on the results. These conditions have to be recorded and followed.

9.6.5   Sterilization processes

Parenteral drug products are required to be sterile. There are principally five different ways to sterilize a product. These are steam, dry heat, radiation, gas and filtration. Selection of which method to use is based on the product that requires sterilization. For example, protein-based drugs are heat-sensitive, so the normal means for sterilizing these products is filtration. The rationale for sterilization validation is to show the reduction in microbial load or destruction of biological indicators.

Steam under pressure at 15 psig (103.4 kPa), 121°C is a very effective sterilant. Bacterial spores that are resistant to dry heat are killed by steam sterilization. The mechanism is thought to be that the steam causes denaturation of proteins and amino acids within the bacterial cells. An autoclave is a typical steam sterilization device. It is validated taking into account the loading pattern of items in the autoclave chamber and the sterilization cycle used. Often, biological indicators such as *Bacillus stearothermophilus* (also known as *Geobacillus stearothermophilus*) and *Clostridium sporogenes* are used to challenge the effectiveness of sterilization.

Dry heat is used to sterilize and depyrogenate components and drug products. The definition of dry heat sterilization is 170°C for at least two hours and depyrogenation cycle at 250°C for more than 30 minutes. Typical equipment includes tunnel sterilizers (force convection, infrared, flame) and microwave sterilizers. An important aspect is the need to ensure air supply is filtered through HEPA filters. Biological indicators such as *Bacillus subtilis* can be used to gauge the performance of sterilization.

Radiation generates high-energy photons, which penetrate microorganisms and cause death through ionization. Commercial radiation sterilization employs gamma-ray radioisotopes such as cobalt-60 and cesium-137. The radiation dose is around 10^3 to 4×10^5 Gy. Radiation may cause degradation in drug products and its effects have to be considered.

Ethylene oxide and hydrogen peroxide are the typical gases for gas sterilization. Their advantage is that they can be used at much lower temperature than steam sterilization: 27–60°C for ethylene oxide and 25–40 °C for hydrogen peroxide. Another advantage is that they do not cause damage to the product or the packaging.

For protein-based drugs, filtration via a 0.2 μm filter is an effective way to achieve sterilization. Factors that determine the filtration efficiency include integrity of filter, pressure, temperature, flow rate, contact time of material with filter, pH, and viscosity. Validation of filters should include chemical compatibility of filter with the product and possibility of contaminant from the filters leaching into the product.

The effectiveness of sterilization can be established by culturing samples of the filtrate in growth medium. Fluid thioglycolate medium and soybean-casein digest medium are normally used. Incubation is 7–14 days at 30–35 °C for fluid thioglycolate medium and 7–14 days at 20–25 °C for soybean-casein digest medium. The absence of microorganism colonies at the end of the growth cycle is an indication of sterility.

Several mathematical functions are used as indicators of microbial destruction. These are D, Z and F values:

> *D value:* The amount of time, at a given temperature, that is required to reduce the microbial population by one order of magnitude (1 log)
>
> *Z value:* The number of degrees of temperature necessary to change the D value by a factor of 10.
>
> *F value:* The equivalent time, in minutes, at a specific temperature delivered to a product to produce a given sterilization effect at a reference temperature and specific Z value.

Both the D and Z values are further illustrated in Figure 9.5.

9.6.6 Stability evaluation

The quality of a drug changes over time under the influence of temperature, humidity and light. It is a requirement that drug products have to be stable during transportation and storage over their projected shelf life. The ICH

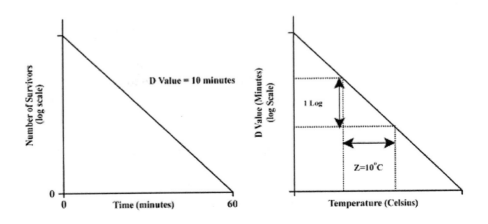

Figure 9.5 Curves showing D and Z values

Harmonized Tripartite Guideline Q1A 'Stability Testing of New Drug Substances and Products' (November 2000) sets out the guidelines for testing the stabilities of new drug substances.

To evaluate the stability of a drug, stress testing is carried out to determine the effects of environmental conditions on the drug. For example, the effect of temperature is assessed over a range of temperatures in 10 °C intervals, humidity at conditions <75% relative humidity, oxidation and photolysis degradation processes and hydrolysis of the drug at different pH levels. These evaluations are to assess any changes in the physical, chemical, biological and microbiological properties of the drug in its container or packaging after it has been transported to various environmental conditions.

The ICH has specified storage conditions to evaluate drug stability as part of the submission data for drug approval (Table 9.6).

9.7 THE FDA'S NEW cGMP INITIATIVE

In August 2002, the FDA announced a new initiative to cGMP. The initiative is called 'Pharmaceutical cGMPs for the 21st Century: A Risk-Based Approach'. It is a two-year program, and there are three goals to this initiative:

- To focus the FDA's cGMP requirements on potential risks to public health and channel additional regulatory attention to manufacturing aspects that pose potential risk

Table 9.6 Storage conditions for evaluating drug stability

Study	Storage condition	Minimum period covered by data at submission
(1) General case		
Long term	25 °C ± 2 °C 60% RH ± 5% RH	12 months
Intermediate	30 °C ± 2 °C 60% RH ± 5% RH	6 months
Accelerated	40 °C ± 2 °C 60% RH ± 5% RH	6 months
(2) Drug substances intended for storage in a refrigerator		
Long term	5 °C ± 3 °C	12 months
Accelerated	25 °C ± 2 °C 60% RH ± 5% RH	6 months
(3) Drug substances intended for storage in a freezer		
Long term	−20 °C ± 5 °C	12 months

RH = Relative humidity.

- To ensure the regulatory work does not impede innovations in the pharmaceutical industry
- To enhance consistency in approach to assure production quality and safety among the FDA's centers and field groups.

A steering committee has been formed and the FDA will be working on this initiative with industry groups . The five principles for guiding the initiative are:

- Risk-based orientation
- Science-based policies and standards
- Integrated quality systems orientation
- International cooperation
- Strong public health protection.

The Risk-Based Approach will merge science-based policies and standards with an integrated quality system. This is to ensure that the FDA's resources are directed to address those areas that are considered to have higher risks; for example, companies with previous compliance problems, new companies with unknown history, and processes requiring aseptic procedures.

There are three steps to implementing the Risk-Based Approach:

- The immediate steps include holding scientific workshops with key stakeholders, re-examine and clarify the scope and interpretation of Part 11 (see Section 9.6.3), develop technical dispute resolution processes, and harmonize inconsistencies between the different centers of the FDA.
- The intermediate steps are to utilize new scientific developments and analysis tools to focus on higher risk areas; and include trained product specialists as members of pharmaceutical inspection teams.
- The long-term steps are to develop and implement science-based risk management to regulatory issues and target inspections in risk areas, while encouraging innovations in pharmaceutical companies with proven regulatory history and control. The FDA is also examining how it can facilitate introduction of process analytical technologies to improve manufacturing efficiencies.

The FDA has established a new CDER Division of Compliance Risk Management. It is working with stakeholders, and aims to develop a risk model by FY 2004. To date, the FDA has released two draft guidance documents: (a) Part 11, *Electronic Records; Electronic Signatures—Scope and Application*, and (b) *Comparability Protocols—Chemistry, Manufacturing and*

Controls Information, which applies to small molecule and veterinary drugs. This protocol allows manufacturers to change manufacturing processes, under certain conditions, without submitting a supplement to the FDA for prior approval. A parallel track to the Risk-Based Approach is the System Approach for GMP inspection. This is discussed in Section 10.3.

9.8 FURTHER READING

Brunkow, R., DeLucia, D., Green, G. et al., *Cleaning and Cleaning Validation: A Biotechnology Perspective*, PDA, Bethesda, MD, 1996.

Carleton, F.J. and Agalloco, J.P. (eds.), *Validation of Pharmaceutical Processes, Sterile Products*, Marcel Dekker, Inc., New York, 1999.

Center for Biologics Evaluation and Research and Center for Veterinary Medicine, *Guidance for Industry for the Submission Documentation for Sterilization Process validation in Application for Human and Veterinary Drug Products*, FDA, Rockville, MD, 1994.

Center for Biologics Evaluation and Research, *Guidance for Industry, Monoclonal Antibodies Used as Reagents in Drug Manufacturing*, FDA, Rockville, MD, 2001, http://www.fda.gov/cber/gdlns/mab032901.htm [accessed Mar 21, 2002].

Center for Biologics Evaluation and Research, *Points to Consider in the Production and Testing of New Drugs and Biologicals Produced by Recombinant DNA Technology*, FDA, Rockville, MD, 1985.

Center for Drug Evaluation and Research and Center for Biologics Evaluation and Research, Guidance *for Industry, ICH Q7A Good Manufacturing Practice Guidance for Active Pharmaceutical Ingredients*, FDA, Rockville, MD, 1997.

Food and Drug Administration, *Guidance for Industry, 21 CFR Part 11; Electronic Records; Electronic Signatures Validation*, FDA, Rockville, MD, 2001.

Food and Drug Administration, *Guide to Inspections Validation of Cleaning Processes*, FDA, http://www.fda.gov/ora/inspect_ref/igs/valid.html [accessed Jan 15, 2003].

Food and Drug Administration, *Points to Consider in the Characterization of Cell Line Used to Produce Biologicals*, FDA, Rockville, MD, 1993.

Gadamasetti, K.G. (ed.), *Process Chemistry in the Pharmaceutical Industry*, Marcel Dekker, Inc., New York, 1999.

International Conference on Harmonization, 'Derivation and characterization of cell substrates used for production of biotechnological/biological products', in *Harmonized Tripartite Guideline*, ICH, 2001.

International Conference on Harmonization, 'Specifications: Test procedures and acceptance criteria for new drug substance and new drug products: Chemical substances', in *Harmonized Tripartite Guideline*, ICH, 1999.

International Conference on Harmonization, 'Specifications: Test procedures and acceptance criteria for biotechnological/biological products', in *Harmonized Tripartite Guideline*, ICH, 1999.

International Conference on Harmonization, 'Viral safety evaluation of biotechnology products derived from cell lines of human or animal origin', in *Harmonized Tripartite Guideline*, ICH, 1997.

International Society for Pharmaceutical Engineering, *GAMP Guide for Validation of Automated Systems*, ISPE, 2001.

Medicines Control Agency, *Rules and Guidance for Pharmaceutical Manufacturers and Distributors*, MCA, 1997.

Office of Regulatory Affairs, *Guide to Inspections of Bulk Pharmaceutical Chemicals*, FDA, Rockville, MD, 1994.

Office of Regulatory Affairs, *Guide to Inspections of Quality Systems*, FDA, Rockville, MD, 1999, http:www.fda.gov/ora/inspect_ref/igs/qsit/qsitguide.htm [accessed Apr 19, 2002].

Vesper, J.L., *Documentation Systems, Clear and Simple*, Interpharm Press. Inc., Buffalo Grove, IL, 1998.

CHAPTER 10

GOOD MANUFACTURING PRACTICE: DRUG MANUFACTURING

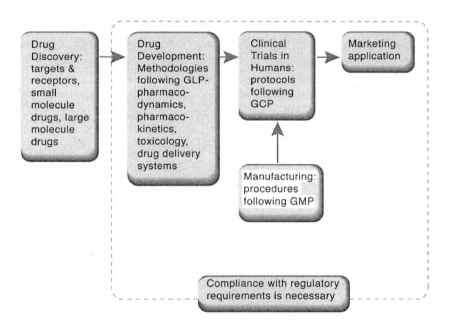

10.1 INTRODUCTION

There are distinct differences in the manufacture of small and large molecule drugs; the former is mainly based on organic chemical synthesis, while the latter relies on biological systems of recombinant DNA (rDNA) technology. In this chapter, we describe the manufacturing processes for these drugs under GMP environments.

Before the large scale manufacturing of drug under a GMP quality system is undertaken, there is a development process, which spans the discovery stage and the commercial production of the drug. From the discovery stage, lead compounds are identified. These lead compounds are tested in a number of stages, from laboratory *in vitro* assays to *in vivo* tests, pharmacology, toxicology, and finally into clinical trials as potential drug candidates. An increasing quantity of the drug material is needed as each stage progresses. The demand for material grows from milligrams to grams and kilograms. A development program is phased in to meet this demand by initially producing drugs on a laboratory scale. It then progresses to pilot plant scale to provide more drug material for clinical trials, and finally implements procedures, processes, equipment and setting up of a manufacturing plant for large-scale commercial production.

Broadly, the drug development program covers the following:

General items

Raw materials: Raw materials have a significant impact on the manufacturing process. Issues such as availability and reliability of supply, reactivity, toxicity, handling, and storage have to be considered. Cost is another factor to take into account. Often, trade-offs between costs, manufacturing processes and yields are considered.

Safety: Production of the requisite drug molecule, called the active pharmaceutical ingredient (API) or bulk pharmaceutical chemical (BPC), may involve materials, solvents or intermediates that are volatile, toxic or even explosive. The development program has to determine the appropriate manufacturing processes to ensure that safety is not compromised and the API can be produced and purified to remove impurities and toxic residues.

Reproducibility of manufacturing processes: The aim of GMP is to ensure the manufacture of potent, pure, and effective drug in a consistent manner. The development program is to evaluate procedures and processes that can be implemented in a large-scale manufacturing environment to ensure the drug product conforms to the intended potency, purity, effectiveness and consistency on a routine basis.

Environmental factors: In addition to conformance to GMP, the manufacturing plant has to comply with local environmental legislation. This may cover materials transportation, handling, storage and disposal. The manufacturing plant is set up with systems for controlling gaseous emission, decontamination of solid waste and treatment of liquid discharge. All these factors are evaluated in the development program.

Small molecule drugs

Organic chemistry synthesis route: The production of API for small molecule drugs requires ingenious and meticulous development of organic synthesis steps. Some drugs may require more than 50 steps to obtain the intended API (There are more than 100 production steps for the manufacture of Roche's new AIDS drug enfuvirtide [Fuzeon], approved by the FDA in March 2003.)

In some cases, drug materials are isolated from natural products. In other cases natural product extraction constitutes the raw material or intermediate for production of the drug via semi-synthetic route. Methods for chemical reactions, product purification, control parameters and analytical procedures are developed and they form the basis for the Chemistry, Manufacturing and Control (CMC) information for regulatory application.

Large molecule drugs

Optimization of protein synthesis route: Protein-based drugs are produced using living systems of microbial or mammalian cells. The development program commences with selection of cell line, cloning methods for genes that express the intended protein molecule, and experimentation of conducive growth environments for high yields and determination of effective purification procedures. Similarly, CMC information is submitted for regulatory application.

Drug development work also includes formulation, stability studies and selection of drug delivery systems, as discussed in Section 5.6. Once the API has been prepared, excipients are added:

- To modify processing properties for the manufacture of finished dosage forms (tablets, capsules, parenterals, etc.)
- As preservatives or buffers to ensure drug stability

- For efficient delivery of the drug to targets.

In API manufacture, whether via chemical synthesis, rDNA technology, or extraction from natural products, there are significant changes (physical and chemical) from the starting materials to the API. In the formulation process, however, the quality and specifications of the API are retained. The addition of excipients to produce the drug product in a finished dosage form does not present physical or chemical changes to the API.

It should be noted that GMP regulations are necessary for approved drug products. Regulatory authorities such as the FDA do not expect total GMP compliance for the manufacture of drugs designated for clinical trials. This is recognized, and ICH Q7A GMP Guidance Section 19, 'APIs for Use in Clinical Trials', sets out the GMP expectations. It states '… controls used in the manufacture of APIs for use in clinical trials should be consistent with the stage of development of the drug product …'. As a sponsor files for an Investigational New Drug (IND), the manufacturing information is presented in the CMC (Section 8.2.2). Initially, for Phase I and II clinical trials, regulatory authorities do not require total GMP compliance in the CMC. However, by Phase III, all quality systems, production processes and validation issues are expected to have been resolved to enable GMP manufacturing of drug products to be carried out routinely.

10.2 GMP MANUFACTURING

Manufacturing of drugs, whether the API or finished dosage form, is required to comply with GMP regulations (see Chapter 9). Figure 10.1 shows the implementation of GMP concepts in drug manufacture.

The first requirement for GMP manufacture is the availability of trained personnel. Other requirements are:

- Raw materials that conform to specifications
- Water, in the form of Purified Water or Water-for-Injection, as required
- An environment with appropriate control for temperature, pressure, relative humidity. For aseptic production, cleanroom conditions monitored for particles and bioburden contamination are necessary
- Equipment that has been validated and maintained with current calibration
- Processes that have been developed and validated to ensure the production of pure and consistent product

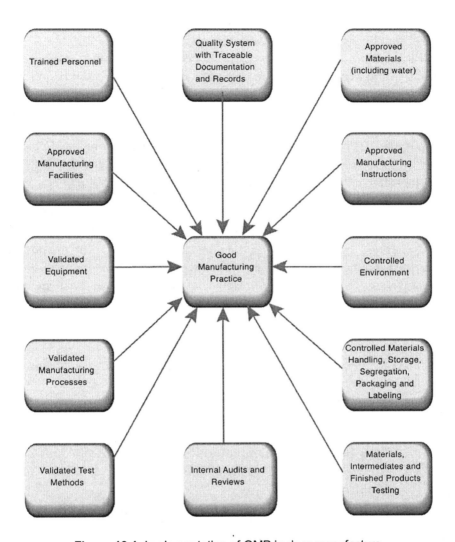

Figure 10.1 Implementation of GMP in drug manufacture

- Operating procedures clearly written down, detailing each manufacturing step
- Approved batch records for registering all relevant information during the manufacturing process
- Quality records to record all tests pertaining to the raw materials, intermediates and finished product

- Validated cleaning procedure to ensure reaction vessels and containers do not carry contaminants.

All these items above must be in place before the manufacturing process begins. In the manufacturing process, deviations from specified conditions and processes may happen. For example, the pH for the reactions may be outside the range stated in the procedure or the reaction process may produce more heat leading to a greater temperature rise than is programmed. These deviations have to be resolved before the following steps can proceed. Similarly, raw materials, intermediates and products that are outside specifications require out-of-specifications investigations. When resolved satisfactorily, the materials, intermediates and products are released. Change controls and corrective actions are required when investigations show failure in controls that need rectification.

QC tests are carried out according to validated analytical methods or established methods from pharmacopeias: *US Pharmacopoeia* and *British Pharmacopoeia*. Exhibit 10.1 lists some of the QC analytical methods performed on drug intermediates and products.

10.3 GMP INSPECTION

Regulatory authorities inspect GMP facilities to ensure drugs are manufactured according to GMP requirements. *The Compliance Program Guidance Manual for FDA Staff: Drug Manufacturing Inspections Program 7356.002* (February 2002) states the strategy for inspection as:

- Evaluating through factory inspections, including the collection and analysis of associated samples, the conditions and practices under which drugs and drug products are manufactured, packed, tested and held, and
- Monitoring the quality of drugs and drug products through surveillance activities such as sampling and analyzing products in distribution.

The FDA carries out the inspections once every two years. The FDA has adopted a systems approach to GMP inspection. A GMP facility is divided into six systems:

- *Quality system:* This consists of procedures and specifications to assure the overall compliance for the facility. Quality control, change control, batch release, internal audits, quality records are part of the Quality System.

Exhibit 10.1 Selected Analytical Methods

High performance liquid chromatography (HPLC): This is a separation method for characterizing or determining the purity of a drug material. The material is passed through a chromatographic column with solid matrix, which binds the material and separates the material according to its physicochemical properties.

Sodium dodecyl sulfate – polyacrylamide gel electrophoresis (SDS-PAGE): This method is used to separate proteins based on molecular weights. SDS is added to the proteins to produce a net negative charge. Under an electric field, the negatively charged proteins migrate to the anode. Smaller molecules migrate longer distances and are separated from larger molecules.

Isoelectric focusing: This is an electrophoretic method in which the proteins are separated based on their charge characteristics. This is accomplished by the proteins moving through a medium with a pH gradient. The protein stops at the point where the pH equals the protein's isoelectric point (pH where the protein has no net charge).

Spectroscopy: Drug compounds absorb visible, infrared and UV radiation at frequencies that are characteristic of the compounds. Quantitative measurements can be calculated from the absorbance readings at specific frequencies or wavelengths.

Circular dichroism: This method is used to determine the enantiomers in racemic mixtures. The isomers rotate polarized light in different directions depending on their chiral characteristics.

Atomic spectroscopy: This method is used to determine the concentration of an element in a drug substance. The intensity of the emission lines of the element measured at specific wavelengths shows its concentration.

Mass spectroscopy: This is based on measurement of the ratio of mass to number of positive or negative charges of the substance to be analyzed. The pattern generated is characteristic of the drug substance. One method is the use of Matrix-Assisted Laser Desorption Ionization – Time of Flight (MALTI-TOF) mass spectroscopy. This gives partial sequences of peptide fragments. From these, the protein identity can be revealed through a database search.

Limulus amebocyte lysate test (LAL): This test is used to detect the presence of endotoxins in the drug substance. It relies on the coagulation reaction between the endotoxin and the blood of a horseshoe crab.

NMR and ELISA methods are discussed in Chapters 3 and 4.

- *Facilities and equipment system:* This includes (1) Buildings and facilities along with maintenance; (2) Equipment IQ, OQ, calibration, maintenance, cleaning and validation of cleaning processes; (3) Utilities such as HVAC, compressed gases, steam and water systems.

- *Materials system:* This is concerned with segregation and storage of raw materials, components and finished products, inventory control and distribution of finished products.
- *Production system:* This includes manufacturing processes, sampling and testing, batch records and process validation.
- *Packaging and labeling system:* This includes control and issuance of labels, packaging operations and validation of these operations.
- *Laboratory control system:* This includes laboratory test methods, stability program and analytical method validation.

The FDA carries out two types of inspections: surveillance inspections and compliance inspections. Surveillance inspections are the biennial inspections. Compliance inspections are to follow-up on previous corrective actions. Compliance inspections also include 'For cause Inspections', which are inspections to audit a specific problem that has come to the FDA's attention, for example, product recall and industry or public complaints. There are two options of inspections: (a) the Full Inspection Option, and (b) the Abbreviated Inspection Option.

The Full Inspection Option is a surveillance or compliance inspection that is thorough and gives the FDA a deep understanding of the cGMP program in a manufacturing facility. This type of inspection is conducted when the FDA has little knowledge about the facility, such as a new facility or where the facility has a history of non-compliance or when the FDA has doubt about the facility's quality system. The Full Inspection Option audits at least four systems in the facility, one of which must be the quality system.

The Abbreviated Inspection Option is a surveillance or compliance inspection. It is a shortened inspection. This is performed when the facility has a satisfactory cGMP compliance record and there are no product problems or there has been little change since the last inspection. At least two systems are audited, including the quality system.

Figure 10.2 shows in simplified form the flow of an FDA inspection and the actions taken. Exhibit 10.2 summarizes the FDA guidelines for the inspection of manufacturers of bulk pharmaceutical chemicals (APIs), biotechnology and finished dosage form drugs. Inspections of biopharmaceutical manufacturing facilities are carried out by Team Biologics, which is a partnership between the Office of Regulatory Affairs and the Center for Biologics Evaluation and Research (CBER) of the Food and Drug Administration (FDA). Team Biologics consists of personnel with

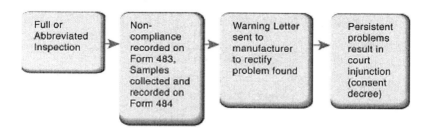

Figure 10.2 FDA inspection and action process

Exhibit 10.2 FDA Guides to Inspections

Guide to Inspections of Bulk Pharmaceutical Chemicals (BPC)—1991

Buildings and Facilities: Contamination/Cross Contamination, Water System/ Water Quality, Aseptic/Sterile Processing.

Equipment: Multipurpose Equipment, Equipment Cleaning and Use Log, Equipment Located Outdoors, Protected Environment, Cleaning of Product Contact Surfaces.

Raw Materials

Containers, Closures, and Packaging Components

Production and Process Controls: Mother Liquors, In-Process Blending/Mixing, Validation of Process and Control Procedures, Reprocessing, Process Change, Impurities.

In-Process Testing: Packaging and Labeling of Finished BPC

Expiration Dating or Re-evaluation Dating

Laboratory Controls

Stability Testing

Reserve Samples

Batch Production Records

Biotechnology Inspection Guide Reference Materials and Training Aids—1991

Cell Culture and Fermentation

    Master Cell Bank and Working Cell Bank

        Origin

        Characterization and History Qualifying Tests

        Storage Conditions and Maintenance

    Media

        Raw materials

        Bovine Serum

        Sterilization

Continued

Exhibit 10.2 *Continued*

Culture Growth
>Inoculation and Aseptic Transfer
>Monitoring of Growth Parameters and Control
>Containment and Containment Control

Ascites Production
>Mouse Colony
>>Characterization and Control of the Mouse Colony
>>Animal Quarters/Environmental Controls
>Manufacturing Processes
>>Animal Identification
>>Tapping Procedure
>>Storage and Pooling of Ascites
>>Purification

Extraction, Isolation and Purification
>Process Types
>Process Validation
>>Documentation
>>Validation
>>Follow-up Investigations
>Process Water/Buffers/WFI
>Plant Environment

Cleaning Procedure
>Detailed Cleaning Procedure
>Sampling Plan
>Analytical Method/Cleaning Limits

Processing and Filling
>Processing
>In-Process Quality Control
>Filling
>Lyophilization

Laboratory Controls
>Training
>Equipment Maintenance/Calibration/Monitoring
>Method Validation

Continued

Exhibit 10.2 *Continued*

> Standard/Reference Material
> Storage of Labile Components
> Laboratory SOPs

Testing

> Quality
> Identity
> Protein Concentration/Content
> Purity
> Potency
> Stability
> Batch-to-Batch Consistency

Environmental Coverage

> Environmental Assessment

Guide to Inspections of Dosage Form Drug Manufacturer

Organization and Personnel

Buildings and Facilities

Equipment

Components and Product Containers

Production and Process Controls: Critical Manufacturing Steps, Equipment Identification, In-Line and Bulk Testing, Actual Yield, Personnel Habits

Sterile Products: Personnel, Buildings, Air, Environmental Controls, Equipment, WFI, Containers and Closures, Sterilization, Laboratory Controls, Production Records.

skills and experience in the biopharmaceutical manufacturing to ensure critical areas are inspected.

If the inspector believes the cGMP has been violated, Form FDA-483 is used to record the observations. Samples may be taken by the FDA inspector for analysis. In this case, Form FDA-484 is issued to the manufacturer for the receipt of samples. A normal practice for the manufacturer is to take more samples for internal analysis and compare with the FDA data when required.

After inspection, the inspector prepares a detailed Establishment Inspection Report (EIR). This is the FDA's primary record for the inspection. Time is given to manufacturer to respond to the deficiencies found and recorded in Form FDA-483. Failure to comply with satisfactory resolution to the deficiencies found will result in the FDA sending out a Warning Letter notifying the manufacturer to comply. If the manufacturer is unable to resolve the deficiency after the deadline set by the FDA, the FDA may proceed to prosecute the manufacturer with an injunction. The injunction is a court order called Consent Decree, and the manufacturer may be required to cease operations until the problem is rectified.

In Europe, inspections are conducted by Member States on behalf of the European Union. For drugs approved under the centralized procedure, inspections are coordinated by the European Agency for the Evaluation of Medicinal Products (EMEA; refer to Sections 7.3 and 8.3.2). For countries that are members of the Pharmaceutical Inspection Cooperation Scheme (PIC/S; Section 7.10), there is mutual recognition of inspections performed by members.

Some typical problems found in GMP inspections are:

- Out-of-specifications: Insufficient investigations to determine root cause of problems and issues are not closed in a timely manner.
- Product sterility: The tests performed are superficial and not validated
- Environment monitoring: Personnel are not monitored, inadequate monitoring, microorganisms are not monitored, there is no identification of contaminants, alert limits for contaminants are set too high
- Raw materials, components and finished product: No or insufficient audit procedure, test methods lack validation
- Training: There is no training plan, training is not documented, investigation of problems in manufacturing does not lead to retraining of staff involved
- Materials: There is no segregation of materials
- Calibration: Lack of scheduling and lapsed calibration validity
- Documentation: Manufacturing steps are not signed off, changes are not explained, obsolete copies of document are used
- Process: Personnel not following set procedures, procedures are not validated
- Internal audit and review: Infrequent internal audit performed, superficial audit insufficient to reveal problems, no follow-up on issues observed at internal audits
- Management: Lack or insufficient commitment on GMP issues.

Examples of some of the typical violations leading to drug product recall according to the FDA (1996) are:

- cGMP deviations
- Sub-potent products
- Product failed *US Pharmacopoeia* dissolution test requirements
- Product failed endotoxin/pyrogen tests
- Presence of contaminants in product
- Label mix-up on the product
- Stability data do not support expiration date
- Product lacks stability
- Product failed content uniformity
- Product failed pH test requirements.

The new initiative from the FDA, *Pharmaceutical Current Good Manufacturing Practices (cGMPs) for the 21st century: A Risk Based Approach*, will have a major effect on the conduct of GMP inspections (see Section 9.7). In early 2003, the FDA has identified three categories of potentially higher-risk drug manufacturing sites for prioritizing inspections:

- Sites making sterile drugs
- Sites making prescription drugs
- Sites of new registrants not previously inspected by the FDA.

By 2004, the FDA intends to develop a more detailed model for cGMP inspections centered on the risk-based approach.

10.4 MANUFACTURE OF SMALL MOLECULE APIs (CHEMICAL SYNTHESIS METHODS)

10.4.1 Conventional synthesis techniques

The manufacturing process for a small molecule API is shown in Figure 10.3. Typically, the chemical reactions are performed in large reaction vessels. For commercial production of an API, the reaction vessel can typically range from 1000 L to 20 000 L in volume (Figure 10.4).

The reaction vessel is normally made of glass-lined stainless steel with a jacket for heating and cooling and consists of:

- Charge-hole for addition of solid raw materials
- Metered-pump input for liquids
- Supply of gases as reactants or inert blanket
- Stirrer for mixing the raw materials
- Condenser unit for solvent reflux

- Vents with filters for gas emission or depressurization
- Transfer line for discharge/separation of reactants/products
- Probes for measuring the temperature, pH and pressure
- Sampling ports for withdrawals of samples for analysis.

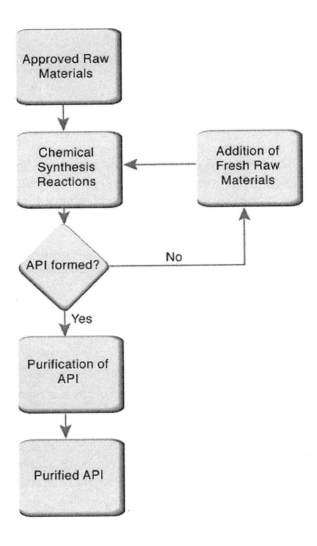

Figure 10.3 Chemical synthesis of small molecule APIs

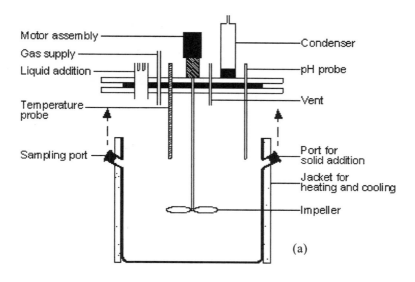

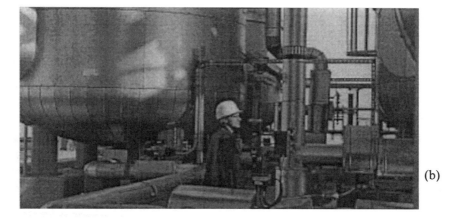

Figure 10.4 Reaction vessel for the manufacture of an API; (a) Schematic drawing, (b) Photo courtesy of Vega Grieshaber KG, Germany.

Production of the API begins with the selection of a synthetic route, as determined in the development program. Raw materials are added into a reaction vessel. These raw materials as reactants are heated or cooled in the reaction vessel (normal range is from –15 °C to 140 °C; purpose-built vessels are needed for extreme reactions that require lower or higher temperature controls or pressurization of reaction processes). The chemical synthesis reactions are monitored and controlled via sensor probes (pH, temperature, and pressure) with in-process feedback controls for adjustments when necessary. Samples are withdrawn at defined intervals for analysis to determine the reaction progress. Catalysts, including enzymes, may be added to speed up and direct the reaction along a certain pathway.

It is important to maintain a uniform reaction environment within the vessel chamber by using a stirrer to agitate and mix the reactants. Gaseous discharge is vented through filters to the outside environment. As the reactions may generate substantial heat (exothermic) and pressure, or may even be potentially explosive, special precautionary features are designed into the vessel.

At the end of the synthesis reactions, the product can be pumped to another vessel or container via transfer lines. If the chemical reactions proceed to completion with negligible trace quantities of impurities, the next stage of production may commence in the same reaction vessel with addition of fresh raw materials. This process is called telescoping.

The finished product is centrifuged and purified via a number of processes, including filtration, fractional distillation, condensation, crystallization and chromatographic separation techniques. The purified API is tested and then it is ready to be formulated into the finished dosage form, as discussed in Section 10.6. Exhibit 10.3 illustrates some of the typical reagents for API manufacture and Exhibit 10.4 presents selected chemical reactions as examples of the synthesis processes for drug manufacture. Purification processes for drug materials are described in Exhibit 10.5.

The production of the API and finished dosage form is required to comply with GMP regulations discussed in Chapter 9 and Section 10.2. The quality system, quality control and validation of equipment and processes have to be developed and adhered to in the manufacturing process. Proper records and documentation are required to be kept in the forms of batch records, test records and manufacturing procedures. Reaction vessels and associated equipment must be calibrated, validated and cleaned to acceptable levels before being used; this is especially the case for multi-product plants where more than one API is manufactured.

As an example, we present in Exhibit 10.6 the synthesis of paclitaxel (Taxol, Bristol-Myers Squibb), an important anticancer drug for breast and ovarian cancer and Kaposi sarcoma. It illustrates the complexity in the synthesis of drug molecules.

Exhibit 10.3 Typical Reagents for API Manufacture

Solvents

Water (Purified Water or Water-for-Injection grade)

Toluene, methanol, ethanol, ether, acetate, dimethyl sulfoxide, tetrahydrofuran, hexane, cyclohexane, dichloromethane, acetonitrile, acetone

Oxidizing agents

Hydrogen peroxide, chromic acid, potassium permanganate, manganese dioxide, ozone

Reducing agents

Hydrogen, lithium aluminum hydride, sodium borohydride, di-isobutyl aluminum hydride, iron metal

Acids

Sulfuric acid, hydrochloric acid, phosphoric acid, methanesulfonic acid, acetic acid, formic acid

Bases

Sodium hydroxide, ammonia, triethylamine, pyridine, butyl lithium, sodium hydride, *α*-methylbenzylamine

Halogenation reagents

Halogens, *N*-bromo- and *N*-chlorosuccinimide, thionyl chloride, phosphorus oxychloride

Alkylating agents

Dimethyl sulfate, methyl iodide, methyl tosylate

Sulfur reagents

Thiols and sulfides, hydrogen sulfide, sodium sulfide, sodium thiocyanate, thiourea, sodium metabisulfide

Phosphorus reagents

Phosphorus halides

Boron reagents

Diborane, boron trifluoride, dialkyl borinates, aryl boronic acids.

SOURCE Lee, S. and Robinson, G., *Process Development: Fine Chemicals from Grams to Kilograms*, Oxford Chemistry Series, Oxford University Press, Oxford, 1995.

Exhibit 10.4 Selected Chemical Reactions as Examples for API Manufacture

Halogenation

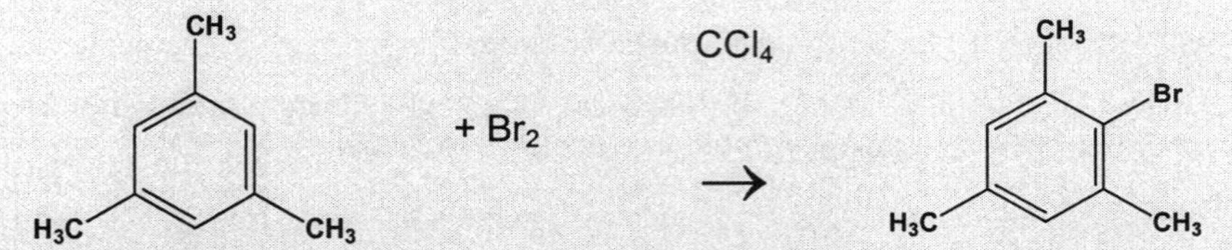

Alkylation

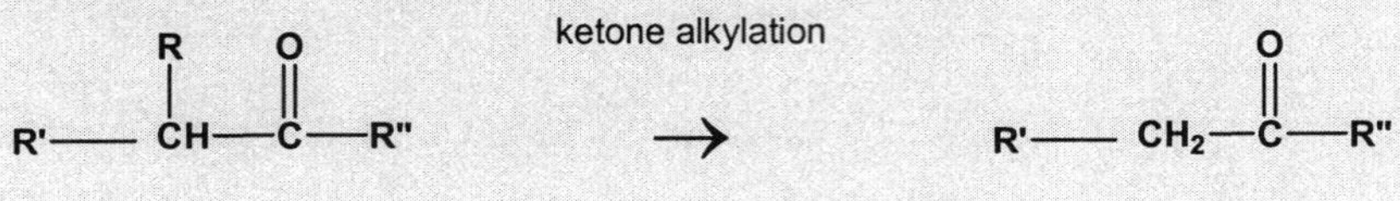

ketone alkylation

Acylation

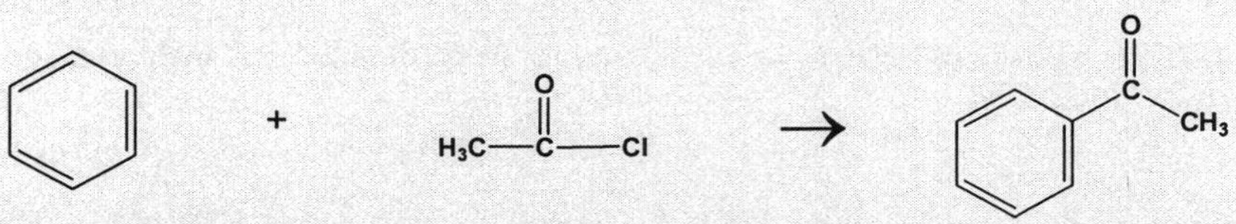

Grignard reaction

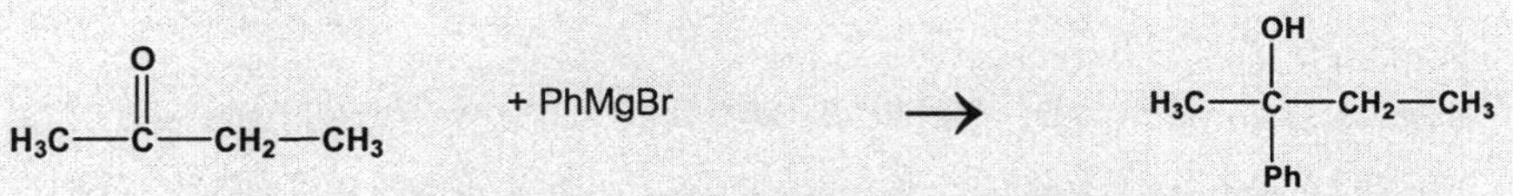

SOURCE Hornback, J.M., *Organic Chemistry*, Brooks/Cole Publishing Company, CA, 1998.

Exhibit 10.5 Purification of an API

Filtration/fractional distillation/condensation

Filters are used to remove solid particles from a solvent. The use of $0.2\,\mu m$ filters can remove microbial contamination. Filtered solutions can be fractionally distilled and condensed to obtain the API.

Crystallization

Crystallization is used to separate the API from its solvent and impurities, or to separate racemic mixtures in solution. Crystallization occurs from a supersaturated solution. Important conditions are the temperature, concentration, stirring rate and heating and cooling rate. Seeding with the desired API can assist in providing nucleation sites for the preferential crystallization of the API.

SOURCE Carstensen, J.T., *Advanced Pharmaceutical Solids, Drugs and the Pharmaceutical Sciences*, Vol. 110, Chapter 6, pp. 89–106, Marcel Dekker, New York, 2001.   *Continued*

Exhibit 10.5 *Continued*

Chromatography
Chromatographic separation relies on the affinity of binding between different components of the API in liquid and the solid column matrix. The API is separated from the impurities by percolating the liquid through chromatographic columns filled with solid phase matrices. The matrices are made of different materials and separate the components on the basis of physicochemical properties such as charges, size and shape, hydrophobic and hydrophilic characteristics, complex formation with certain ions or metals, and interaction with dyes.

Exhibit 10.6 Synthesis of Paclitaxel (Taxol)

An introduction to Taxol (Bristol-Myers Squibb) is presented in Exhibit 3.4. The active pharmaceutical ingredient (API) is paclitaxel. The chemical name is $5\beta,20$-Epoxy-$1,2\alpha,4,7\beta,10\beta,13\alpha$-hexahydroxytax-11-en-9-one 4,10-diacetate 2-benzoate 13 ester with ($2R$, $3S$)-N-benzoyl-3-phenylisoserine.

Early production of 1 kg of paclitaxel required extraction from about 13 000 kg of the Pacific yew tree bark. This process was refined, and paclitaxel is now produced by a semi-synthetic route. The starting material, 10-deacetyl baccatin III (10-DAB) is obtained from the needles of *Taxus baccata* (European yews) or *T. wallichiana* (Himalayan yews). The yield is around 1000 kg of needles to produce 1 kg of 10-DAB.

SOURCE Cabri, W. and Di Fabio, R., *From Bench to Market: The Evolution of Chemical Synthesis*, Oxford University Press, Oxford, 2000.

10.4.2 Chiral synthesis techniques

Production of synthetic drug often gives rise to racemic mixtures of API enantiomers, i.e. they are mirror images of each other (see Section 3.5). The first problem is if the production process generates equal amounts of the enantiomers and only one enantiomer is active. In this case, only half the yield is effective for drug application. Another problem is that often one isomer is effective and the other may be benign or create undesirable side effects when interacting with biological receptors that are chiral in themselves. Examples of the differing effectiveness of chiral drugs are presented in Exhibit 10.7.

Manufacturing of chiral drugs has become increasingly important; first to improve potency, secondly to improve yield, and thirdly to extend the patent life for approved drugs based on racemic mixtures. Stereoselective synthetic methods are used to produce chiral drugs. There are three basic methods being applied:

Exhibit 10.7 Examples of Chiral Drugs

Thalidomide: The (R)-enantiomer is a sedative and the (S)-enantiomer is teratogenic, i.e. causes fetal deformity.

Propranolol: An antihypertensive drug: the (S)-enantiomer is 130-fold more potent than the (R)-enantiomer, a β-adrenoceptor antagonist.

Dextropropoxyphene: The (2R,3S)-enantiomer marketed as Davron is an analgesic, whereas the (2S,3R)-enantiomer called Novrad is an antitussive.

Dexetimide: Dexetimide has 10 000-fold more affinity for the muscarinic acetylcholine receptor than its enantiomer, levetimide.

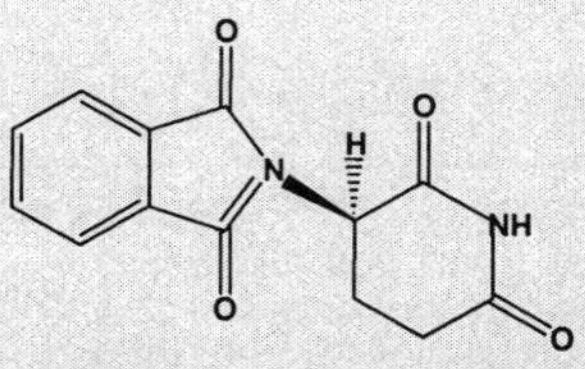

(R)-Thalidomide 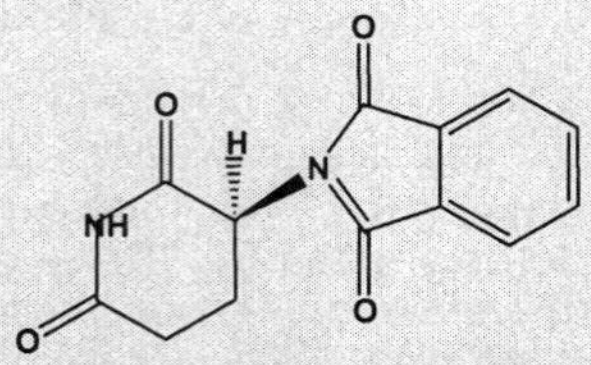   (S)-Thalidomide

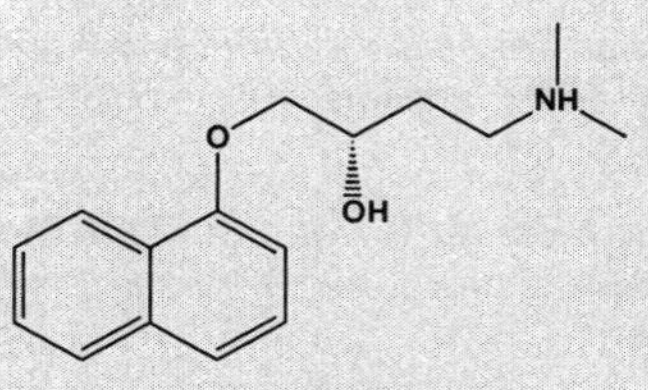

(S)-Propranolol 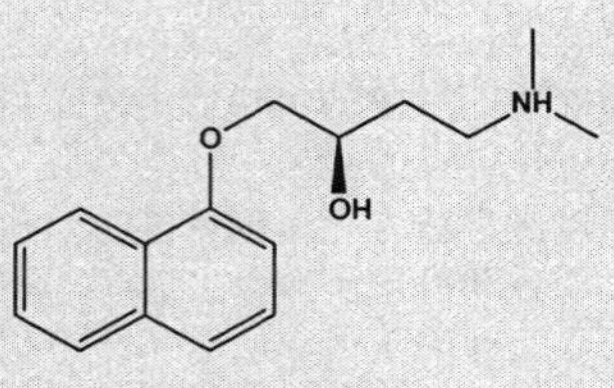   (R)-Propranolol

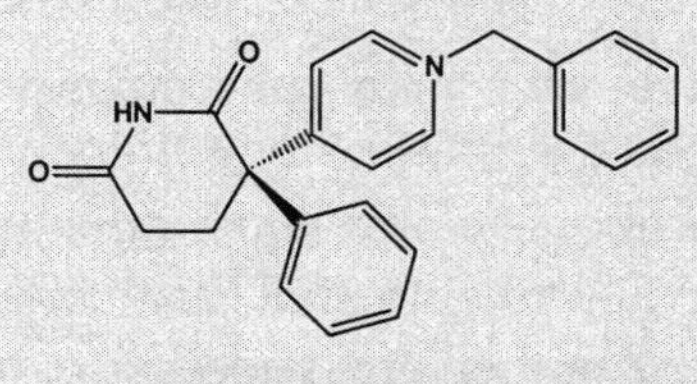

(S)-(+)-Dexetimide 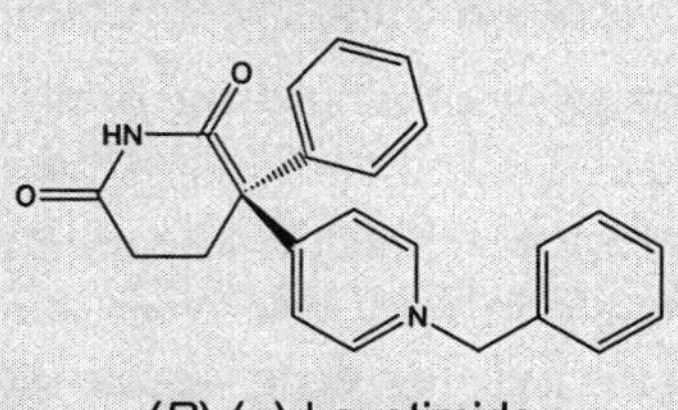   (R)-(−)-Levetimide

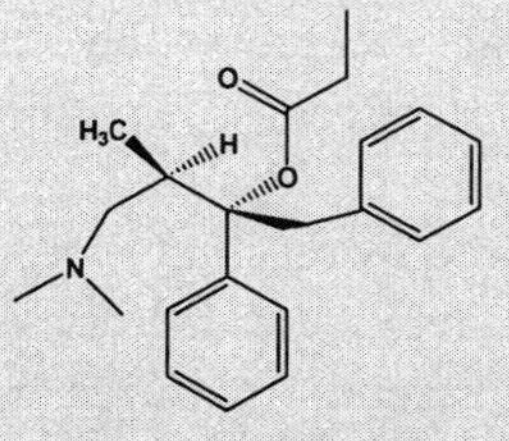

Darvon 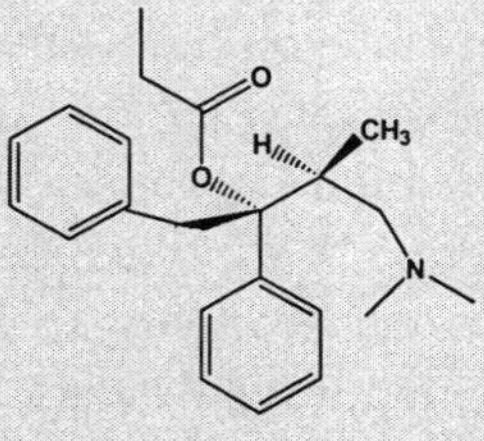   Novrad

- Enzyme and non-enzyme catalysts
- Chiral building blocks
- Chiral auxiliary.

Enzyme and non-enzyme catalysts

By nature, enzymes themselves are chiral and they catalyze a variety of chemical reactions with stereoselectivity. These reactions include oxidations, reductions, and hydrations. Examples of enzymes are oxidases, dehydrogenases, lipases, and proteases. Metoprolol, an adrenoceptor-blocking drug, is produced using an enzyme-catalyzed method.

Non-organic and organometallic catalysts are also used to channel the reactions towards the chiral synthesis pathway. The drug called levodopa, (S)-3,4-dihydroxyalanine, is an effective drug against Parkinson's disease. It is stereoselectively manufactured using catalysts such as rhodium or ruthenium complexes.

Chiral building blocks

Some drugs are made using chiral building blocks to generate the required chiral centre in the drug. The introduction of chiral centers ensures that the reaction proceeds in the desired direction. The preparation of enalapril, an ACE inhibitor, is an example of the use of chiral building blocks.

Chiral auxiliary

A chiral auxiliary is an intermediate formed by the attachment of a pure enantiomer to an achiral substrate. The attachment, called a chiral auxiliary, restricts the approach of reactants to react in specific ways to produce the chiral molecule. The antibacterial drug, aztreonam, is synthesized using the chiral auxiliary method.

10.5 MANUFACTURE OF LARGE MOLECULE APIs (RECOMBINANT DNA METHODS)

The manufacturing process for a typical large molecule protein-based API is shown in Figure 10.5. The production of these APIs uses 'factories' that are living cells in the form of cell lines, which can grow indefinitely under appropriate conditions. As discussed in Section 4.3.3, monoclonal antibodies are conventionally produced using hybridoma cell lines. Other protein-based drugs are produced using a variety of cell lines: from bacterial or fungal to insect and mammalian cell lines.

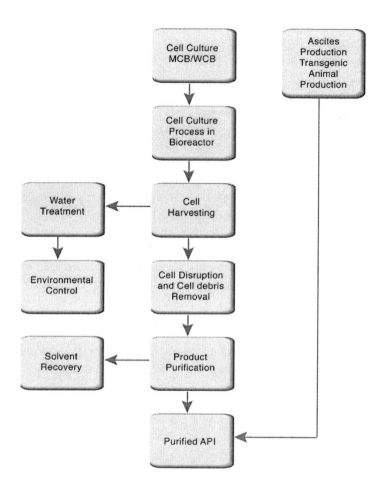

Figure 10.5 Cell culture production of biopharmaceutical drug
SOURCE   Adapted from Food and Drug Administration, *Biotechnology Inspection Guide: Reference Materials and Training Aids*, FDA, Rockville, MD, 1991.

Currently, about equal numbers of the approved protein drugs are derived from microbial and mammalian cells, although more drugs are expected to be produced from mammalian cell lines in the future. There are pros and cons for each type of cells as production 'factories' for the protein drugs:

Microbial cells (for example E. coli cells)
Advantages: Cells grow rapidly on relatively inexpensive media; the

fermentation technology for growing microbial cells is well established.
Disadvantages: The protein expressed is accumulated within the cell matrix
(intracellular); protein does not undergo post-translational modifications;
likely presence of lipopolysaccharides (pyrogens) to contaminate product,
and the need for more extensive chromatographic purification.

Mammalian cells (for example Chinese hamster ovary and baby hamster kidney cell)

Advantages: Post-translational modification of protein product can be
performed; extracellular expression of proteins, which requires less complex
purification processes.
Disadvantages: Cells have complex nutritional requirements; higher
production cost; cells grow more slowly and are susceptible to physical
damage; requires specially designed bioreactors.

The recombinant technique involves transfecting cells with DNA that
codes for the production of the intended protein. The process of transfection
is shown in Exhibit 10.8. Once transfected, the cells (microbial or
mammalian) grow and divide as clones and express the intended protein
through instructions from the foreign DNA genes introduced into the cells.

A master cell bank (MCB) is set up which forms the first generation of
these clones. They are stored in hundreds of vials under liquid nitrogen
freezers ($-150\,°C$ or below) to preserve them indefinitely. From the MCB, a
vial is taken and another generation of clones is produced, these constitute
the working cell bank (WCB), and they too are maintained in liquid nitrogen
freezers. Subsequently, a vial is taken from the WCB for each batch of
production. This two-tier system of MCB and WCB can supply production
needs indefinitely. For example, 200 vials each of the MCB and WCB for a
production rate of 10 batches per year will last 4000 years.

Cells from the WCB are cultured initially in flasks, which contain nutrient
medium. The medium may contain the following:

- Amino acids
- Vitamins A, D, E and K
- Ionic salts (Na^+, K^+, Mg^{2+}, Ca^{2+}, Cl^-, SO_4^{2-}, PO_4^{3-}, HCO_3^-)
- Glucose (as a source of energy)
- Organic supplements (proteins, peptides, nucleoside, citric acid, lipids, cholesterols)
- Hormones, growth factors, antibodies and antibiotics.

Exhibit 10.8 Recombinant DNA Techniques – Genetic Engineering

The first step is the isolation of DNA genes that code for the production of the desired protein. The next stage is the insertion of these genes (foreign DNA) into a vector, or carrier. Common vectors used are the bacteriophage (a virus) and the bacterial plasmids, which are circular bacterial DNA.

Both the foreign DNA and plasmid are cleaved by an enzyme called a restriction endonuclease. They are mixed and then joined together using another enzyme called ligase.

The plasmid with the inserted DNA genes is transfected (introduced) into bacterial or mammalian cells. Methods used include electroporation, microinsertion or chemical mediated transfection. When these cells are cultured in medium with nutrients, they grow and divide. In the growth process, the foreign genes express proteins within the cell (intracellular) or outside the cells (extracellular). At the end of the growth cycle, the cells are killed and the proteins are extracted and purified as the protein drug material. The process is illustrated below, where the cells act as 'factories' for producing the protein of interest.

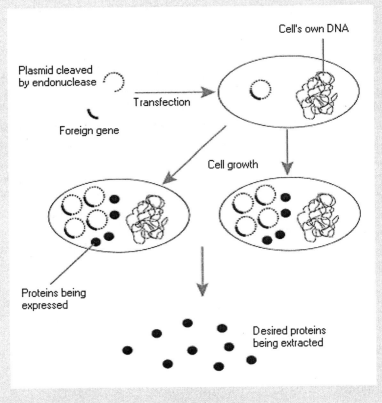

In certain cases, serum (fetal bovine serum [FBS]) is added to promote the growth of cells. However, the Bovine Spongiform Encephalopathy (BSE) problem has necessitated tight control on the quality of FBS (refer to Exhibit 10.9). This increases production and downstream processing costs. For new cell lines being developed, serum-free and protein-free media are used to circumvent the possibility of virus contamination from animal sources and the variation that may arise from use of serum from animal herd.

Exhibit 10.9 Bovine Spongiform Encephalopathy

Bovine spongiform encephalopathy (BSE or 'mad cow disease') is a progressive neurological degenerative disease in cattle. It is caused by a mutated protein called a prion. BSE was first reported in the United Kingdom in 1986. Creutzfeldt-Jakob disease (CJD) is a rare disease that occurs in humans. Evidence to date indicates it is possible for humans to acquire CJD after consuming BSE-contaminated cattle products.

A number of measures have been taken to contain BSE. Thousands of cattle have been culled and there are controls prohibiting the feeding of mammalian proteins to ruminant animals (cows, sheep and goats). There are also surveillance programs set up to monitor CJD in humans.

The FDA and European regulatory authorities have strongly recommended drug manufacturers not use materials derived from ruminant animals in countries where BSE has been reported. Manufacturers of protein drugs that require fetal bovine serum (FBS) for cell growth use FBS from countries such as the US, Australia and New Zealand—countries considered safe from BSE. As precautionary measures, newly developed cell lines for production of protein drugs are focusing on serum-free and protein-free growth medium.

Most cells grow well under a fermentation process at a pH of around 7.0 to 7.4. However, as cells grow CO_2, is produced. To maintain optimal growth, the media are often buffered with, for example, phosphate buffered saline. Cells go through different phases of growth (Figure 10.6). The cell viability, density and consumption of nutrients are constantly monitored (Figure 10.7).

When the cells grow to a certain density (number of cells per milliliter, around $1\text{--}3 \times 10^6$ cells/mL) and have an acceptable viability (normally >90% survival rate), they are inoculated into larger vessels called bioreactors. There may be several steps for growth in different size bioreactors before a final production bioreactor is used, which may be as large as 10 000 to 20 000 L.

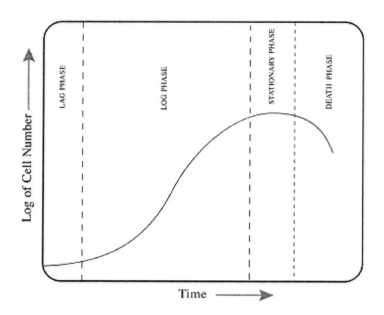

Figure 10.6 Stages of cell growth

Cells grow under different conditions that have been optimized in the development stage. Some cells prefer to anchor onto solid substrates. In this case, microcarrier beads or hollow fibers are used to provide attachment for the cells. Some other cells grow best in suspension within the media. Yet, in other cases, continuous supply and harvesting of the cells are optimal; these are the perfusion techniques. The advantages and disadvantages of these methods are described in Exhibit 10.10. Cells are monitored for growth, viability, consumption of nutrient, discharge of metabolites and use of oxygen and carbon dioxide.

As cells grow, proteins are secreted. At the end of the growth cycle, the proteins are harvested. For cells that produce intracellular proteins, the cell membranes are lysed to free the proteins. The proteins are purified, normally via several stages through chromatographic columns (Exhibit 10.11). The purified protein as an API is tested to ensure it meets specifications. Once it passes the requisite specifications, it is ready to be processed into the finished form (see Section 10.6).

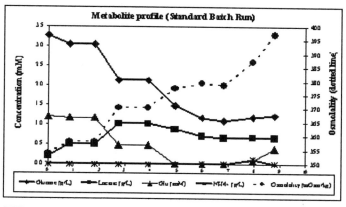

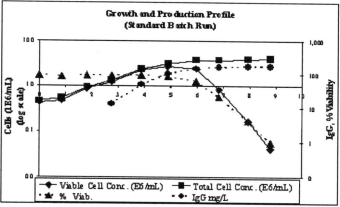

Figure 10.7 Monitoring of cell growth and generation of metabolite over time

Exhibit 10.10 Cell Culture Methods

Suspension process (stirred/sparged tank)

Advantages: Easy to operate in batch and fed-batch; easy to obtain cell sampling to determine cell concentration and viability; easy to scale up.

Disadvantages: Sensitive to shear force from stirrer; foaming when serum is added to media.

Anchorage-dependent process (microcarriers, hollow fiber)

Advantages: Established technology; easy to scale up.

Disadvantages: Cells only grow when attached to solid substrates; cells require additional attachment factor; more cleaning validation issues and high disposal cost; more difficult to operate than Suspension Process.

Exhibit 10.11 Purification using Chromatographic Techniques

Ion exchange: Separation is based on selective, reversible adsorption of charged molecules to an immobilized ion exchange group of opposite charge. An ion exchanger consists of an insoluble porous matrix to which charged groups have been covalently bound. Anion exchanger group: DEAE, Diethylaminoethyl; QAE, Quaternary aminoethyl; Q, Quaternary ammonium. Cation exchanger group: Carboxymethyl, sulfopropyl.

Affinity: Product to be purified binds to an affinity ligand that is coupled to a matrix. The ligand is specific for a particular type of protein/peptide molecule, or group of such molecules. The targeted product binds to the ligand under specific conditions of high or low ionic strengths and at a certain pH. After the unbound impurities are removed, the product can be eluted by using a gradient of increasing or decreasing ionic strength or by changing the pH.

Hydrophobic: Proteins and peptides differ from one another in their hydrophobic properties. Salt solutions are used to mediate the binding of molecules to a hydrophobic matrix substituted with a hydrophobic ligand.

Reversed phase: This technique is based on hydrophobic regions on the surface of proteins and the hydrophobic groups covalently attached to the surface of the matrix. Organic solvents are required for elution. It is suitable for peptides and proteins up to 2.4×10^4 Da.

Gel filtration: Separation is in accordance to size. Large molecules elute in void volumes and are eluted earlier. Small molecules penetrate pores of the matrix and elute later because of increase in path length.

Cells grow from a single vial (1–5 mL) to thousands of liters in bioreactors. Many generations of cell division and growth are involved. It is important that in this process, which may last weeks to months, the cells do not mutate and faithfully express the intended protein. Cells at the completion of production are collected as an end of production cell bank (EPCB), and analyzed to verify that the protein is produced properly.

Exhibit 10.12 presents the production of etanercept (Enbrel, Immunex), a new generation drug for the treatment of rheumatoid arthritis.

10.6 FINISHED DOSAGE FORMS

10.6.1 Examples of different dosage forms

A finished dosage form is a drug formulated with an API and excipients in a form that is suitable for administering to patients. Some of the reasons for preparing finished dosage forms are:

Exhibit 10.12 Etanercept (Enbrel)

Etanercept (Enbrel, Immunex) is a dimerized protein molecule that consists of a portion of the tumor necrosis factor receptor coupled to the Fc portion of human IgG1 (see Section 4.3). It has 934 amino acids and a molecular weight of approximately 150 kDa.

Etanercept is produced by recombinant technology in a Chinese hamster ovary mammalian cell expression system. The WCB are grown in proprietary media system. The cells are cultured initially in flasks and then inoculated into the bioreactor vessel. The product is purified in a number of chromatographic steps, followed by viral inactivation and viral filtration steps.

The finished form is a sterile, lyophilized powder formulated with trimethamine, mannitol and sucrose as excipients.

SOURCE   Center for Biologics Evaluation and Research, *Chemistry, Manufacturing and Controls Review, BLA 980286, TNFR:Fc, Immunex*, FDA, Rockville,   MD,   1998;   Immunex,   *Enbrel*, http:///www.immunex.com/search/searchresults.jsp [accessed Jan 10, 2003].

- An exact quantity of the effective drug is incorporated into the formulation
- Drug products are easier to handle and this increases compliance in taking or administering the drug
- Preservatives and stabilizers can be added to the API to improve shelf life and result in less stringent storage conditions
- Taste, color and odor of the API can be masked by additions of excipients
- Delivery vehicles (Section 5.6) can be used to provide more specific targeting of the drug to receptors
- Extended drug effect can be maintained with controlled release formulations
- Different types of delivery mechanisms can be achieved for effective drug action, e.g. intravenous injection, inhalation, sublingual application.

Table 10.1 lists the finished dosage forms for various routes of drug administration. The choice of which finished dosage form to administer to a patient depends on a number of factors. These factors include the nature of the disease, time required for onset of drug action, age of patient, site of intended receptor, and health status of patients. In general, where possible, drug manufacturers provide several dosage forms for an API to enable it to be applied in different ways for achieving reliable and effective therapy.

Table 10.1 Finished dosage form application

Route of administration	Finished dosage form
Oral	Tablets, capsules, solutions, syrups, gels, powders
Sublingual	Tablets, lozenges
Parenteral	Solutions, suspensions
Topical	Ointments, creams, pastes, powders, lotions, solutions, aerosols
Inhalational	Aerosols, sprays
Rectal	Solutions, ointments, suppositories
Vaginal	Solutions, ointments, tablets, suppositories
Urethral	Solutions

SOURCE Ansel, H.C., *Introduction to Pharmaceutical Dosage Forms*, 3rd edn., Lea & Febiger, London, 1981, p. 48.

Solids Solid dosage forms are the most common means for presenting the drug product for patient administration. Most APIs are in crystallized or powder forms. They are ground to predetermined sizes using mills or pulverizers. The APIs and excipients are then mixed using blenders or tumblers.

Tablets are manufactured through a compression process. Excipients such as binders, lubricants, colorants, flavorings and disintegration modifiers are added. The production process has to ensure that tablets have the required mechanical strength and do not crumble. Tablets may be coated or uncoated. Uncoated tablets consist of granules of API and excipients compressed into tablets. Various substances are applied to coat tablets, from sugar to waxes, gums, plasticizers and flavorings. Effervescent tablets contain acids or carbonates, which, when mixed with water, release carbon dioxide to disperse the drug materials. Release modifiers are added to tablets to alter the time and duration of drug release. Enteric coatings are used to protect drugs from being dissolved in the acid environment of the stomach.

Capsules consist of shells for enclosing drug materials. Hard gelatin shells are made of gelatin, sugar and water. Soft gelatin shells have additional glycerin or sorbitol to soften the wall. Powder or liquid can fill the capsule shells. Hard capsules consist of two prefabricated shell sections. Drug API and excipients in solid form or paste are placed in one section and it then is capped with the other section. Soft capsules are mainly filled with liquids and sealed in one operation. There are modified-release capsules for delayed-release or sustained-release application. Another type is the specially formulated shells that are resistant to acid in stomach, for drug release in the intestine.

An important specification for solid dosage form manufacture is the dissolution factor. The product is formulated and manufactured such that it will have the specified dissolution profile for maximum effectiveness.

Liquids   The liquid dosage form comes in several categories: solution, emulsion and suspension. They are prepared by dissolving the API in solvents such as water (purified water), alcohol, glycerin or glycol. Flavorants, colorants, antioxidants, preservatives and agents for stabilizing, emulsifying and thickening are often added to the solution to prepare the required liquid formulation. Important criteria in the manufacture of liquid dosage form are the uniformity of dispersion and the effectiveness of preservatives.

Parenterals   The most important criterion for parenterals is that they have to be sterile for injection or infusion administration. Excipients are added to make parenterals isotonic with blood, improve solubility, and control pH of the solution. The solvent vehicles include water-for-injection, sterile sodium chloride, potassium chloride, or calcium chloride solution, and nonaqueous solvents such as alcohol, glycol and glycerin. Preservatives, antioxidants and stabilizers are normally added to enhance the properties of the drug product.

Manufacturing is performed in cleanroom conditions. Sterilization processes in the forms of heat, steam, gas or radiation are applied to ensure microorganisms are destroyed in the drug product. For protein-based drugs that can be damaged by the normal sterilization processes, the product is manufactured under aseptic conditions. Both sterility and pyrogen (microbial substances that causes fever) tests are performed to ensure parenteral drug products are safe to be injected.

Inhalants   Inhalants are pressurized dosage forms whereby powder or liquid drug substances are delivered in fine dispersions of aerosols or sprays by propellants. Typically, the particle size of the API is in the range of 2– 20 µm for delivery to the respiratory system, and larger sizes for topical applications. Excipients such as preservatives, stabilizers and diluents are added. The manufacturing of inhalants involves filling the container with the API, propellant, liquid (if required) and excipients. The container is capped with a valve assembly and actuator for control of dosage. Production issues are the effectiveness of preservatives, container leakages and control of dosage delivery.

Ointments and creams   Ointments are applied to the skin for topical treatment or to be absorbed into the blood system for delivery to target areas. They are semisolid preparations obtained by mixing the API with selected ointment bases depending on intended use. These bases include petrolatum, paraffin, mineral oil, lanolin and glycols. Preservatives are often added to ensure the ointments will maintain the recommended shelf life.

Creams are less viscous than ointments. They are dispersions of the API in emulsions. Both oil-in-water and water-in-oil emulsions have their applications.

10.6.2 Packaging and labeling

The finished dosage forms are packaged into blister packs, bottles, vials, syringes, aerosol containers or tubes. Nowadays, packaging has tamper-proof designs to ensure the integrity of the packaging. Labeling of the packaging is in accordance with information submitted to regulatory authorities. Exhibit 10.13 describes the FDA regulations for packaging and labeling of intermediates, APIs and finished dosage forms.

Exhibit 10.13 Packaging and Labeling of APIs and Intermediates (ICH (1997) Guide for API: Good Manufacturing Practice). Also Including Finished Dosage Forms

- Written procedures for receipt, identification, quarantine, sampling, examination, testing, release, and handling of packaging and labeling materials
- Records of shipment and packaging
- Containers suitable for intended use, not be reactive, additive or absorptive to intermediates or API and protect contents from deterioration and contamination
- Access to labels limited to authorized personnel
- Reconciliation of quantities of labels issued and used
- Procedures to ensure correct packaging and labels are used
- Labeling operations should prevent mix-ups
- Examination of containers and packages to ensure use of correct labels
- Transport materials with seals that will alert recipient possibility of alteration if seal has been breached.

10.7 FURTHER READING

Ansel, H.C., *Introduction to Pharmaceutical Dosage Forms*, 3rd. edn., Lea & Febiger, Philadelphia, 1981.

British Pharmacopoeia (2002).

Cabri, W. and Di Fabio, R., *From Bench to Market: The Evolution of Chemical Synthesis*, Oxford University Press, Oxford, 2000.

Campbell, M.K., *Biochemistry*, 3rd edn., Harcourt Brace & Company, FL, 1999.

FDAnews, *Surviving an FDA inspection*, Washington Business Information, Inc., Virginia, 2001.

Food and Drug Administration, *Biotechnology Inspection Guide Reference Materials and Training Aids*, FDA, Rockville, MD, 1991.

Food and Drug Administration, *Guide to Inspections of Bulk Pharmaceutical Chemicals*, FDA, Rockville, MD, 1991.

Food and Drug Administration, *Guide to Inspections of Dosage Form Drug Manufacturers*, FDA, Rockville, MD, 1993.

Food and Drug Administration, *The Compliance Program Guidance Manual for FDA Staff: Drug Manufacturing Inspections Program 7356.002*, FDA, Rockville, MD, 2002.

International Conference on Harmonization, *Derivation and Characterization of Cell Substrates Used for Production of Biotechnological/Biological Products*, ICH, 1997.

International Conference on Harmonization, *Specifications: Test Procedures and Acceptance Criteria for Biotechnological/Biological Products*, ICH, 1999.

International Conference on Harmonization, *Specifications: Test Procedures and Acceptance Criteria for New Drug Substances and New Drug Products: Chemical Substances*, ICH, 1999.

International Conference on Harmonization, *Viral Safety Evaluation of Biotechnology Products Derived from Cell Lines of Human or Animal Origin*, ICH, 1997.

King, F.D. (ed.), *Medicinal Chemistry Principles and Practice*, Royal Society of Chemistry, Cambridge, UK, 1999.

Klegerman, M.E. and Groves, M.J., *Pharmaceutical Biotechnology: Fundamentals and Essentials*, Interpharm Press, Inc., Buffalo Grove, IL, 1992.

Krogsgaard-Larsen, P., LilJefors, T. and Madsen, U. (eds.), *Textbook of Drug Design and Discovery*, 3rd edn, Taylor & Francis, London, 2002.

Lee, S. and Robinson, G., *Process Development: Fine Chemicals from Grams to Kilograms*, Oxford Science Publications, Oxford, 1995.

Repic, O., *Principles of Process Research and Chemical Development in the Pharmaceutical Industry*, John Wiley & Sons, Inc., New York, 1998.

Thomas, G., *Medicinal Chemistry, An Introduction*, John Wiley & Sons, Ltd., Chichester, 2000.

US Pharmacopoeia 26 and National Formulary 21, The Official Compendia of Standards, 2003.

Walsh, G., *Biopharmaceutical: Biochemistry and Biotechnology*, John Wiley & Sons, Chichester, 1998.

Welling, P.G., Lasagna, L. and Banakar, U.V. (eds.), *The Drug Development Process: Increasing Efficiency and Cost Effectiveness*, Marcel Dekker, Inc., New York, 1996.

CHAPTER 11

FUTURE PERSPECTIVES

1.1 PAST ADVANCES AND FUTURE CHALLENGES

Drug discovery and development underwent astounding changes in the last decade. These have been fuelled by advances in many areas, especially cell and molecular biology, recombinant DNA technology, genomics, proteomics, bio- and chemical informatics, as well as laboratory equipment and automation. In tandem with these advancements, there were changes in regulatory requirements, with the aim to approve drugs in an efficient manner for those in need of the medication. Great strides have also been made in the harmonization of regulations to adopt some form of international regulatory standards, in the hope of lowering regulatory costs and expediting approvals. New and more efficient manufacturing technologies and processes have enabled purer and more potent drugs to be produced.

Against this backdrop of advances, the pharmaceutical industry also faces unprecedented challenges in many areas. The pipelines for new drugs are drying up, in spite of huge investments allocated for research and development. Drugs are not being discovered and developed fast enough to fill the pipeline. The prospects of generating more blockbuster drugs are not encouraging. Some new technologies, such as combinatorial chemistry and high throughput screening, have yet to live up to expectations of speeding up drug discovery. Clinical trials have become more complex, lengthy and expensive. In addition, there are ethical, social, political and intellectual property issues that need due consideration. There are many more diverse questions, such as gene therapy, cloning, intellectual property, sustainable biodiversity, transgenic production systems, bioterrorism, cost of treatment, and quality of life, that challenge the industry to face them squarely.

In this chapter, we discuss some of these issues and the likely course of events that may unfold in the decades ahead.

11.2 SMALL MOLECULE PHARMACEUTICAL DRUGS

There are two distinct routes to the discovery of small molecule drugs: (a) from natural products and (b) from rational design.

11.2.1   Drugs from natural products

Proponents of drugs from natural products argue that natural products provide a vast diversity of chemical compounds. These compounds with myriad chemical compositions and structures serve as reservoirs for many pharmacologically active lead compounds to be discovered.

As described in Exhibit 3.2, there are now regulations enacted to protect the environment with respect to natural product collection. Bioprospecting from natural habitats has to take into account the 1993 *Convention on Biological Diversity*.

Hitherto, the normal source of collections has been from terrestrial habitats. However, marine bioprocessing represents a vast untapped area that is likely to be intensified. Exhibit 11.1 describes the diversity and life forms in this habitat.

It can be envisioned that laboratory equipment and assay systems will continue to play crucial roles in natural product drug discovery. Although high throughput technologies have not yet delivered more drug candidates, there will continue to be a push for even higher density screening

Exhibit 11.1 Marine Bioprospecting

There are 34 fundamental phyla of life: 17 occur on land and 32 in the sea (including some overlaps). There is more chemical diversity among marine life forms. Most of these are from invertebrate organisms—sponges, tunicates and mollusks. Some of the compounds from marine life forms are extremely potent, given that these organisms have to defend themselves from attacks in vast volumes of water that dilute the compound.

The range of climatic conditions, from tropical waters to cold arctic ocean, shallow continental shelves to great ocean depths with high pressure and low oxygen content, means that there is a potentially huge supply of life forms with extensive biodiversity.

SOURCE Willis, R.C., Nature's pharma sea, *Modern Drug Discovery*, 5, pp. 32–38 (2002).

throughputs. Further miniaturization of liquid dispensing and more specific and sensitive assay systems will continue to be developed. Larger compound libraries and more comprehensive databases will be another natural progression to widen the boundaries of chemical diversities, with the hope that drug candidates will be included within these boundaries.

11.2.2 Drugs from rational design

The use of a combination of technologies such as X-ray crystallography, NMR, bioinformatics, computational chemistry and combinatorial chemistry has yet to realize the full potential to design safe and effective drugs with high success rates. The use of microarrays and proteomics to identify targets that cause diseases will help to define the focus on these targets. A variety of technology platforms is then used to simulate drug compound-target interactions with the aim of interrupting or diverting disease pathways.

An often-quoted limitation of rational drug design is the lack of biodiversity and chemical space (the various possible chemical compositions in nature, estimated to be as high as 10^{100} different compounds) in the libraries of compounds examined. The use of advanced software, together with artificial intelligence for simulation, is an important tool to extend the chemical space and provide a greater diversity of chemical structures for use as scaffolds to test for potential drug candidates. There are likely to be more useful rules such as the Lipinski's rule (see Section 3.3.4) being implemented to test the scaffolds and functional groups to be attached. The development of intelligent information-rich systems will be a key to the success of rational design technological platforms. Combinatorial chemistry with chiral selectivity will help to design and generate potent drugs more expeditiously.

Imatinib   mesylate   (Gleevec,   Novartis),   zanamivir   (Relenza, GlaxoSmithKline) and oseltamivir (Tamiflu, Roche) are examples of drugs (Exhibit 3.11 and Exhibit 3.7) that show the successful contributions of rational drug design. Recently, the X-ray structure of angiotensin-converting enzyme (ACE) was reported (see Exhibit 11.2), and this may pave the way for more effective ACE inhibitors to be developed for the treatment of hypertension and heart disorders.

Exhibit 11.2 X-ray Structure of Angiotensin-Converting Enzyme

Angiotensin-converting enzyme is an important enzyme for the regulation of blood pressure. It exists in two forms. The somatic form has 1277 amino acids. The sperm cell form has 701 amino acids. The somatic form consists of two domains: the carboxy-terminal (C) domain and the amino-terminal (N) domain. The sperm cell form consists of only the C domain. Studies have shown that the C domain is the dominant angiotensin-converting site for controlling blood pressure and cardiovascular functions.

The structure of testicular ACE (sperm cell form) was determined using X-ray crystallography. It has 27 helices, six short strands of β-structure and six glycosylation sites.

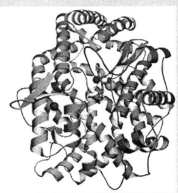

The structure with an inhibitor, lisinopril, revealed the exact nature of the binding of the drug to the active site. With this detailed analysis, more efficacious drugs are expected to be developed to bind to the active site and control blood pressure.

SOURCE Reprinted with permission from Natesh, R., Schwager, S.L., Sturrock, E.D. and Acharya, K.R., Crystal structure of the human angiotensin-converting enzyme-lisinopril complex, *Nature*, 421, pp. 551–554 (2003).

11.3 LARGE MOLECULE BIOPHARMACEUTICAL DRUGS

The biopharmaceutical industry for producing large molecule protein-based drugs has grown exponentially in the past 25 years (Exhibit 11.3).

Exhibit 11.3 Biopharmaceuticals

Insulin was the first recombinant drug, approved in 1982. There are now about 150 biopharmaceuticals approved for treatment of a variety of disorders. The value is US$30 billion (<7% of total drug market) and currently about 500 biopharmaceuticals are undergoing clinical trials.

It is expected that biopharmaceuticals will grow to 25% of the total drug market by 2010.

The knowledge base of life sciences doubles every 14 months. Molecular biology has contributed to many types of proteins being expressed in different cell systems. Manufacturing processes for producing consistent, pure and potent biopharmaceuticals are now widely available.

To date, most approved protein-based drugs are for therapeutic or replacement therapies. They are recombinant versions of natural proteins such as insulin and erythropoietin. Their characteristics and functions are relatively well defined and known. The next phase of biopharmaceuticals, such as antibodies and vaccines, is more complex and requires more tests and characterizations. Controls for the reliability, contamination and fidelity of expression systems will be high on the agenda in the coming decade.

The high cost of biopharmaceuticals has been due in part to the stringent requirements of aseptic manufacturing processes, process control and stability issues of the proteins. Some efforts are likely to be directed at developing more robust protein expression systems, better control parameters for efficient and reliable manufacturing processes, and more stable formulations. Production of biopharmaceuticals using transgenic plants and animals may also lower manufacturing costs (see Section 11.12). Most forecasts predict that we are at the threshold of seeing many more effective and potent biopharmaceuticals for a variety of treatments.

11.4 TRADITIONAL MEDICINE

There has been a revival in the use of traditional medicine (TM) in the last decade. TM is also called Complementary or Alternative Medicine (CAM). It is likely that this revival trend will continue when there are still unmet needs to be filled by 'Western' drugs. The quandary with Western drugs is that pharmaceutical firms have to ensure a reasonable return on shareholders' investment. With many drug discovery and development programs costing billions of dollars, most pharmaceutical firms concentrate on blockbuster drugs with large market potential. The way is thus left open for the treatment of many therapies to be filled by other means such as TM.

Another perceived view about Western drugs is the adverse effects. It is sometimes viewed that Western medicine is akin to a sledgehammer method rather than the more holistic approach using TM. Costs of Western medicine can be prohibitive as well, especially for patients in countries where there are no comprehensive healthcare systems. For example, treatment with pegylated interferon for hepatitis C can cost tens of thousands of dollars per year. Limitations of Western drugs in some cases, such as resistance to antibiotics, also highlight the problems and pave way for people to consider TM. See Exhibit 11.4 on how GlaxoSmithKline made available its AIDS drugs to the third world nations.

Exhibit 11.4   AIDS Drugs in the Third World

GlaxoSmithKline, under pressure for not doing more to help the AIDS sufferers in South Africa, relented and handed over the rights to the manufacture of its AIDS drugs to a South African firm. GlaxoSmithKline waived its royalty rights and the South African drug firm will pay 30% of net sales to government organizations fighting HIV and AIDS. The drugs are the antiretroviral drugs zidovudine (AZT, Retrovir) and lamivudine (3TC, Lamivir), and a combination drug of the two, Combivir. This action will help to supply badly needed drugs to the Third World countries; it also sets up the precedent of differential strategies for the manufacture and supply of drugs in the world.

SOURCE Reuters, 8 October 2001.

For TM to be accepted into mainstream medical treatment, a likely scenario is the application of scientific methodologies and controls for TM development, evaluation and production. Many of the tools for high throughput screening (HTS) and assay systems can be used to test the efficacy of TM, similar to the irrational approach of screening natural products. Pharmacology studies have to be conducted in accordance with Good Laboratory Practice (GLP).

Some regulatory authorities have foreseen the future impact of TM and set up appropriate guidelines. The EU has legislations for traditional herbal products. Another example is the Therapeutic Goods Administration of Australia, which has set up a complementary medicine section that controls the regulatory practices for TM.

The conditions for growing and harvesting of traditional herbs are sources of variability and contamination. Good Agricultural Practice (GAP) is required to minimize contamination to the raw herbs and ensure consistent levels of active ingredients. Factors such as climatic variations and processing conditions may also affect the quality of TM. Better characterization methods, as well as Good Manufacturing Practice (GMP), are needed for the scientifically based development and production of reliable, consistent and efficacious TM.

Exhibit 11.5 shows the strategy drawn up by the World Health Organization for TM.

Exhibit 11.5 The WHO Traditional Medicine Strategy, 2002-2005

There are four objectives:

Policy: Integrate TM/CAM with national health care systems, as appropriate, by developing and implementing national TM/CAM policies and programs.

Safety, efficacy and quality: Promote the safety, efficacy and quality of TM/CAM by expanding the knowledge base on TM/CAM, and by providing guidance on regulatory and quality assurance standards.

Access: Increase the availability and affordability of TM/CAM, as appropriate, with an emphasis on access for poor populations.

Rational use: Promote therapeutically sound use of appropriate TM/CAM by providers and consumers.

SOURCE World Health Organization, *WHO Traditional Medicine Strategy*, WHO, 2002, http://www.who.int/medicines/library/trm/trm_strat_eng.pdf [accessed Mar 20, 2003].

11.5 INDIVIDUALIZED MEDICINE

The challenge is that, one day, drugs will be tailor-made for individuals and adapted to each person's own genetic makeup. In this way, the drugs will be used optimally and adverse events minimized, if not eliminated. Environment, diet, age, lifestyle, and state of health can all influence a person's response to drugs, but understanding an individual's genetic makeup is thought to be the key to creating personalized drugs.

An individual's blood samples can be collected and analyzed. Through the study of single nucleotide polymorphisms and pharmacogenomics, the genes that cause diseases can be pinpointed. The results will show the individual's disease condition or predisposition to some diseases. In this way, treatment or preventive measures can be prescribed.

It is envisaged that cheaper and more affordable drugs may also result as drugs are designed for specific groups of people. Clinical trials may be shortened considerably and save millions of dollars. Large patient population groups to trial a drug may no longer be required. These drugs can also be introduced faster into the market to treat people in need of these tailor-made medications.

Exhibit 11.6 shows how differences in genetic make-up affect the effectiveness of a drug on individuals.

Exhibit 11.6 Drug and Genetic Variations

In one study, researchers from Vanderbilt University in Nashville, US, compared responses to a β-blocker called atenolol among 34 patients. All patients had genetic variations affecting one of the building blocks of the receptor that binds to β-blocker drugs, which affected the way the receptor responded to the binding of the drug.

Thirteen had one type of genetic variation, Gly389, and 21 had another variation called Arg389.

Patients with the Arg389 variant achieved a significantly lower resting blood pressure and heart rate with the drug than did Gly389 patients, suggesting that the drug was more effective for them. However, this finding held true only at rest, and not during exercise.

SOURCE HeartCenterOnline, *Response to Blood Pressure Drugs in the Genes*, http://www.heartcenteronline.com/myheartdr/News_about_the_heart/Response_t o_blood_pressure_drugs_in_the_genes.html [accessed Aug 18, 2002].

11.6 GENE THERAPY

Currently, there is still a gap for the potential of gene therapy to be fulfilled. Gene therapy clinical trials have been conducted for diseases such as severe combined immunodeficiency disease (SCID, 'bubble baby' syndrome), sickle cell anemia, cystic fibrosis, familial hypercholesterolemia and Gaucher disease.

The aim of gene therapy is to supply healthy genes to replace those that are missing or flawed. One key to the success of gene therapy is the vectors that are used to transport the genes (see Section 4.6). Another critical success factor is the understanding of the effects and functions of genes. Of the estimated 35 000 human genes, we know the functions of relatively few. Although some diseases such as sickle cell anemia and cystic fibrosis are caused by single genes, there are other diseases that may be the result of multiple gene disorders, and the relationships of these genes have to be studied.

There are two types of gene therapy: somatic cell and germ cell gene therapy. Somatic cells are non-reproductive cells and, as such, somatic cell gene therapy affects the individual only. The change in gene is not passed on to the next generation. Germ cell gene therapy involves changes to the reproductive cells, the sperm and egg, with the result that the new genes are passed on to future generations. Although most researchers support research on somatic cell gene therapy, there are differences in opinion concerning germ cell gene therapy. For example, the ethical questions are:

- If gene therapy can remedy missing or faulty genes, why can it not be applied to germ cell gene therapy to stop the fault from passing onto future generations?
- Gene therapy is costly. Who decides which patient receives the therapy? Who pays for the treatment?

Exhibit 11.7 describes a recent gene therapy trial that resulted in unexpected outcomes, which the regulatory authorities have to consider. A recent report of gene therapy for treatment of Alzheimer's disease is also included.

11.7 CLONING AND STEM CELLS

We can divide cloning into therapeutic cloning and reproductive cloning. Therapeutic cloning is synonymous with stem cell research. Under proper control and environment, embryonic stem cells can potentially be directed to grow and develop into different tissues that are invaluable for replacing damaged or diseased tissues and organs. Reproductive cloning is the replication of another living being with genes from only one individual. An example is the cloning of Dolly the sheep in 1996 (Exhibit 11.8).

As discussed in Section 4.7, stem cells have the potential to treat medical conditions beyond the scope that can be offered by drugs alone. However, there are many scientific and ethical hurdles to overcome. On the scientific

Exhibit 11.7 Gene Therapy Trials

SCID gene therapy trial

Infants with severe combined immunodeficiency disease (SCID, 'bubble boy' syndrome) have a gene defect that leads to a complete lack of white blood cells. Without treatment, these infants die from complications of infectious diseases during the first few years of life. The only treatment currently approved for this condition is a bone marrow transplant.

Gene therapy offers another potential avenue to 'fix' the defective gene. The therapy itself is by no means straightforward. In a French gene therapy trial, two children with SCID were successfully treated. However, both these children unexpectedly developed a leukemia-like condition. On this news, the FDA put a temporary clinical hold on the gene therapy trial until further investigations are carried out.

SOURCE   *FDA places temporary halt on gene therapy trials using retroviral vectors in blood stem cells,* FDA Talk Paper, 2003, http://www.fda.gov/bbs/topics/ANSWERS/2003/ANS01190.html [accessed Mar 12, 2003].

Recent gene therapy study

In a recent gene therapy study, a gene for the expression of a protein called neprilysin was introduced into transgenic mice. Neprilysin regulates amyloid levels, which are implicated in Alzheimer's disease (Exhibit 11.9). The results showed a 50% reduction in the levels of amyloid.

SOURCE Brown, M., Gene therapy success for Alzheimer's?, *BioMedNet*, May, 2003, http://news.bmn.com/news/story?day=030501&story=2 [accessed May 20, 2003].

Exhibit 11.8 Dolly the Sheep (1996–2003)

In February 1997, the Scottish scientist, Ian Wilmut, and colleagues at the Roslin Institute announced the birth of a cloned sheep called Dolly in July 1996. They had removed the nucleus from the egg cell of a sheep and replaced it with the nucleus from an adult sheep. Dolly was born from a surrogate mother sheep and is an exact clone of the adult sheep, unlike offspring from the reproductive process, in which the offspring inherits the genes from both parents.

Dolly suffered from premature arthritis in 2002 and had to be put down in February 2003 at the age of 6½, because of progressive lung disease common in older sheep. It is not known whether Dolly's premature death is related to cloning; her life was about half the normal sheep lifespan of 12 years. The cause of Dolly's death is being investigated.

part, stem cell research activities will intensify over the next decade. These challenges can be broadly divided into (a) determining how to develop stem cells into specific tissues, and (b) implanting these tissues into the body without rejection by the recipient's immune system. On the ethical front, it is expected that there will be more debates on the ethical issues of stem cell research. Most scientists consent to therapeutic cloning (stem cell research) but not reproductive cloning. The ethical issue of stem cell research concerns the harvesting of cells from embryos that are a few days old. This action destroys the embryos. Some questions are:

- What is the legal and religious status of the embryos?
- Who has the right to give informed consent?
- Under what conditions can this consent be given?

In April 2003, the members of the Europe Parliament voted to impose severe restrictions on the use of stem cells taken from human embryos. They also called for an outright ban on human reproductive cloning. The decision has to be approved by the 15 Member States before it becomes law. If adopted, it will have a serious effect on embryonic stem cell research.

11.8 OLD AGE DISEASES AND AGING

We are living in an aging society. The United Nations estimates that the world will have two billion people over the age of 60 by 2050. With the aging population, there are old age diseases that we have to face and treat with more effective therapies. Hypertension, strokes, Alzheimer's disease, heart diseases, type 2 diabetes, Parkinson's disease and osteoporosis are some examples (Exhibit 11.9).

Exhibit 11.9 Old Age Diseases

Hypertension
Hypertension, or high blood pressure, is the elevation of arterial blood pressure. For an adult, a systolic pressure above 140 mmHg or diastolic pressure above 90 mmHg is considered hypertension. The cause for hypertension may be narrowing or hardening of blood vessels, kidney diseases, or other unknown origins. Some commonly used drugs for the treatment of hypertension are angiotensin-converting enzyme (ACE) inhibitors, angiotensin II receptor blockers, and calcium antagonists (calcium-channel blockers). ACE inhibitors the enzyme from hydrolyzing angiotensin I to angiotensin II. The angiotensin II receptor blockers block the effects of angiotensin, and calcium antagonists are used to reduce heart rate and relax blood vessels.

Continued

Exhibit 11.9 *Continued*

Stroke
A stroke occurs when there is an interruption of blood supply to the brain. An ischemic stroke occurs when a clot prevents blood flow in the brain. A hemorrhagic stroke is when there is a rupture of a blood vessel in the brain. In either case, the brain cells in the affected area die. This area is called an infarct. Medical treatment is required to arrest the damage. More effective treatment can be administered within six hours of the onset of stroke. A stroke may result in weakness, paralysis, impairment of speech and memory, or even death. Medical treatment includes the use of anticoagulants to treat stroke victims.

Alzheimer's disease
This disease is due to the accumulation of β-amyloid protein in the brain. The protein is believed to trigger brain degeneration through cell deaths of the neurons. Alzheimer's disease is characterized by loss of memory and intellectual performance, and slowness in thought. In the US, a class of drugs called cholinesterase inhibitors is approved to treat Alzheimer's disease. In Europe, a drug called memantine is approved for treatment of Alzheimer's disease, and it is under review by the FDA.

Diabetes
Refer to Exhibit 4.9 for a description of diabetes.

Parkinson's disease
Parkinson's disease is a progressive neurological disorder. It is due to the degeneration of neurons in the part of the brain that controls movement. The degeneration of neurons causes a decrease in the level of dopamine, a neurotransmitter chemical necessary for the proper transmission of signals. Patients experience tremors in limbs, rigidity, difficulty in movements, and loss of facial expression. Recent clinical trials show the promise of a new drug, called Glial Derived Neurotrophic Factor, which controls dopamine producing nerve cells.

Osteoporosis
Osteoporosis is the loss of structural bony tissue, and gives rise to brittleness in bones. This may lead to fractures of hips, spines and wrists. Osteoporosis can begin at a young age if a person does not receive enough calcium and vitamin D. A person reaches maximum bone strength between 25 and 30 years of age; after that, the bone strength decreases by about 0.4% per year. After menopause, bone strength reduces by about 3% per year. Drugs such as estrogen, calcitonin, alendronate, raloxifene, and risedronate are approved for the treatment of postmenopausal osteoporosis.

For some of these diseases, such as hypertension and heart disease, drugs such as ACE inhibitors and β-blockers are available for treatment. For some other diseases, such as Alzheimer's disease, more effective drugs have yet to be discovered.

It is also expect that, in the coming decades, there will be more research on aging. Exhibit 11.10 describes some recent findings concerning aging.

Exhibit 11.10 Aging

Aging is another research area that challenges scientists to understand and perhaps devise means to slow the process. An increasing number of scientists believe that aging is due to the prolonged process of oxidative damage. It has been found that oxygen radicals attack cell proteins and membranes, with the mitochondria being the most susceptible.

An antioxidant enzyme, superoxide dismutase (SOD), breaks down oxygen radicals and renders them harmless. Fruit flies and rats with mutated genes for SOD expression live longer than normal by as much as 40%. Can this antioxidant really prolong human lifespan? There are no proven data to show that consuming copious amounts of antioxidant will help. One possible reason is that the human body can only accept a certain level of antioxidant; excessive amounts are excreted. A recent article by noted scientists in the field of aging has warned against the false belief of slowing aging by consuming hormones or antioxidants.

SOURCE Olshansky, S.J., Hayflick, L. and Carnes, B.A., No truth to the fountain of youth, *Scientific American*, June, pp. 92–95 (2002); Hopkin, K., Your new body—making Methuselah, *Scientific American*, September, pp. 32–37 (1999).

11.9 LIFESTYLE DRUGS

As society becomes more affluent, there are demands for 'lifestyle' drugs, to treat non-life threatening conditions, or even to make a person feel more confident or look better. It is likely that there will be a proliferation of lifestyle drugs in the future.

The major areas for lifestyle drugs are:
- Obesity treatment
- Aging: enhance muscular tone and youthful vitality
- Aging: anti-wrinkles
- Memory enhancement
- Sexual dysfunction
- Smoking cessation
- Hair loss therapy.

We have witnessed lifestyle drugs in the form of orlistat (Xenical, Roche) prescribed for obesity management (Exhibit 2.10), and growth hormones have been promoted for enhancement of muscle tone and youthful vitality

(Exhibit 4.8). Botulinum toxin (Botox) is being injected as an anti-wrinkle treatment (Exhibit 11.11), and a vitamin A derivative (Retin-A gel, Tretinoin) is prescribed for the treatment of facial wrinkles. Drugs such as tacrine and donepezil, which work by attacking enzymes that breakdown acetylcholine, have been approved for boosting memory. Sildenafil (Viagra, Pfizer) is used to treat sexual dysfunction (Exhibit 3.15).

Currently, bupropion (Zyban, GlaxoSmithKline) is the only approved drug for helping in ceasing cigarette smoking, and finasteride (Propecia, Merck) has been approved by the Food and Drug Administration (FDA) for the treatment of male baldness.

Based on the current trend, we can only expect that, in the coming decades, more lifestyle drugs will be approved.

Exhibit 11.11 Botox

Botox is a toxin produced by the bacterium *Clostridium botulinum*. When Botox is injected into facial tissues, it is absorbed by the nerve endings of muscle fibers. Nerve transmissions are interrupted and consequently the muscle relaxes. The relaxed muscle is then no longer effective to pull the facial lines to show the wrinkles.

Treatment with Botox is temporary. Once the nerve endings return to normal, the muscle will resume its contractual pull on the wrinkles.

11.10   PERFORMANCE-ENHANCING DRUGS

In this competitive world, especially in the sports field, athletes try their best to outperform each other. Unfortunately, some athletes resort to the use of performance-enhancing drugs to have a competitive edge. Table 11.1 is a list of banned performance-enhancing drugs published by the World Anti-Doping Association and the International Olympic Committee. This list is effective from 1 January 2003 to 31 December 2003.

Despite measures such as regular screenings and threats of suspensions, some athletes continue to take risks and consume these banned drugs. It is clear that to wrestle with banned drugs requires better detection technology together with more stringent monitoring and legal control. Undoubtedly, stamping out banned drugs in the sports arena will be very difficult and protracted.

Table 11.1 List of drugs banned in sport

Prohibited classes	Prohibited drugs
A. Stimulants <u>a</u>	Amiphenazole, amphetamines, bromantan, caffeine, carphedon, cocaine, epiphedrines, fencamfamin, penterazol, pipradrol and related substances
A. Stimulants <u>b</u>	Formoterol, salbutamol, salmeterol, terbutaline and related substances
B. Narcotics	Buprenorphine, dextromoramide, diamorphine (heroin), methadone, morphine, pentazocine, pethidine and related substances
C. Anabolic agents <u>a</u>	Clostebol, fluoxymesterone, metandienone, metenolone, nandrolone, 19-norandrostenediol, 19-norandrostenedione, oxandrolone, stanosolol, and related substances
<u>b</u>	Androstenediol, dehydroepiandrosterone (DHEA), androstenedione and related substances
Other anabolic agents	Clenbuterol, salbutamol
D. Diuretics	Acetazolamide, bumetanide, chlortalidone, etacrynic acid, furosemide, hydrochlorothiazide, mannitol, mersalyl, spironolone, triamterene and related substances
E. Peptide hormones, mimetics and analogues	Chorionic gonadotrophin, Pituitary and synthetic gonadotrophins, Corticotrophins, growth hormone, insulin-like growth factor, erythropoietin and insulin
F. Agents with anti-estrogenic activity	Aromatase inhibitors, clomiphene, cyclofenil, tamoxifen and related substances
G. Masking agents	Diuretics, epitestosterone, probenecid, plasma expanders

SOURCE World Anti-Doping Agency and International Olympic Committee, *Prohibited Classes of Substances and Prohibited Methods 2003*, WADA, 2003.

11.11 CHEMICAL AND BIOLOGICAL TERRORISM

The anthrax case in the United States (11 infected, 5 died) in late 2001, ricin (a potent poison that inhibits protein synthesis) found in early 2003 in the United Kingdom and France, and sarin (an organophosphate nerve gas) poisoning in Japan in 1995 (11 deaths, 5500 people affected) highlighted that terrorism with biological and chemical materials is real. Both chemical and biological terrorism can cause tremendous medical, social, commercial, legal and political upheavals and problems. In late 2002, the Russian authorities used a gas based on opiate fentanyl to secure the release of hostages held by Chechen rebels in a Moscow theatre.

Governments in many countries are collaborating to examine ways to improve response preparedness in the event of chemical and biological terrorism. Both the European Agency for the Evaluation of Medicinal Products (EMEA) and the FDA have implemented counter-terrorism strategies. These include streamlining of regulatory approvals for vaccines and therapeutics for diseases that are possible biological weapons, such as anthrax, botulism, smallpox, plague, tularemia, and hemorrhagic fevers. A list of potential toxic chemicals has also been prepared. Other anti-terrorism solutions are to improve the networks of health reports so that outbreaks can be detected early and precautionary measures taken within a short time. In addition, there are considerations on stockpiling of antibiotics and vaccines, although this is a complex matter because of the multitudes of microorganisms and chemicals that may be deployed.

In June 2002, the FDA amended its regulations for the approval of certain drugs based on animal efficacy data. For those drugs that are intended to protect or treat individuals exposed to lethal or disabling toxic substances or organisms, marketing approval may be granted based on evidence of effectiveness from appropriate animal studies when human efficacy studies are not ethical or feasible. Under this 'animal efficacy rule', the FDA approved pyridostigmine bromide for US military personnel. This drug increases survival rate after exposure to Soman nerve gas poisoning. Another medication approved is a lotion called Reactive Skin Decontamination Lotion, which is a liquid decontamination lotion for topical application to remove or neutralize chemical warfare agents and T-2 fungal toxin. Exhibit 11.12 provides some basic information about sarin and anthrax.

Exhibit 11.12 Bioterrorism Agents

Anthrax

Anthrax is a toxin with three separate components: a 'protective antigen' (PA), an 'edema factor' (EF) and a 'lethal factor' (LF).

The LF is the most disruptive to cellular functions, and disables intracellular signaling molecules. It prevents macrophages from releasing tumor necrosis factor (TNF) and interleukin cytokines, although the production of TNF and cytokines in the macrophages is not impeded. The host's immune system is compromised and is unable to eliminate the anthrax bacillus.

Ultimately, the macrophages die, releasing the enormous built-up stores of TNF and cytokines, triggering a septic shock-like collapse of multiple organ systems.

Exhibit 11.12 *Continued*

Scientists at the Harvard Medical School have prepared a recombinant form of a receptor. The idea is to use this cloned receptor as a decoy and mop up the anthrax molecules in circulation. This has been confirmed in laboratory experiments, but is yet to be trialed on animals.

SOURCE Stubbs, M.T., Anthrax X-rayed: New opportunities for biodefence, *Trends in Pharmacological Sciences*, 23, pp. 539–541 (2002).

Sarin

Pure sarin is a colorless, odorless, volatile and highly lethal compound. It inhibits the enzyme action of cholinesterase, causing the production of excessive amounts of acetylcholine, which in turn affects the central nervous system. Diazepam and pralidoxime iodide are prescribed for victims affected by sarin.

11.12   TRANSGENIC ANIMALS AND PLANTS

The production of drugs under GMP conditions is costly, especially for protein-based drugs, which require aseptic handling. Manufacturers have looked to transgenic animals and plants as possible 'factories' for the production of cost-effective protein-based drugs.

To produce protein-based drugs, DNA genes that code for the expression of the desired protein are inserted into animals or plants. These animals or plants treat the DNA as part of their own genome. As the animals or plants grow, the protein is expressed. Most of the proteins are collected in milk or in eggs for animals; and in fruits or tubers for plants. The proteins are then extracted, purified and formulated as the protein-based drugs. There are several potential issues. First, animals or plants may produce proteins that have different protein sequences, structures and glycosylation patterns than the proteins from human origin. This would render the drug less effective. Secondly, other biological materials from the animals or plants that are potential contaminants for humans may be present. This would require stringent steps for their removal. Thirdly, transgenic animals or plants have to be separated from natural animals and plants to prevent cross-contamination. Fourthly, both the animals and plants have to be kept under close surveillance to ensure they are free of diseases.

Exhibit 11.13 describes a recent work about the potential of edible vaccines.

Exhibit 11.13 Edible Vaccine

Researchers from the University of Maryland in Baltimore, the Boyce Thompson Institute for Plant Research in Ithaca, NY, and Tulane University in New Orleans have performed the first human trial of edible vaccine. Potatoes were genetically engineered to produce a diarrhea-causing toxin secreted by the bacterium *Escherichia coli*.

Of the 14 volunteers for the Phase 1 study, 11 were given the transgenic potatoes containing the toxin as vaccine and three had ordinary potatoes. Blood and stool samples were collected from the volunteers to evaluate the vaccine's ability to stimulate both systemic and intestinal immune responses. Ten of the 11 volunteers who ingested the transgenic potatoes had fourfold rises in serum antibodies at some point after immunization, and six of the 11 developed fourfold rises in intestinal antibodies. The potatoes were well tolerated and no one experienced serious adverse effects.

Research on other edible vaccines is in the pipeline: (a) potatoes and bananas that might protect against Norwalk virus, a common cause of diarrhea, and (b) potatoes and tomatoes that might protect against hepatitis B.

SOURCE   MolecularFarming.com, *Molecular Farming of Edible Vaccines*, http://www.molecularfarming.com/ediblevaccine.html [accessed Feb 24, 2003].

11.13   REGULATORY ISSUES

Regulatory requirements are dynamic. They are introduced or amended as circumstances change. The amendment by the FDA to the animal efficacy rule (Section 11.11) and the initiative for a new risk-based approach to cGMP (Section 9.7) are examples of dynamic responses to changing environment and conditions. In Europe, the recognition and adoption of regulatory controls for traditional medicine is another positive development. The formation of the International Conference on Harmonization (ICH) in harmonizing drug regulations, such as the ICH Q7A document, has helped to establish a common denominator for regulatory requirements of GMP for many countries. The other common technical documents also assist to streamline regulatory processes.

As gene therapy and stem cell research progress, we can expect more regulatory requirements to be developed to ensure proper safeguards are implemented. Similarly, xenotransplantation and control of biopharmaceutical products will experience specific regulatory controls as new advances are made. Exhibit 11.14 presents the FDA's current oversight on gene therapy.

Exhibit 11.14 FDA's Oversight on Gene Therapy

The FDA has not yet approved for sale any human gene therapy product. However, gene-related research and development is continuing to grow and the FDA is very involved in overseeing this activity. Since 1989, the FDA has received about 300 requests from medical researchers and manufacturers to study gene therapy and to develop gene therapy products. Presently, the FDA is overseeing approximately 210 active Investigational New Drug (IND) gene therapy studies.

Several gene therapies have received orphan drug designation; these are treatments for cystic fibrosis, Gaucher disease and metastatic brain tumor.

SOURCE   Food and Drug Administration, Center for Biologics Evaluation and Research, www.fda.gov/cber/ [accessed Mar 3, 2003].

11.14   INTELLECTUAL PROPERTY RIGHTS

Intellectual property rights (IPR) are an important asset for the pharmaceutical industry. Most successful companies have suites of patents to protect their IPR. The effect of IPR protection is amply demonstrated by the Prozac case. Fluoxetine (Prozac, Eli Lilly) was a blockbuster drug for many years. During the first half of 2001, when Prozac was protected by patent, the sales were US$1.3 billion. Within one year of patent expiration, generics from other companies were released to the market. The sales of Prozac were reduced to US$380 million for the first half of 2002.

Pharmaceutical companies are adopting strategies to protect their products. These range from new claims for the drugs, reformulations or isolation of the effective enantiomer (see Section 3.5.). Lifecycle management of drugs and IPR protection are strategies that pharmaceutical firms will focus on more closely in the coming decades. This is especially the case where pharmaceutical firms try to exclude the encroachment of generics for as long as possible. We describe in Exhibit 11.15 the legal battle between AstraZeneca, the manufacturer of Prilosec, and other companies trying to manufacture omeprazole generics. A brief description of the FDA's rules for generics is presented in Exhibit 11.16 to explain how the prevailing system works.

It should be noted that at times pharmaceutical firms have to waive their IPR for a certain segment of the market. This is shown in Exhibit 11.17.

Exhibit 11.15 Prilosec's Legal Battle

The AstraZeneca patent on omeprazole expired in October 2001. AstraZeneca went to court to seek extended patent protection for a special formulation of omeprazole. The special formulation consists of a subcoating layer inserted between the core of the drug's active ingredient, and the outer coating. The subcoating is formulated to protect the drug from being broken down quickly by the harsh acids in the stomach.

In October 2002, a US federal judge ruled that three generic companies have infringed on AstraZeneca's patent. However, a fourth company that has its own patent for coating the drug was cleared to market the drug in generic form.

SOURCE Debaise, C., *Wall Street Journal*, October 12 (2002).

Exhibit 11.16 The FDA's Rule on Generics

To encourage generic production, the FDA allows submission of an Abbreviated New Drug Application (ANDA) by a generic manufacturer before the expiration of the patented drug. For the FDA to commence review of the ANDA, the generic drug applicant must certify that the patent for the existing drug is invalid and the generic product does not infringe it. The generic drug applicant must also notify the patent holder that it has filed the ANDA application. If the patent holder files an infringement suit against the generic applicant within 45 days of the ANDA notification, the patent holder is given a one-time 'stay' of a generic drug's entry into the market for resolution of a patent challenge unless, before that time, the patent expires or is determined to be invalid or not infringed. This 30-month stay gives the patent holder time to assert its patent rights in court before a generic competitor is permitted to enter the market.

SOURCE Center for Drug Evaluation and Research, *FDA Generic Drugs Final Rule and Initiative*, FDA, Rockville, MD, 2003, http://www.fda.gov/oc/initiatives/generics/default.htm [accessed Apr 10, 2003].

Exhibit 11.17 Sleeping Sickness in Africa

Sleeping sickness is caused by the presence of parasitic protozoans (*Trypanosoma gambiense* or *T. rhodesiense*) in the blood. The parasite causes drowsiness, lethargy and eventually death if patient is untreated. As many as 55 million people in 36 African countries are exposed to this disease. In the late 1990s, the WHO persuaded companies such as Bristol-Myers Squibb, Aventis and Bayer to waive their patent rights and donate drugs for treating sleeping sickness to Africans. In addition, these companies agreed to contribute US$5 million per year for five years for monitoring, treatment and research and development of sleeping sickness.

SOURCE Wickware, P., Resurrecting the resurrection drug, *Nature Medicine*, 8, pp. 908–909 (2002).

11.15   CONCLUDING REMARKS

As we embark on a new millennium, a reflection on the last 100 years shows the tremendous progresses made in drug discovery and development. With better sanitation and health care, life expectancy has increased from an average of 50s at the beginning of the 20th century to high 70s now. The drug market continues to expand, even during times of economic downturn. With the introduction of many new technologies and processes, we can expect more effective and specific drugs in the decades ahead. However, a worrying trend has also appeared. It is the declining number of new drugs approved in the past five years, in spite of the billions of dollars spent on research and development (Figure 11.1). In the first four months of 2003, the FDA approved four new molecular entities (NMEs) under New Drug Application (NDA) and four new biologics under Biologics License Application (BLA).

Pharmaceutical firms have to re-examine their strategies to devise means to increase their drug pipelines for continuous streams of products. The high failure rates of New Investigational Drugs during clinical trials (Exhibit 5.7) necessitate the development of better assay systems and animal models that correlate closely with human pharmacodynamics and pharmacokinetics. The study of pharmacogenomics will be crucial to address this issue.

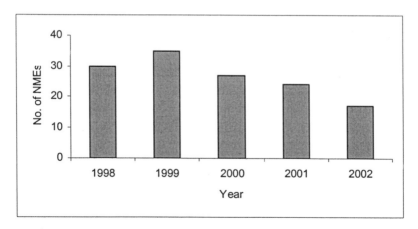

Figure 11.1 The number of new molecular entities (NMEs) approved by the CBER from 1998 to 2002. SOURCE Food and Drug Administration, Center for Biologics Evaluation and Research, http://www.fda.gov/cber/ [accessed Apr 2, 2003].

In addition, the pharmaceutical industry is no longer isolated from society as a whole. It has to factor in considerations for social, political and ethical issues. The attitudes and concerns of society have to be taken into account. The cost of drugs and their availability to the Third World nations are other important aspects for consideration. Furthermore, pharmaceutical firms need to be proactive and vigilant to comply with changes in regulations and government policies. New areas of research, such as gene therapy and stem cells, have opened up many ethical issues to be resolved. Production of protein-based drugs using transgenic animals and plants raises potential topics for ethical and political debates.

These challenges require investment, commitment and ingenious solutions. Ultimately pharmaceutical firms and research organizations, together with government authorities and representatives from society, will have to collaborate and address these challenges. The results will be the development of novel and efficacious drugs and therapies to treat patients and lead to improvements in the quality of life.

11.16   FURTHER READING

Dove, A., Uncorking the biomanufacturing bottleneck, *Nature Biotechnology*, 20, pp. 777–779 (2002).

Drews, J., Strategic trends in the drug industry, *Drug Discovery Today*, 8, pp. 411–420 (2003).

Fleming, E. and Ma, P. Drug life-cycle technologies, *Nature Reviews Drug Discovery*, 1, pp. 751–752 (2002).

Franz, S., Screening the right candidate, *Nature Reviews Drug Discovery*, http://www.nature.com/drugdisc/nj/articles/nrd1082.html (2003).

Gershell, L. and Atkins, J.H., A brief history of novel drug discovery technologies, *Nature Reviews Drug Discovery*, 2, pp. 321–327 (2003).

Gibbs, W.W., A diabetes switch?, *Scientific American*, June, p. 16 (1999).

Happier, Hornier, Hairier, *Nature Biotechnology*, 21, 1 (2003).

Harvey, A.L. (ed.), *Advances in Drug Discovery Techniques*, John Wiley & Sons, New York, 1998.

Hopkin, K., Your new body—making Methuselah, *Scientific American*, September, pp. 32–37 (1999).

Jones, D., Anticoagulants, the clot thickens, *Nature Reviews Drug Discovery*, 2, p. 251 (2003).

Jurgen, D., *In Quest of Tomorrow's Medicine*, Springer-Verlag, New York, 1999.

Larru, M., Adult stem cells: An alternative to embryonic stem cells?, *Trends in Biotechnology*, 19, p. 487 (2001).

Larvol, B.L. and Wilkwerson, L.J., In silico drug discovery: Tools for bridging the NCE gap, *Nature Biotechnology*, 16, pp. 33–34 (1998).

Natesh, R., Schwager, S.L., Sturrock, E.D. and Acharya, K.R., Crystal structure of the human angiotensin-converting enzyme-lisinopril complex, *Nature*, 421, pp. 551–554 (2003).

Olshansky, S.J., Hayflick, L. and Carnes, B.A., No truth to the fountain of youth, *Scientific American*, June, pp. 92–95 (2002).

Roden, D.M. and George Jr., A.L., The genetic basis of variability in drug responses, *Nature Reviews Drug Discovery*, 1, pp. 37–44 (2002).

Schwartz, L., Preece, P.E. and Hendry, R.A., *Medical Ethics, A Case-Based Approach*, Saunders, Edinburgh, 2002.

Stubbs, M.T., Anthrax X-rayed: New opportunities for biodefence, *Trends in Pharmacological Sciences*, 23, pp. 539–541 (2002).

Ulrich, R. and Friend, S.H., Toxicogenomics and drug discovery: Will new technologies help us produce better drugs?, *Nature Reviews Drug Discovery*, 1, pp. 84–88 (2002).

Walters, W.P. and Namchuk, M., Designing screens: How to make your hits a hit, *Nature Reviews Drug Discovery*, 2, pp. 259–266 (2003).

Walters, W.P., Stahl, M.T. and Murcko, M.A., Virtual screening–an overview, *Drug Discovery Today*, 3, pp. 160–178 (1998).

Wechsler, J., The push for generics challenges manufacturers, *Pharmaceutical Technology*, July, pp. 26-34 (2003).

Willis, R.C., Nature's pharma sea, *Modern Drug Discovery*, 5, pp. 32–38 (2002).

World Anti-Doping Agency and International Olympic Committee, *Prohibited Classes of Substances and Prohibited Methods 2003*, WADA, 2003.

World Health Organization, *WHO Traditional Medicine Strategy*, WHO, 2002, http://www.who.int/medicines/library/trm/trm_strat_eng.pdf [accessed Mar 20, 2003].

APPENDIX 1

HISTORY OF DRUG DISCOVERY AND DEVELOPMENT

A1.1 EARLY HISTORY OF MEDICINE

Drug discovery and development has a long history and dates back to the early days of human civilization. In those ancient times, drugs were not just used for physical remedies but were also associated with religious and spiritual healing. Sages or religious leaders were often the administrators of drugs. The early drugs or folk medicines were mainly derived from plant products, and supplemented by animal materials and minerals. These drugs were most probably discovered through a combination of trial and error experimentation and observation of human and animal reactions as a result of ingesting such products.

Although these folk medicines probably originated independently in different civilizations, there are a number of similarities, for example, in the use of same herbs for treating similar diseases. This is likely to be a contribution by ancient traders, who in their travels might have assisted the spread of medical knowledge.

Folk medicines were the only available treatments until recent times. Drug discovery and development started to follow scientific techniques in the late 1800s. From then on, more and more drugs were discovered, tested and synthesized in large-scale manufacturing plants, as opposed to the extraction of drug products from natural sources in relatively small batch quantities. After World War I, the modern pharmaceutical industry came into being, and drug discovery and development following scientific principles was firmly established.

Although pharmaceutical drugs are now widely used worldwide, many ethnic cultures have retained their own folk medicines. In certain instances, these folk medicines exist side by side and are complemented by pharmaceutical drugs.

The following are some snapshot examples of how drugs were discovered from the early human civilizations.

A1.1.1 Chinese medicine

Traditional Chinese medicine (TCM) is believed to have originated in the times of the legendary emperor Sheng Nong in 3500 BC. The dynasty system and meticulous recording have helped to preserve the TCM scripts of old China. Some important medical writings are *Shang Han Lun* (Discussion of Fevers), *Huang Di Nei Jing* (The Internal Book of Emperor Huang) and *Sheng Nong Ben Cao Jing* (The Pharmacopoeia of Sheng Nong—a legendary emperor). Exhibit A1.1 relates a legend about the discovery of a herb for treating injuries.

The Chinese pharmacopoeia is extensive. Some of the active ingredients from Chinese herbs have been used in 'Western' drugs; for example, reserpine from *Rauwouofia* for antihypertensive and emotional and mental control, and the alkaloid ephedrine from *Mahuang* for the treatment of asthma.

Exhibit A1.1 A Legend about San Qi

Chinese legend described that the legendary emperor Sheng Nong one day tried to kill a snake by beating it. The snake returned a few days later, apparently none the worse after the beating. He beat it again and left it mortally injured. Again, the snake returned several days later. This time, after the beating, he observed that the snake crawled back into the bush and ate a plant material. This plant is now called San Qi (*Panax notoginseng*) and is used for treating external injuries. It is an ingredient for the well-known TCM herbal formula known as Yunnan Bai Yao.

SOURCE Reid, D., *Chinese Herbal Medicine*, Shambhala Publications, Boston, 1996.

A1.1.2 Egyptian medicine

Ancient papyrus provided written records of early Egyptian medical knowledge. The Ebers papyrus (from around 3000 BC) provided 877 prescriptions and recipes for internal medicine, eye and skin problems, and gynecology. Another record, from the Kahun papyrus of around 1800 BC, detailed treatments for gynecological problems. Medications were based mainly on herbal products such as myrrh, frankincense, castor oil, fennel, sienna, thyme, linseed, aloe and garlic.

A1.1.3 Indian medicine

The Indian folk medicine, called Ayurvedic medicine, can be traced back 3000–5000 years, and was practiced by the Brahmin sages of ancient times. The treatments were set out in sacred writings called Vedas. The material medica are extensive and most are based on herbal formulations. Some of the herbs have appeared in Western medicines, such as cardamom and cinnamon. Susruta, a physician in the fourth century AD, described the use of henbane as antivenom for snakebites.

A1.1.4 Greek medicine

Some of the Greek medical ideas were derived from the Egyptians, Babylonians, and even the Chinese and Indians. Castor oil was prescribed as a laxative; linseed or flex seed were used as a soothing emollient, laxative and antitussive. Other treatments include fennel plant for relief of intestinal colic and gas, and asafetida gum resin as an antispasmodic. The greatest Greek contribution to the medical field is perhaps to dispel the notion that diseases are due to supernatural causes or spells. The Greeks established that diseases result from natural causes. Hippocrates, the father of medicine, at about 400 BC is credited with laying down the ethics for physicians. Exhibit A1.2 describes the mythology of Asclepius, the Greek God of Medicine.

Exhibit A1.2 Asclepius: Greek God of Medicine

In Greek mythology, Asclepius, the god of medicine, studied medicine under Chiron. He excelled over Chiron, and his medical skills were reputed to be able to bring back the dead. This incurred the wrath of Pluto, the god of the underworld, and the envy of other gods. They complained to Zeus, who also thought that he alone should have the power of life and death. Zeus slew Asclepius with a thunderbolt. However, Asclepius' daughters, Panacea and Hygeia, survived and carried on to tend to the sick.

SOURCE Leadbetter, R., *Asclepius*, http://www.pantheon.org/articles/a/asclepius. html [accessed May 31, 2001].

A1.1.5 Roman medicine

As great administrators, the Romans instituted hospitals, although these were used mainly to cater for the needs of the military. Through this work, organized medical care was made available. The Romans also extended the pharmacy practice of the Greeks. Dioscorides and Galen were two noted physicians in Roman days. Dioscorides' *Materia Medica* contains descriptions of treatments based on 80% plant, 10% animal and 10% mineral products.

A1.2 DRUG DISCOVERY AND DEVELOPMENT IN THE MIDDLE AGES

The Middle Ages, from around AD 400 to 1500, witnessed the decline of the Roman influences. This was also the time when plagues scourged many parts of Europe. Diseases such as bubonic plague, leprosy, smallpox, tuberculosis and scabies were rampant. Many millions of people succumbed to these diseases.

A1.2.1 The early Church

There are some references to herbs in the Bible. However, the Church's main contribution to medicines is the preservation and transcription of Greek medical manuscripts and treatises. This enabled the knowledge developed in the ancient times to be continued and later used in the Renaissance period.

A1.2.2 Arabian medicine

Through trades with many regions, the Arabians learned and extended medical knowledge. Their major contribution is perhaps the knowledge of medical preparations and distillation methods, although the techniques were probably derived from the practices of alchemists. Avicenna, around AD 900–1000, recorded a vast encyclopedia of medical description and treatment. Another noted physician was Rhazes, who accurately described measles and smallpox.

A1.3 FOUNDATION OF CURRENT DRUG DISCOVERY AND DEVELOPMENT

The Renaissance period laid the foundation for scientific thoughts in medicinal preparations and medical treatments. There were many advances made in anatomy, physiology, surgery and medical treatments, including public health care, hygiene and sanitation.

A1.3.1 Smallpox

In 1796, Edward Jenner successfully experimented with smallpox inoculations (Exhibit A1.3). This paved the way for the use of vaccination against some infectious diseases.

A1.3.2 Digitalis

In the late 1700s, William Withering introduced digitalis, an extract from the plant foxglove, for treatment of cardiac problems.

A1.3.3 Scurvy

John Hunter (1768) noted that scurvy was caused by the lack of vitamin C. He prescribed the consumption of lemon juice to treat scurvy.

A1.3.4 Rabies

Louis Pasteur (1864) discovered that microorganisms cause diseases, and he devised vaccination against rabies. This was achieved through the use of attenuated rabies virus.

A1.4 BEGINNINGS OF MODERN PHARMACEUTICAL INDUSTRY

Despite the advances made in the 1800s, there were only a few drugs available for treating diseases at the beginning of the 1900s. These were:

- Digitalis: extracted from a plant called foxglove, digitalis stimulates the cardiac muscles, and was used to treat cardiac conditions
- Quinine: derived from the bark of the Cinchona tree, and used to treat malaria
- Ipecacuanha: extracted from the bark or root of the Cephaelis plant, and used to treat dysentery
- Aspirin: extracted from bark of willow tree, and used for the

treatment of fever

- Mercury: used to treat syphilis.

More systematic research was being performed to discover new drugs from the early 1900s.

Paul Ehrlich used an arsenic compound, arspheamine, to treat syphilis. Gerhard Domagh found that the red dye Prontosil was active against streptococcal bacteria. Later, French scientists isolated the active compound to be sulfanilamide, and this gave rise to a new range of sulfa drugs against hosts of bacteria.

A1.4.1 Penicillin

In 1928, Alexander Fleming discovered that *Penicillium* mould was active against staphylococcus bacteria. Ernst Chain rediscovered this fact some 10 years later, when he collaborated with Howard Florey. By 1944, large-scale production of penicillin was available through the work of Howard Florey and Ernst Chain. This work foreshadowed the commencement of biotechnology, where microorganisms were used to produce drug products. A description of the discovery and large-scale manufacturing of penicillin is given in Exhibit A1.4.

Exhibit A1.4 The Development of Penicillin

In the 1930s, Howard Florey and Ernst Chain worked with a team of scientists at Oxford University in Britain. Ernst Chain discovered an earlier paper by Alexander Fleming on the anti-bacterial properties of penicillin.

The Florey–Chain team's investigation showed that penicillin interferes with the cell wall of bacteria. Bacteria cells ruptured instead of continuing to grow. In 1938, their animal test, on eight mice given lethal doses of infectious bacteria, showed stunning results. The four mice with penicillin survived, whereas four controls with no medication died. Their first human patient who suffered from infection showed early improvement with penicillin, but died subsequently when the stock of penicillin was exhausted.

The team worked on the technology for large-scale production of penicillin. Commercial quantities were available before the end of World War II and saved millions of lives, especially soldiers wounded in the war.

SOURCE   Torok, S., *Howard Florey—the Story: Maker of the Miracle Mould*, http://www.abc.net.au/science/slab/florey/story.htm [accessed Jun 2, 2002].

A1.5 EVOLUTION OF DRUG PRODUCTS

In the early days, until the late 1800s, most drugs were based on herbs or extraction of ingredients from botanical sources.

The synthetic drugs using chemical methods were heralded at the beginning of the 1900s, and the pharmaceutical industry was founded. Many drugs were researched and manufactured, but mostly they were used for therapeutic purposes rather than completely curing the diseases.

From the early 1930s, drug discovery concentrated on screening natural products and isolating the active ingredients for treating diseases. The active ingredients are normally the synthetic version of the natural products. These synthetic versions, called new chemical entities (NCEs) have to go through many iterations and tests to ensure they are safe, potent and effective.

In the late 1970s, development of recombinant DNA products utilizing knowledge of cellular and molecular biology commenced. The biotechnology industry became a reality.

The pharmaceutical industry, together with the advances in gene therapy and understanding of mechanisms of causes of diseases, and the research results from the Human Genome Project, have opened up a plethora of opportunities and made possible the development and use of drugs specifically targeting the sites where diseases are caused.

A1.6 FURTHER READING

Harvey, A.L. (ed.), *Advances in Drug Discovery*, John Wiley & Sons and Interpharm, US, 2000.

Medicines–The Discovery Process, Zeneca Pharmaceuticals Education Liaison Group, London.

The Pharmaceutical Century: Ten Decades of Drug Discovery, ACS Publications, November 17, 2000, http://pubs.acs.org/journals/pharmcent/ [accessed Jun 8, 2002].

APPENDIX 2

CELLS, NUCLEIC ACIDS, GENES AND PROTEINS

A2.1 Cells
A2.2 Nucleic Acids
A2.3 Genes and Proteins
A2.4 Further Reading

A2.1 CELLS

Cells are the basic units for all living organisms. All cells are bounded by a membrane, and bacterial and plant cells have a cell wall. The membrane protects the cell from the outside environment. It consists of a lipid bilayer (Figure A2.1). The function of the membrane is to control materials that enter and exit the cell and enable biochemical reactions to take place within the cell.

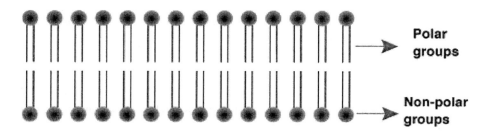

Figure A2.1 Lipid bilayer cell membrane

A2.1.1 Prokaryote cell

Simple single-cell organisms, such as bacteria and algae, are called prokaryotes (see Figure A2.2). Prokaryotes do not have a well-defined nucleus.

The genetic material, deoxyribonucleic acid (DNA), is concentrated in the nuclear region. DNA controls the functions of the cell. Ribosomes, granular structures that consist of ribonucleic acid (RNA) and proteins, are distributed in the cytosol (soluble part of the cell excluding the nuclear region).

Prokaryote cells divide and grow into two daughter cells. In the division process, the DNA replicates and each daughter cell receives one copy.

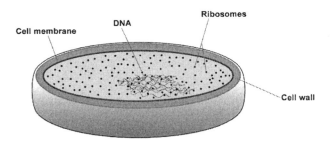

Figure A2.2 A prokaryote cell

A2.1.2 Eukaryote cell

Complex multicellular cells, such as those of plants and humans, are termed eukaryotes. The cell structure is considerably more complex than that of the prokaryote cells (see Figure A2.3 for a human eukaryote cell; plant cells are not shown: they have well-defined cell wall and different structure).

Within the cell membrane is the cytoplasm. This is where many biochemical reactions take place. The most important structure within the human cell is the nucleus. It is bounded by a nuclear membrane and is separated from other organelles (non-cellular structures in a cell that serve specific functions) in the cytoplasm.

DNA is organized into strands within the chromosomes inside the nucleus. There are 46 chromosomes in the human cell, 23 from maternal (egg) and 23 from paternal (sperm) origin (see Exhibit A2.1). All human cells contain a full set of chromosomes and identical genes. However, different sets of genes are expressed, or turned on, in different cells, leading to the various types of cells, such as nerve cells and muscle cells.

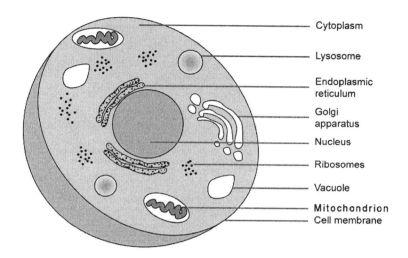

Figure A2.3 A human eukaryote cell

Organelles in the cytoplasm are:

- *Mitochondrion:* the powerhouse of the cell, where oxidation processes take place to provide energy for the cell
- *Endoplasmic reticulum (ER):* a single membrane system of two distinct types, rough and smooth. The rough ER has ribosomes attached to the membrane, whereas the smooth ER does not
- *Ribosomes:* sites where protein synthesis takes place
- *Golgi apparatus:* involved in gathering and dispatching of proteins and lipids
- *Lysosomes:* membrane-bound sacs filled with enzymes for processing nutrients
- *Vacuole:* a space within the cytoplasm that consists of wastes and materials taken in by the cell, for example, bacteria engulfed by white blood cell.

A2.2 NUCLEIC ACIDS

A2.2.1 DNA

DNA is a polymer composed of monomeric nucleic acids called nucleotides. A nucleotide consists of a nitrogenous base, sugar and phosphoric acid (whereas a nucleoside consists of only the base and sugar; see Figure A2.4).

Exhibit A2.1 Cells and Chromosomes

Cells can be divided into germ cells and somatic cells. Germ cells are reproductive cells, for example, ova or sperm. Germ cells contain genetic characteristics that are passed on to the next generation. Somatic cells do not contribute their genes to future generations; they are the tissue cells such as nerve cells and muscle cells.

Within the cell is the nucleus with the chromosomes. DNA strands are housed within the chromosomes, together with some proteins. The 46 human chromosomes are grouped into 22 pairs and two sex chromosomes. Numbering of chromosomes is based on sizes, chromosome 1 being the largest and 22 the smallest.

In addition to the 22 pairs, a female cell contains two X chromosomes and a male cell contains an X and a Y chromosome. When a female egg (carrying an X chromosome) combines with male sperm having an X chromosome, a female offspring is born. When the egg combines with a sperm having a Y chromosome, a male offspring results.

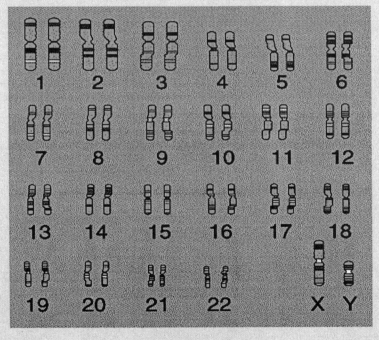

SOURCE Access Excellence Resource Center, *Understanding Gene Testing*, http://www.accessexcellence.org/AE/AEPC/NIH/gene03.html [accessed Jan 30, 2003].

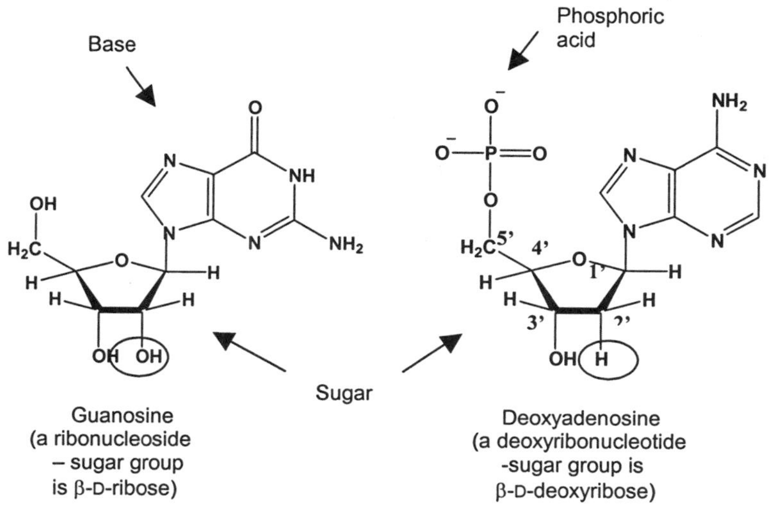

Figure A2.4 Nucleoside and nucleotide. Circled areas show the presence and absence of oxygen atom in the ribose and deoxy ribose sugars

There are two types of bases: pyrimidines and purines (Figure A2.5). The pyrimidine bases include cytosine, thymine and uracil. Cytosine is found in both DNA and RNA. Thymine only occurs in DNA, and uracil is substituted for thymine in RNA. The purine bases are adenine and guanine, both of which are found in DNA and RNA.

Nucleotides are joined into a chain formation, as illustrated in Figure A2.6(a). In DNA, two nucleotide chains intertwine around each other in a double helix formation (Figure A2.6(b)). The backbone of the two strands is the phosphate-sugar linkage.

Alignment of the two strands is via the interactions of the bases: adenine (A) of one strand pairs up with thymine (T) of the complementary strand (with two hydrogen bonds); similarly, guanine (G) pairs up with cytosine (C) (with three hydrogen bonds) as shown in Figure A2.6(c).

There are 10 base pairs in a complete turn of the helix, which spans a distance of 3.4 nm. The outside diameter of the helix is about 2 nm. By convention, the double stranded DNA sequence is written from left to right; the 5′ end (position 5 of the sugar group) is assigned to the top left hand strand.

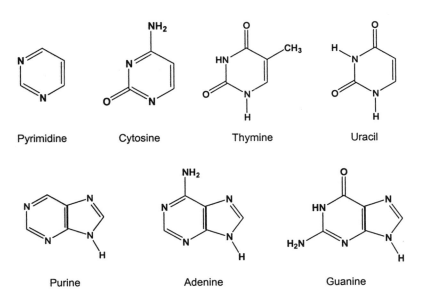

Figure A2.5 Nucleic acid bases

A2.2.2 RNA

RNA is made up of nucleotides similar to DNA, except that the sugar is β-D-ribose compared to DNA's β-D-deoxyribose (Figure 2.4). There are two-stranded RNAs, but normally RNA exists in single strand.

There are three kinds of RNA: messenger RNA (mRNA), transfer RNA (tRNA) and ribosomal RNA (rRNA). All three RNAs are involved in the synthesis of proteins using amino acids.

Information for making a protein is passed from the DNA to the mRNA. This is likened to the master copy (DNA) of a building plan residing in a document room (nucleus) being photocopied onto a duplicate (mRNA). The duplicated plan (mRNA) is then taken to a building site (ribosome) for protein construction. DNA determines the nucleotide sequence of the mRNA; the process of transferring the order of sequence is called transcription. Amino acids (there are 20 naturally occurring amino acids; see Table A2.1) for the construction of protein are brought to the ribosome by tRNAs. The role of rRNA is to combine with protein to form ribosomes, the site where protein synthesis takes place. The order of amino acids in the protein is controlled by mRNA via a process called translation. A schematic representation of the protein synthesis process is shown in Figure A2.7.

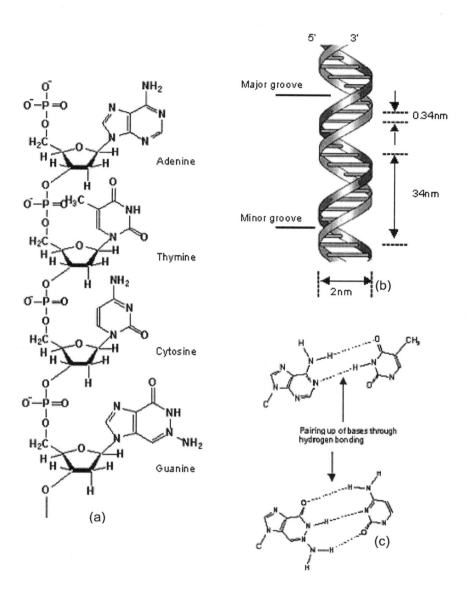

Figure A2.6 (a) Single strand nucleotide, (b)DNA in double helix formation and (c) the pairing up of bases on two separate strands via hydrogen bonding to form the double helix.

Table A2.1 The 20 Naturally Occurring Amino Acids

Name	Abbreviation	Name	Abbreviation
Alanine	Ala	Leucine	Leu
Arginine	Arg	Lysine	Lys
Asparagine	Asn	Methionine	Met
Aspartic Acid	Asp	Phenylalanine	Phe
Cysteine	Cys	Proline	Pro
Glutamic Acid	Glu	Serine	Ser
Glutamine	Gln	Threonine	Thr
Glycine	Gly	Tryptophan	Trp
Histidine	His	Tyrosine	Tyr
Isoleucine	Ile	Valine	Val

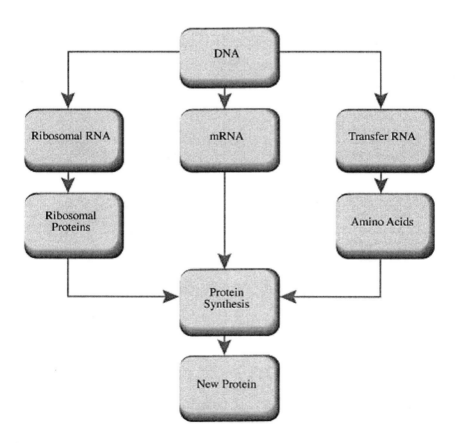

Figure A2.7 Protein synthesis process

A2.3   GENES AND PROTEINS

A2.3.1 Genes

Genes are our hereditary units. Each gene contains the instruction for the synthesis of protein. The summation of all the genes within a cell is called the genome. Instructions for synthesis of proteins are stored in the DNA through specific arrangements of the base sequence. The sequence is made up of the four bases: adenine, thymine, guanine and cytosine (A, T, G and C). These instruction codes are arranged in three-letter words called codons. Each word specifies which amino acid is to be used for constructing the proteins. Genes are not found in a continuous fashion in the DNA sequence. Sequences that are expressed (used to make proteins) are called exons. Intervening sequences, which do not code for proteins, are called introns. Promoters and repressors are present along the DNA sequence to control the expression or suppression of a gene. Information from the exons is transcribed from DNA to mRNA. There are many ways to process transcription, and so one gene can code for multiple versions of mRNA, leading to multiple proteins.

To transcribe information from DNA to mRNA, one strand of the DNA is used as a template. This is called the anticoding, or template, strand and the sequence of mRNA is complementary to that of the template DNA strand (Figure A2.8) (i.e. C→G, G→C, T→A and A→U; note that T is replaced by U in mRNA). The other DNA strand, which has the same base sequence as the mRNA, is called the coding, or sense, strand. There are 64 ($4 \times 4 \times 4$) possible triplet codes of the four bases; 61 are used for coding amino acids and three for termination signals. As there are 20 amino acids for the 61 codes, some triplets code for the same amino acid. A table of the genetic code is presented in Exhibit A2.3.

A2.3.2 Proteins

Proteins are the workhorses in our bodies, and carry out all the essential processes and functions. They may come in the forms of enzymes for catalyzing reactions, hormones for transmitting information between cells, receptors for receiving signals and antibodies for defending us from invading organisms. Proteins are made up of chains of amino acids. Amino acids have a carboxyl group (COO^-) at one end and an amino group (NH_3^+) at another. Peptide bonds are formed by joining one carboxyl group with an amino group (Figure A2.9).

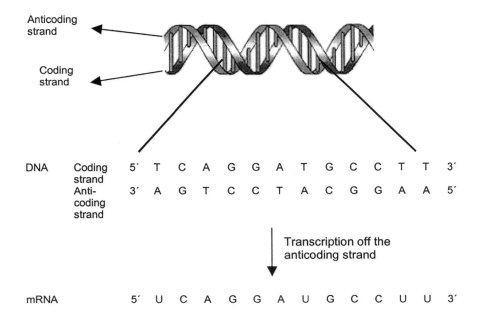

DNA   Coding   5′ T C A G G A T G C C T T 3′
       strand
       Anti-   3′ A G T C C T A C G G A A 5′
       coding
       strand

Transcription off the anticoding strand

mRNA   5′ U C A G G A U G C C U U 3′

Figure A2.8 Transcription from DNA to mRNA

Exhibit A2.3 The Genetic Code Dictionary

The triplet codon genetic codes of mRNA are translated into amino acids as shown below.

UUU→Phe	UCU→ Ser	UAU→Tyr	UGU→Cys
UUC→Phe	UCC→Ser	UAC→Tyr	UGC→Cys
UUA→Leu	UCA→Ser	UAA→Stop	UGA→Stop
UUG→Leu	UCG→Ser	UAG→Stop	UGG→Trp
CUU→Leu	CCU→Pro	CAU→His	CGU→Arg
CUC→Leu	CCC→Pro	CAC→His	CGC→Arg
CUA→Leu	CCA→Pro	CAA→Gln	CGA→Arg
CUG→Leu	CCG→Pro	CAG→Gln	CGG→Arg
AUU→Ile	ACU→Thr	AAU→Asn	AGU→Ser
AUC→Ile	ACC→Thr	AAC→Asn	AGC→Ser
AUA→Ile	ACA→Thr	AAA→Lys	AGA→Arg
AUG→Met	ACG→Thr	AAG→Lys	AGG→Arg

Exhibit A2.3 *Continued*

GUU→Val	GCU→Ala	GAU→Asp	GGU→Gly
GUC→Val	GCC→Ala	GAC→Asp	GGC→Gly
GUA→Val	GCA→Ala	GAA→Glu	GGA→Gly
GUG→Val	GCG→Ala	GAG→Glu	GGG→Gly

SOURCE   Klegerman, M.E. and Groves, M.J., *Pharmaceutical Biotechnology, Fundamentals and Essentials*, Interpharm Press, Inc., Buffalo Grove, IL, 1992.

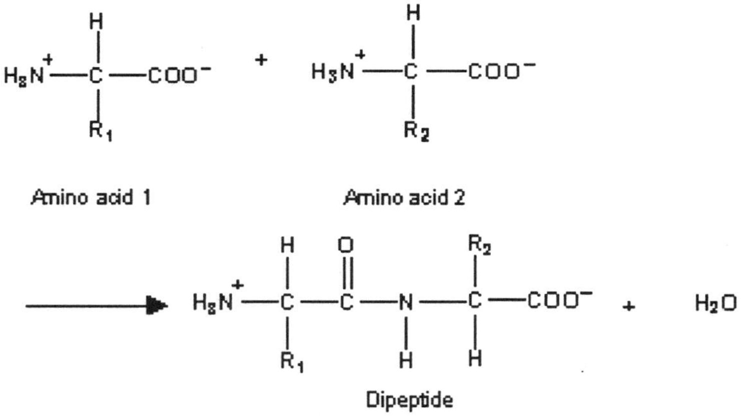

Figure A2.9 Formation of a peptide bond

The translation of genetic information from the mRNA data in Figure A2.8 gives rise to the amino sequence shown below, using the translation table from Exhibit A2.3 as a guide:

UCA   GGA   UGC   CUU

Ser   Gly   Cys   Leu

Through the formation of polypeptide bonds between amino acids, very long chains of sequences are obtained. Generally, proteins consist of hundreds and thousands of amino acids. For example, human hemoglobin has four polypeptide chains, of which two are α-chains and two are β-chains. There are 141 amino acids in each α-chain with a sequence of:

Val Leu Ser Pro Ala .... Thr Ser Lys Tyr Arg

The β-chain has 146 amino acids with the sequence:

Val His Leu Thr Pro .... Ala His Lys Tyr His

Proteins are not linear molecules. From the linear sequences (primary structures) of amino acids, the interactions of various components of the amino acids via H-bonding, disulfide bonding and electrostatic influences can result in the proteins forming into helices or sheets (secondary structures). They can further become folded into large three-dimensional structures called tertiary structures. These tertiary structures may aggregate into even larger units through non-covalent bonding and give rise to quaternary structures (Figures A2.10 and A2.11).

A2.2.3 Human Genome Project, genomics and proteomics

The Human Genome Project was launched in 1990. It is a US$3 billion project involving 350 laboratories around the world. In 2001, a draft copy of the sequence of the three billion base pairs was published. By April 2003, 99% of the human genome had been sequenced. The project goals are:

- *Identify* all the approximately 30 000 genes in human DNA
- *Determine* the sequences of the three billion chemical base pairs that make up human DNA
- *Store* this information in databases
- *Improve* tools for data analysis
- *Transfer* related technologies to the private sector
- *Address* the ethical, legal, and social issues that may arise from the project.

Scientists are continuing to determine the 30 000–40 000 genes that control our lives. Genomics helps scientist to understand biochemistry in our body and thereby develop better drugs to treat diseases.

The real value in the genome sequence is to find out the regions of the genome that encode proteins. Proteomics, the study of the structures and functions of proteins, further enhances our understanding of proteins and their functions, leading to insights on how they are affected in normal and disease conditions.

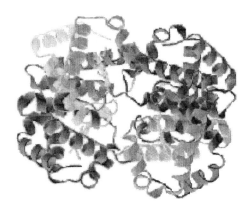

Figure A2.10 Protein structure: Human deoxyhemoglobin. SOURCE: Reprinted with permission from Protein Data Bank, PDB ID: 1A3N, J. Tame, B. Vallone, http://www.rcsb.org/pdb/cgi/explore.cgi?job=graphics;pdbId=1A3N;page=0&opt =show&size= 250 [accessed Apr 16, 2003].

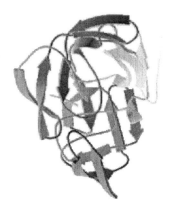

Figure A2.11 Protein structure: HIV-1 Protease complexed with a tripeptide inhibitor. SOURCE Reprinted with permission from Protein Data Bank, PDB ID:1A30, J. M. Louis, F. Dyda, N. T. Nashed, A. R. Kimmel, D. R. Davies, Hydrophilic peptides derived from the transframe region of Gag-Pol inhibit the HIV-1 protease, *Biochemistry* 37 *pp.* 2105 (1998), http://www.rcsb.org/pdb/cgi/explore.cgi?job=graphics;pdbId=1A30;page=0;pid=4502105307053 0&opt=show&size=250 [accessed Apr 16, 2003].

A2.4 FURTHER READING

Basic Genetics, http://www.dnapatent.com/science/genetics.html [accessed Jul 23, 2002].

Campbell, M.K., *Biochemistry*, Harcourt Brace & Company, FL, 1995.

Human Genome Project Information, http://www.ornl.gov/TechResources/ Human_Genome/home.html [accessed Jul 3, 2002].

Karp, G., *Cell & Molecular Biology—Concept and Experiments*, John Wiley & Sons, Inc., New York, 1996.

Lander, E.S., Linton, L.M., Birren, B. et al., Initial sequencing and analysis of the human genome, *Nature*, 409, pp. 860–921 (2001).

APPENDIX 3

SELECTED DRUGS AND
THEIR MECHANISMS OF ACTION

Generic name (brand name)	Class of drug	Mechanism of action
Acyclovir (Zovirax)	Antiviral agent	Inhibits the replication of viral DNA
Alendronate (Forsamax)	Treatment for osteoporosis	Binds to hydroxyapatite in bone and inhibits osteoclast-mediated bone resorption
Amoxicillin/ Clavulanate (Amoxil/ Augmentin)	Antibiotic	Inhibits bacterial cell wall synthesis
Atenolol (Tenormin)	β-Adrenergic receptor blocker	Competitive blocker of β-Adrenergic receptors in heart and blood vessels
Atorvastatin (Lipitor)	Antilipidemic agent	Inhibits the enzyme HMG-CoA reductase and reduces the biosynthesis of cholesterol
Candesartan (Atacand)	Angiotensin II receptor antagonist	Acts as an angiotensin II receptor antagonist
Celecoxib (Celebrex)	Antiinflammatory, COX-2 inhibitor	Inhibits the synthesis of prostaglangins via the selective inhibition of the enzyme cyclooxygenase-2
Chloroquin (Aralen)	Antimalarial	Inhibits protein synthesis by inhibiting DNA and RNA polymerase
Cimetidine (Tagamet)	H_2 receptor antagonist	Blocks H_2 receptor and reduces secretion of gastric acid and pepsin output
Cisplatin (Platinol)	Platinum-containing anticancer agent	Binds to DNA and prevents separation of the helical strands
Clomipramine (Anafranil)	Tricyclic antidepressant	Affects neuronal transmissions
Codeine (Codral Forte)	Narcotic analgesic	Binds to opiate receptors and blocks pain pathway

Generic name (brand name)	Class of drug	Mechanism of action
Diazepam (Valium)	Antianxiety agent, hypnotic	Acts as central nervous system depressant
Digoxin (Lanoxin, Lanoxicaps)	Cardiac glycoside	Inhibits Na/K/ATPase, increases intracellular calcium and increases ventricular contractibility
Diphenhydra-mine (Benadryl)	H_1 receptor blocker	Blocks the actions of histamine on H_1 receptor
Doxazosin (Cardura)	α-Adrenergic blocker, antihypertensive agent	Blocks α_1-adrenergic receptor, resulting in decrease blood pressure
Fluoxethine (Prozac)	Selective serotonin reuptake inhibitor	Inhibits reuptake of 5-hydroxytryptamine (serotonin) into central nervous system neurons
Ibuprofen (Motrin)	Non-steroidal anti-inflammatory	Inhibits cyclooxygenase, inhibition of inflammatory mediators
Interferon alpha (Roferon-A)	Antineoplastic	Inhibits replication of viruses or tumor cells
Lamivudine (Epivir, Epivir-HBV)	Antiviral	Inhibits HIV reverse transcriptase and DNA polymerase
Loratadine (Claritin)	H_1 receptor blocker	Antagonizes histamine effects
Methylphenidate (Ritalin)	Therapeutic agent for attention deficit hyperactivity disorder	Blocks reuptake of norepinephrine
Omeprazole (Prilosec)	Gastric proton pump inhibitor	Inhibits H^+K^+-ATPase
Paclitaxel (Taxol)	Antineoplastic	Inhibits tumor cell division
Ramipril (Altace)	Angiotensin-converting enzyme (ACE) inhibitor	Inhibits ACE, decreases peripheral arterial resistance
Tamoxifen (Nolvadex)	Antiestrogen agent	Inhibits DNA synthesis by binding to estrogen receptors on tumor cells
Zidovudine, azidothymidine, AZT (Retrovir, Combivir)	Antiretroviral agent	Inhibits HIV replication by blocking reverse transcriptase

SOURCE   Reprinted with permission from The McGraw Hill Companies, Ehrenpreis, S. and Ehrenpreis, E. D., *Clinician's handbook of Prescription Drugs*, McGraw-Hill Companies, Inc., New York, 2001.

APPENDIX 4

PHARMACOLOGY/TOXICOLOGY REVIEW FORMAT

Information for the following pages is adapted from the Food and Drug Administration (2001), *Guidance for Reviewers, Pharmacology/Toxicology Review Format*. It provides in standardized formats the information that reviewers examine in reviewing Investigational New Drugs (INDs) and New Drug Applications (NDAs).

Pharmacology

Primary pharmacodynamics:
    Mechanism of action:
    Drug activity related to proposed indication:
Secondary pharmacodynamics:
Pharmacology summary:
Pharmacology conclusions:
Safety Pharmacology:
Neurological effects:
Cardiovascular effects:
Pulmonary effects:
Renal effects:
Gastrointestinal effects:
Abuse ability:
Other:
Safety pharmacology summary:
Safety pharmacology conclusions:

Pharmocokinetics/Toxicokinetics:

Pharmacokinetic parameters:
Absorption:
Distribution:

Metabolism:
Excretion:
Other studies:
Pharmacokinetic/toxicokinetic summary:
Pharmacokinetic/toxicokinetic conclusions:

Toxicology

Study title:
Key study finding:
Methods:
Dosing:
      Species/strain:
      #sex/group or time point (main study):
      Satellite groups used for toxicokinetics or recovery:
      Age:
      Weight:
      Doses in administered units:
      Route, form, volume, and infusion rate:
Observations and times:
      Clinical signs:
      Body weights:
      Food consumption:
      Ophthalmoscopy:
      Electrocardiography:
      Hematology:
      Clinical chemistry:
      Urinalysis
      Gross pathology:
      Organs weighed:
      Histopathology:
      Toxicokinetics:
      Other:
Results:
      Mortality:
      Clinical signs:
      Body weights:
      Food consumption:
      Ophthalmoscopy:

Electrocardiography:
Hematology:
Clinical chemistry:
Urinalysis
Organ weights:
Gross pathology:
Histopathology:
Toxicokinetics:
Summary of individual findings:
Toxicology summary:
Toxicology conclusions:

Genetic Toxicology:

Study title:
Key findings:
Methods:
    Strains/species/cell line:
    ⎵ Dose selection criteria:
        Basis of dose selection:
        Range finding studies:
    Test agent stability:
    Metabolic activation system:
    Controls:
        Vehicle:
        Negative controls:
        Positive controls:
        Comments:
    Exposure conditions:
        Incubation and sampling times:
        Doses used in definitive study:
        Study design:
    Analysis:
        Number of replicates:
        Counting method:
    Criteria for positive results:
Summary of individual study findings:
    Study validity:
    Study outcome:

Genetic toxicology summary:
Genetic toxicology conclusions:

Carcinogenicity

Study title:
Key study findings:
Study type:
Species/strain:
Number/sex/group; age at start of study:
Animal housing:
Formulation/vehicle:
Drug stability/homogeneity:
Methods:
      Doses:
      Basis of dose selection:
      Restriction paradigm for dietary restriction studies:
      Route of administration:
      Frequency of drug administration:
      Dual controls employed:
      Interim sacrifices:
      Satellite pharmacokinetic or special study groups:
      Deviations from original study protocol:
      Statistical methods:
Observations and times:
      Clinical signs:
      Body weights:
      Food consumption:
      Hematology:
      Clinical chemistry:
      Organ weights:
      Gross pathology:
      Histopathology:
      Toxicokinetics:

Results:
      Mortality:
      Clinical signs:
      Body weights:

Food consumption:
Hematology:
Clinical chemistry:
Organ weights:
Gross pathology:
Histopathology:
    Non-neoplastic:
    Neoplastic:
Toxicokinetics:
Summary of individual study findings:
    Adequacy of the carcinogenicity study & appropriateness of the test
        model:
    Evaluation of tumor findings:
Carcinogenicity summary:
Carcinogenicity conclusions:
    Recommendations for further analysis:
Labeling recommendations:

Reproductive and Developmental Toxicology

Study title:
Key study findings:
Methods:
    Species/strain:
    Doses employed:
    Route of administration:
    Study design:
    Number/sex/group:
    Parameters and endpoints evaluated:
Results:
    Mortality:
    Clinical signs:
    Body weights:
    Food consumption:
    Toxicokinetics:
For fertility studies:
    In-life observations:
    Terminal and necroscopic evaluations:
For embryo fetal development studies:

In-life observations:
Terminal and necroscopic evaluations:
  Dams: Offspring:
For peri-postnatal development studies:
  In-life observations:
    Dams: Offspring:
  Terminal and necroscopic evaluations:
    Dams: Offspring:
Summary of individual study findings:
Reproductive and developmental toxicology summary:
Reproductive and developmental toxicology conclusions:
Labeling recommendations:

ACRONYMS

ABS	acrylonitrile butadiene styrene
ACE	angiotensin-converting enzyme
ADME	absorption, distribution, metabolism and excretion
AIDS	Acquired Immune Deficiency Syndrome
ANDA	Abbreviated New Drug Application
APC	antigen-presenting cell
API	active pharmaceutical ingredient
AUC	area under curve
BHK	baby hamster kidney
BLA	Biologics License Application
BPC	bulk pharmaceutical chemical
BSL	biosafety level
CAM	complementary or alternative medicine
CBER	Center for Biologics Evaluation and Research (FDA)
CD	cluster of differentiation
CDER	Center for Drug Evaluation and Research (FDA)
cDNA	complementary DNA
CFR	Code of Federal Regulation (FDA)
CFTR	cystic fibrosis transmembrane conductance regulator
cGMP	current Good Manufacturing Practice
CIP	Clean-In-Place
CMC	chemistry, manufacturing and control
COP	Clean-Out-of-Place
CPAC	Central Pharmaceutical Affairs Council (Japan)
CPMP	Committee for Proprietary Medicinal Products (EMEA)
CRF	Case Report Form
CRO	Clinical Research Organization
CTC	Clinical Trial Certificate
CTD	Common Technical Document
CTN	Clinical Trial Notification
CTX	Clinical Trial Exemption
CVMP	Committee for Veterinary Medicinal Products (EMEA)
DDR	Department of Drug Registration (China)
DED	Drug Evaluation Division (China)
DMF	Drug Master File

DNA	deoxyribose nucleic acid
DQ	design qualification
ED	effective dose
EIR	Establishment Inspection Report
ELA	Establishment License Application
ELISA	enzyme linked immunosorbent assay
EMEA	European Agency for the Evaluation of Medicinal Products
EPAR	European Public Assessment Report
EPCB	end of production cell bank
EPO	erythropoietin
EST	expressed sequence tag
ESTRI	Electronic Standards for Transmission of Regulatory Information
EU	European Union
Fab	antigen-binding fragment
FACS	fluorescence-activated cell sorter
FBS	fetal bovine serum
Fc	constant fragment
FDA	Food and Drug Administration (United States)
Fv	variable fragment
GAMP	Good Automated Manufacturing Practice
GAP	Good Agricultural Practice
GCP	Good Clinical Practice
GLP	Good Laboratory Practice
GM-CSF	granulocyte macrophage colony stimulating factor
GMP	Good Manufacturing Practice
GPCR	G-protein coupled receptor
GRAS	generally recognized as safe
HAMA	human anti-mouse antibody
HEPA	high efficiency particulate air
hGH	human growth hormone
HGP	Human Genome Project
HIV	Human Immunodeficiency Virus
HPLC	High Performance Liquid Chromatography
HTS	high throughput screening
HVAC	heating, ventilation and air-conditioning
ICH	International Conference on Harmonization
IDDM	insulin-dependent diabetes mellitus
IEC	independent ethics committee

IFN	interferon
IGF	insulin-like growth factor
IL	interleukin
IND	Investigational New Drug
IQ	installation qualification
IRB	Independent Review Board
ISO	International Organization for Standardization
LAL	limulus amebocyte lysate
LD	lethal dose
MA	marketing authorization
MAb	monoclonal antibody
MAC	maximum allowable carryover
MCA	Medicines Control Agency (United Kingdom)
MCB	master cell bank
M-CSF	macrophage colony stimulating factor
MedDRA	Medical Dictionary for Regulatory Activities Terminology
MHLW	Ministry of Health, Labor and Welfare (Japan)
mRNA	messenger RNA
MSE	bovine spongiform encephalopathy
NCE	New Chemical Entity
NDA	New Drug Application
NIDDM	non-insulin dependent diabetes mellitus
NIH	National Institutes of Health (United States)
NME	new molecular entity
NMR	nuclear magnetic resonance
NOE	nuclear overhauser effects
NSAID	non-steroidal anti-inflammatory drug
OOS	out of specification
OPSR	Organization for Pharmaceutical Safety and Research (Japan)
OQ	operational qualification
OTC	over-the-counter
PCT	Patent Cooperation Treaty
PD	pharmacodynamics
PDGF	platelet-derived growth factor
PDUFA	Prescription Drug User Fee Act (United States)
PGHS	prostaglandin H_2 synthase
PIC/S	Pharmaceutical Inspection Cooperation Scheme
PK	pharmacokinetics

PLA	Product License Application
POU	point of use
PQ	performance qualification
PTC	point to consider
QA	quality assurance
QC	quality control
rDNA	recombinant DNA
RNA	ribose nucleic acid
RO	reverse osmosis
SAR	structure–activity relationship
SCID	severe combined immune deficiency
SDA	State Drug Administration (China)
SNP	single nucleotide polymorphism
SOP	standard operating procedure
SPA	scintillation proximity assay
SPC	Summary of Product Characteristics
SSM	standard safety margin
TCM	traditional Chinese medicine
TGA	Therapeutic Goods Administration (Australia)
TM	traditional medicine
TNF	tumor necrosis factor
TOC	total organic carbon
tRNA	transfer RNA
UHTS	ultra high throughput screening
URS	user requirement specification
WCB	working cell bank
WFI	water-for-injection
WHO	World Health Organization
WTO	World Trade Organization

GLOSSARY

adrenaline:
> A hormone that prepares the body for 'fright, flight or fight'; also called epinephrine.

adverse event:
> An unanticipated event that involves risk to the subject and that results in harm to the subject or others.

affinity:
> A measure of the binding of an antibody to an antigen.

amide:
> An organic compound containing an (O–C–N) group.

amine:
> An organic compound with the general formula of $R_{3-x}NH_x$ where R is a hydrocarbon group and $0 < x < 3$.

amino acid:
> An organic compound containing an amino group (–NH$_2$) and a carboxyl group (–COOH).

aminotransferase:
> An enzyme that catalyzes the transfer of an amino group to an acid.

amyloid:
> A glycoprotein that is deposited extracellularly in tissues.

angiotensin:
> A peptide. There are two forms of angiotensin: I and II. Angiotensin I is converted to angiotensin II by an enzyme, angiotensin-converting enzyme. Angiotensin II constricts blood vessels to increase blood pressure.

antibody:

>   A protein secreted by B cells when they are stimulated by an antigen. Antibodies act specifically against particular antigens in an immune response.

assay:

>   A test or trial.

avidity:

>   Strength of binding, especially the binding of an antibody to an antigen.

Bacillus:

>   Rod-shaped bacteria.

bacteriophage:

>   A type of virus that destroys bacteria; also called phage.

cell line:

>   A collection of cells that will proliferate indefinitely when provided with appropriate space to grow and fresh medium to feed on.

cyclase:

>   An enzyme that forms a cyclic compound.

cytochrome:

>   A substance that contains iron and acts as a hydrogen carrier for the eventual release of energy in aerobic respiration.

cytometry:

>   The method of counting cells using a cytometer.

Dalton:

>   A unit of measurement equal to the mass of a hydrogen atom.

electrophoresis:

>   The differential movement of molecules through a gel under the influence of an electric field.

endotoxin:

A poison release by a bacterium when the cell wall is broken.

entropy:

A measure of disorder.

epinephrine:

See *adrenaline*.

esophagitis:

Inflammation of the esophagus.

ethical drugs:

Patented prescription drugs.

ex vivo:

Outside a living body.

expression:

Information from a gene is transcribed and translated, which results in the production of a protein.

generics:

Copies of drugs for which the patents have expired.

genome:

The entire DNA of a cell.

genomics:

The study of genes and gene function.

glycoconjugate:

A carbohydrate that is linked to a lipid or protein.

glycoprotein:

See *glycosylation*.

glycosylation:
During and after protein synthesis, the protein molecule can undergo modifications. Glycosylation is the attachment of a carbohydrate to the –OH group of serine and threonine (*O*-glycosylation) or the amide – NH_2 group of asparagine (*N*-glycosylation) of the protein, to form a glycoprotein.

hepatic:
Relating to the liver.

hydrophilic:
Soluble in water.

hydrophobic:
Insoluble in water.

IgG:
Immunoglobulin G, a class of antibody.

in vitro:
Within a glass, in a test tube—an artificial environment.

in vivo:
Within a living body.

intercellular:
Between cells.

intracellular:
Within cell.

ischemia:
A low supply of oxygen due to low blood flow.

kinase:
An enzyme that catalyzes the transfer of a phosphate group.

ligand:

    A molecule that binds to another molecule.

ligase:

    An enzyme involved in DNA replication.

Limulus amebocyte lysate:

    A reagent for determining the quantity of bacterial endotoxins. It is obtained from the aqueous extracts of circulating amebocytes of the horseshoe crab.

liposome:

    A spherical vesicle formed by a lipid enclosing an aqueous part.

log P:

    Logarithmic function of the partition coefficient.

lupus erythematosus:

    A chronic inflammatory disease of connective tissue, affecting the skin and internal organs.

lymphoma:

    A malignant tumor of the lymph nodes.

multiple sclerosis:

    A disease of the nervous system.

myclodysplasia:

    Abnormal or defective formation of the bone marrow.

Mycoplasma:

    Minute primitive bacteria without a rigid cell wall. *Mycoplasma pneumoniae* causes atypical pneumonia in humans.

myeloma cells:

    Malignant tumor cells.

nucleic acid:
>   A molecule composed of nucleotides joined together.

nucleotide:
>   A compound consisting of a nitrogen-containing base, a sugar and a phosphate group.

oligonucleotide:
>   Molecule containing up to 20 nucleotides joined by phosphodiester bonds. Above this length, the term 'polynucleotide' is used.

otitis media:
>   Inflammation of the middle ear.

pathogenesis:
>   The mechanism and cellular events leading to the development of a disease.

peroxidase:
>   An enzyme that catalyzes the oxidation of substances in the presence of hydrogen peroxide.

pH:
>   The negative logarithm of H_3O^+ ion concentration. The scale ranges from 1 to 14; less than 7 is acidic and more than 7 is basic.

phagocytosis:
>   The engulfment of a particle or a microorganism by leukocytes.

pharmacogenomics:
>   The study of how an individual's genetic inheritance affects the body's response to drugs.

phosphatase:
>   An enzyme that catalyzes the hydrolysis of phosphoric acid esters.

phosphorylation:
>   The addition of a phosphate group to a compound.

plasmid:

A cytoplasmic DNA that is capable of autonomous replication.

Pneumococcus:

The bacterium *Streptococcus pneumoniae*, which is associated with pneumonia.

polypeptide:

A molecule consisting of many joined amino acids, but not as complex as a protein.

prophylactic:

An agent that is used to prevent the development of a disease or condition.

prostaglandin:

A protein that has many functions, including mediation of the inflammatory process.

protease:

An enzyme that acts on proteins.

proteomics:

The study of protein expression of normal and diseased cells and tissues.

pyrogen:

A substance or agent that causes fever.

re-stenosis:

Recurrent stenosis, a condition where the blood vessel or heart valve is narrowed.

restriction enzyme:

An enzyme that cuts DNA into short segments.

retrovirus:

An RNA virus.

saccharide:
   A carbohydrate.

single nucleotide polymorphism:
   Difference at one nucleotide in a DNA sequence among individuals.

subcutaneous:
   Beneath the outer skin.

target:
   A specific protein or enzyme upon which a drug acts.

therapeutic index:
   A measure of the relative desirability of a drug, the ratio is given by LD_{50}/ED_{50}.

therapeutic:
   Treatment and healing of disease.

transcription:
   The process of transfer of genetic information from DNA to RNA.

translation:
   The process of transfer of information from RNA into manufacture of protein.

vector:
   A carrier.

xenotransplantation:
   The transplantation of cells, tissues or organs from non-human animal sources into humans.

REFERENCES Martin, E.A. (ed.), *Concise Medical Dictionary*, 5th edn., Oxford University Press, Oxford, 1998; *On-Line Medical Dictionary*, http://cancerweb.ncl.ac.uk/omd/index.html.

INDEX

Note: The alphabets "e", "f" and "t" following a page number denotes the exhibit, figure and table, respectively on the referenced page.